**HISTORY OF MEDICINE**
IN SOUTHEAST ASIA

T0141674

# TRANSLATING
# THE BODY

The *History of Medicine in Southeast Asia* Series promotes academic research in all aspects of the history of medicine and health in Southeast Asia from the ancient to modern times. In order to foster closer fellowship among medical historians and greater cooperation among scholars and students, especially those practicing in the region, it provides a forum for the international exchange of research on various topics from the history of traditional medicine to the postcolonial fate of biomedicine in the region. Both monographs and edited volumes will be considered.

**Series Editor:** Laurence Monnais

# TRANSLATING THE BODY

## Medical Education in Southeast Asia

*Edited by*

*Hans Pols, C. Michele Thompson &*
*John Harley Warner*

NUS PRESS
SINGAPORE

*Published by*:

NUS Press
National University of Singapore
AS3-01-02, 3 Arts Link
Singapore 117569
Fax: (65) 6774-0652
E-mail: nusbooks@nus.edu.sg
Website: http://nuspress.nus.edu.sg

ISBN: 978-981-4722-05-6 (Paper)

**National Library Board, Singapore Cataloguing in Publication Data**

Name(s): Pols, Hans | Thompson, C. Michele | Warner, John Harley.
Title: Translating the body: medical education in Southeast Asia / edited by
    Hans Pols, C. Michele Thompson & John Harley Warner
Other title(s): Medical education in Southeast Asia.
Description: Singapore: NUS Press, National University of Singapore,
    [2017] | Series: History of medicine in Southeast Asia series.
Identifier(s): OCN 966601101 | ISBN 978-981-47-2205-6 (paperback)
Subject(s): LCSH: Medical education--Southeast Asia. | Traditional medicine
    --Southeast Asia--History. | Medicine, Chinese--Southeast Asia--History.
Classification: DDC 615.880959--dc23

*Cover image*: National Archives Overseas (ANOM, France), FR CAOM 30Fi126/10 Economic Agency of France overseas, mobile medical team, outdoor consultation by the French Red Cross, 1945/54.

Printed by: Markono Print Media Pte Ltd

# Contents

*List of Illustrations*                                                    vii

Introduction                                                                 1

1.  Nel Stokvis-Cohen Stuart (1881–1964) and Her Role                       38
    in Educating Female Nurses and Midwives in the
    Dutch East Indies
    *Liesbeth Hesselink*

2.  Trouble with "Status": Competing Models of British and                  67
    North American Public Health Nursing Education and
    Practice in British Malaya
    *Rosemary Wall and Anne Marie Rafferty*

3.  Cattle for the Colony: Veterinary Science and Animal                     95
    Breeding in Colonial Indochina
    *Annick Guénel*

4.  Women's Health in Laos: From Colonial Times to                          116
    the Present
    *Kathryn Sweet*

5.  Learning to Heal the People: Socialist Medicine and                     146
    Education in Vietnam, 1945–54
    *Michitake Aso*

6.  The Expansion and Transformation of Medical Education                   173
    in Indonesia During the 1950s in Jakarta and Surabaya
    *Vivek Neelakantan*

7. "Cambodian Pathology": Imagining Modern Biomedicine     194
   in the Cambodian-Soviet Medical Journal, *Revue Médico-*
   *Chirurgicale de l'Hôpital de l'Amitié Khméro-Soviétique*
   (1961–71)
   *Jenna Grant*

8. Epidemics, Empire, and Education: Contested Discourses     230
   on the 1918 Influenza Pandemic in the Philippines
   *Francis A. Gealogo*

9. Medical Education "from Below": Self-medication, Medical     250
   Pluralism, and Therapeutic Citizenship in Colonial Vietnam
   *Laurence Monnais*

10. The Invention of Medical Tradition in Thailand:     273
    Thai Traditional Medicine and Thai Massage
    *Junko Iida*

11. Honoring the Teachers, Constructing the Lineage:     295
    A *Wai Khru* Ritual among Healers in Chiang Mai, Thailand
    *C. Pierce Salguero*

*Bibliography*     319

*Contributors*     345

*Index*     351

# List of Illustrations

## Chapter 1

Figure 1    The young couple in front of their house in Semarang;    41
on the sign her office hours for private patients.

Figure 2    A delivery in the hospital supervised by Stokvis-Cohen    43
Stuart; her first pupil Mien holds the newborn baby.

Figure 3    The students at work in the boarding school    46
(*pondok moerid*).

Figure 4    A *mantri* nurse (near the window) with some male    48
nursing students.

Figure 5    The midwife-nurse Raden Ajeng Soelastri opens    53
a course for mothers in Yogyakarta.

Figure 6    The students and a European nurse with babies in the    57
garden of the Semarang hospital.

## Chapter 2

Figure 1    Number of nurses in territories with the highest    69
number of Overseas Nursing Association nurses,
1925–35.

Figure 2    Elizabeth Darville in Penang, second from right, with    79
staff of the Government Health Center at Tanjong
Tokong, Penang rural area, including a Chinese health
nurse, third from right.

## Chapter 3

Figures 1 and 2    Brochure produced by the veterinary service    103
and distributed by the government of
Cochinchina. Its purpose was to urge farmers to
report bovine contagious diseases (particularly
rinderpest and bovine pasteurellosis) to the
local authorities as soon as these occurred
in the villages, by informing farmers of the
benefits of vaccinations.

## Chapter 6

Figure 1    Breaking the ice: President Soekarno receives    182
Professor Francis Scott Smyth from the University of
California, San Francisco on August 25, 1952.

## Chapter 7

Figure 1    Page from the dance program for the inauguration of    201
the Khmer-Soviet Friendship Hospital, August 29, 1960.

Figure 2    Radiologic devices, from *Cambodge d'Aujourd'hui*    203
(July–August 1960): 37.

Figure 3    *Annales Médico-Chirurgicales de l'Hôpital de l'Amitié*    204
*Khméro-Soviétique* (1968).

Figure 4    Topics in the *Revue* according to number of pages,    206
1961–70/71 (*Pulmonology includes tuberculosis).

Figure 5    Before/After: photographs of patients with strabismus,    212
from Karach and Tep Than, "Traitement Opératoire du
Strabisme Concomitant," *Revue Médico-Chirurgicale
de l'Hôpital de l'Amitié Khméro-Soviétique* (1962):
260–5.

Figure 6    Normal/Pathological: Microphotographs of uterine    213
cells, from Inn Sunlay and Alexandrova, "Les
hémorragies Utérines Dysfonctionnelles," *Annales
Médico-Chirurgicales de l'Hôpital de l'Amitié
Khméro-Soviétique* (1966): 42–9.

Figure 7   Equipment and devices: Treatment of Intestinal          214
           Parasites with Oxygen, from Ngo Béng Tuot and
           Daniline, "Utilisation d'oxygène dans le Traitement de
           la Parasitose Intestinale," *Revue Médico-Chirurgicale
           de l'Hôpital de l'Amitié Khméro-Soviétique* (1961): 53–5.

Figure 8   Inside/Outside: Images from Karach and Kozlova,          215
           "Les Corps Étrangers dans l'orbite," *Revue Médico-
           Chirurgicale de l'Hôpital de l'Amitié Khméro-
           Soviétique* (1962): 270–2.

## Chapter 10

Figure 1   Inscriptions on the walls at Wat Pho.                    276

Figure 2   Statues of hermits at Wat Pho.                          276

## Chapter 11

Figure 1   Layout of courtyard on the day of the celebration.       301

Figure 2   View of altar pagoda, with main icons, offerings,        302
           and *khan khru*.

Figure 3   *Bai si* and other items on the offering table.          303

Figure 4   Devotional activities around the pagoda.                 304

Figure 5   Monks seated under the overhang for the *paritta* ritual.  306

INTRODUCTION

# Translating the Body: Medical Education in Southeast Asia

*John Harley Warner, Hans Pols and C. Michele Thompson*

Medical education has at its core the acquisition of a new culture. Students trained in biomedicine today, for example, can attest to how becoming a physician involves not only mastering new knowledge and technical skills but also a fundamental transformation in values, affect, and identity. Students and teachers alike commonly refer to the first year of medical school as above all a matter of learning a new language. New explanatory frameworks for understanding the body cast in this new idiom can, in turn, set them apart from the interpretive frameworks held by others who have not been initiated into the healer's culture, including patients. Medical education, accordingly, involves fundamentally a kind of cultural translation, practiced not only in transactions between teachers and students, but also between doctors and patients, and between public health officers and the wider populace targeted in public health education campaigns.

Receiving a European- or North American-style medical education in late-colonial or postcolonial Southeast Asia was until recently an even more profoundly transformative experience, as conceptions of the body rooted in the beliefs of Western science often differed significantly from indigenous knowledge and commonly held explanatory frameworks. At the same time, for European and North American medicine to be embraced even selectively by the general population, modern conceptions of the human body needed to be translated into local languages and related to vernacular views of health, disease, and healing. This process of medical translation developed in the context of colonialism, which

1

sought to remake colonized societies in a multitude of ways. "In the colonial context the universal claims of science always had to be represented, imposed, and translated into other terms," Gyan Prakash has argued. "Translation in the colonial context meant trafficking between the alien and the indigenous, forcing negotiations between modernity and tradition, and rearranging power relations between the colonizer and the colonized."[1] So too, Vicente Rafael has highlighted the effects of colonialism and power differences on translation in general, calling translation "a kind of conquest" that irrevocably transforms the recipient language.[2]

The effects of such translation efforts have varied, depending on the strategies employed by both Western-trained health care professionals and local healers; prevalent perspectives on health, disease, and the human body; generally accepted healing traditions; and common health behaviors. The contributors to this volume chart and analyze the organization of Western-style medical education in Southeast Asia, public health education campaigns in the region, and the ways in which practitioners of what came to be newly conceived of as "traditional medicine" organized themselves in response. Medical education and public health education were part of larger processes of social change initiated during the colonial era and continued after independence—processes that involved transmission, assimilation, and transformation.[3] These efforts had significant but often unpredictable effects on local understandings of health and hygiene, practices around the care of the human body, and the organization of health care.

We use "translating the body" as a shorthand to call attention to the processes through which medical ideas, practices, and epistemologies are formulated in pedagogical contexts, selectively taken up, and sometimes refashioned, processes involving both interpretation and transmission. Translation, regarded in this way, is a linguistic but also a cultural operation, and in approaching medical education, we follow recent work in translation studies that underscores the translation not merely of words but of cultures. As one literary critic has put it, "translation necessarily marks the border crossing where, if anywhere, one culture passes over to the other, whether to inform it, to further its development, [or] to capture or enslave it."[4] Translation from one language into another played a particularly prominent role in colonial and early postcolonial medical education in Southeast Asia, as medical teachers, practicing healers, and public health officers translated Western medicine into local vernaculars for students, for patients, and for wider publics.

At the same time, it is important to recognize that the work of translation did not rest solely with teachers.[5] The instruction of Malay-speaking students in Dutch, or of Vietnamese students in French or Russian, for example, placed the lion's share of the linguistic work of translation on the students. More than this, translating Western medical ways of knowing, explaining, and managing the body in sickness and in health is best seen at the level of culture more than of language per se—the translation of cosmologies. Differences in words were but the most immediately legible sign of the deeper work involved in transmitting across cultures modes of thought and a new medical lexicon for reading the body.

In this volume, we bring together 11 contributions that analyze how medical knowledge and pedagogic methods which originated outside Southeast Asia were selectively taken up and creatively transformed in the training of physicians, nurses, and midwives as well as in public health education campaigns. Spanning the late-colonial to postcolonial periods, they illustrate the long history of pedagogic ideas, practices, and institutions, drawing attention not only to the profound changes catalyzed by decolonization but also to continuities in medical education even across times of rapid social and political change. They underscore the many ways in which students acquired attitudes, skills, routines, and professional identities that were derived partly from models of medical education originating in Europe and North America. They analyze not only the circulation of knowledge but also the transfer and transformation of educational practices that were central to teaching medical insights and their application under new circumstances. The concept of education often carries value-laden connotations, which include a sense of high purpose, moral transformation, and *Bildung*. While we do not want to dismiss those meanings of formal education in the transmission of ideas and practices regarding health, healing, and the body, we want to be explicit about looking beyond them. Throughout this book, our ambition is to blur the boundaries among education, school learning, apprenticeship, promotion, advertising, and propaganda.

We have accordingly embraced a broad concept of education that emphasizes the wider circulation of health beliefs and practices in the many different societies that comprise Southeast Asia. Our concern is with both the shaping of health practitioners and the fashioning of health citizenship.[6] The contributors in this volume pay attention to the multiplicity of vehicles for education, which include formal training programs, classroom and clinical teaching, apprenticeships, journals, textbooks, newspapers, and advertisements; the promotional techniques of public health campaigns that sought to change health attitudes and health behaviors; the daily work of doctors, nurses, midwives, and veterinarians who served as selective cultural conduits; and the advertising and selling of health products in pluralistic medical marketplaces. As we approach it, medical education comprises all the means through which people were persuaded to think differently about their own bodies, their ailments, and the relationship between their health and their environments, and in particular how they were induced to change health behaviors (such as self-treatment, choice of healers and therapies, and disease avoidance practices). The concern here is with the multitude of ways in which the body has been translated, the transformative effect of translating into local linguistic and cultural idioms, and the difficulties translators and interpreters often encounter.

## The Selective Transmission of Medical Precept

Western physicians often believed that in order to bring about health improvements, colonized populations had to be educated in the principles of health and hygiene as well as to change a variety of everyday behaviors. They assumed that, in the process, their audience would abandon what they regarded as outdated folk beliefs and superstitious ideas in favor of modern, scientific understandings of the body. The first generation of historians to study medical education and the transmission of Western medical and scientific insights to colonized populations tended to apply a diffusion or deficit model, which viewed the transfer of Western ideas as a one-way process.[7] More recent research by historians of medicine has demonstrated the inadequacy of the diffusion model to describe the process of educating colonial subjects about the body, and has revealed the vastly more complex processes at play.[8] Both at the popular level and, at times, the professional level as well, Western ideas interacted with a rich variety of indigenous medical traditions. At the same time, Western ideas on health, disease, and the body changed over time and were far from monolithic, and British, Dutch, French, American, and Soviet approaches to health and medicine, each with its own specific character, were not uniform in the medical lessons they sought to transfer to the region. Each set of ideas placed emphases differently and entailed various models of health education and ideas about the organization of health care. The interaction of these different sets of Western concepts and approaches common in the many different areas in Southeast Asia led to a multiplicity of ideas about health, disease, and the body.

The prominence of indigenous medical teachers in colonial and postcolonial Southeast Asia and the centrality of the role they were expected to play in promoting imported medical ideas and practices draws attention to the people they were intended to teach, and the medical education of the wider Southeast Asian population is a prominent theme explored in this volume. Within the history of medicine, three historiographic movements have, in particular, encouraged this focus. One is the deliberate move away from passive diffusion models for the transmission of medical beliefs and practices, supplanting the notion that good knowledge tends to move to where it is needed with models of active transmission that emphasize the agency of individual people—gendered, raced, classed, and sometimes vocal—who selectively took up some medical precepts while actively rejecting others. Another is the impulse to re-write the history of medicine from the patient's perspective, both to understand the experience of illness and health care and to explain how and why popular health ideas, behaviors, and expectations have changed over time. And a third is the growing recognition that any understanding of the cultural authority of biomedicine must pay close attention not only to transformations in scientific knowledge and choices made by states, the medical professions, and philanthropic agencies, but also to the appraisals made by diverse subjects and citizens who held the power to convert claims to possession of particular kinds of medical expertise into authentic cultural authority.

These three historiographic maneuvers inform the questions that the contributors to this book ask about the wider medical education of the Southeast Asian populace. How did not only specific health precepts but also wider ideas, epistemological commitments, and practices regarding maintaining health, preventing disease, and curing illness circulate, and how were they transformed in the process? To what extent can changes in medical belief and behavior be mapped onto larger political, social, cultural, and economic transformations, including programs for development and modernization? How and why did the educational credentials of European- and Western-trained indigenous healers translate (or fail to translate) into cultural authority? And what was the role of other indigenous healers in this process of translation that was itself an educational initiative? What were the multiple vehicles for health education—especially the daily work of doctors, nurses, midwives, and veterinarians who served as cultural conduits; the selling of health products and ideas alike in pluralistic medical marketplaces; popular health lectures, newspapers, journals, advertisements, films, and the vast array of promotional techniques of public health campaigns? And how did they operate in everyday life? How was it that people came to think differently about their own bodies? How are ideas about health and the body related to the developmental aims of newly formed states?

The first historical studies of medicine in the colonies tended to emphasize the heroic efforts of Western physicians who, sometimes risking their own lives, discovered the cause of tropical scourges and found ways to implement preventive measures to safeguard the lives of colonial administrators, soldiers, traders, and, at times, indigenous populations. Narratives of the role of Walter Reed in discovering the role of the mosquito vector in the transmission of yellow fever by conducting risky experiments on his soldier-volunteers in American-occupied Cuba is a proverbial example of this genre.[9] Sanitation measures helped the Americans succeed in building the Panama Canal; later, it was said that "the canal had been dug with a microscope."[10] In these early accounts, hardly any attention is given to medical education. The physicians who arrived in the areas to be colonized were fully prepared—at least so it seemed—and they did not even contemplate educating the inhabitants of the colonies about the principles of medicine as they saw them. In the 1980s, partly because of the influence of the work of Michel Foucault, the role of medicine in the colonies began to be analyzed as part of a larger project of civilizing, disciplining, and controlling colonial populations. In one of the first collections exploring the role of Western medicine in colonial empires, for example, Roy MacLeod characterized medicine as "an instrument of empire" and "an imperializing cultural force"; investigating its role, he claimed, could shed light on "the experience of European medicine overseas."[11] In most of this early research, the inhabitants of the colonies only appeared as the objects of Western medical intervention—either acceding to it or finding creative ways of circumventing unwanted hygienic measures. Why they at times embraced Western medical interventions and at other times rejected them was not examined much further in these early studies. More recent works such as that of David Arnold, Cristiana Bastos, Mariola Espinosa, Annick Guénel, Ann Jannetta, Laurence Monnais, Steven Palmer, C. Michele Thompson, and Megan Vaughan, have examined precisely this question but without extended discussions of the place of medical education, in its myriad forms, in the translation of medical ideas and ideals.[12]

## Vernacularization and the Ambitions of Education

Closely situated in time and place—focusing on the Philippines, Indonesia, Malaysia, Thailand, Laos, Cambodia, and Vietnam—the chapters in this book are insistent about the specificity of local cultural contexts and meanings. Rightly eschewing a universalizing, homogenizing depiction of Southeast Asian medical education, they all situate their local stories on an international stage, underscoring the relationship between individual colonial and national experiences and wider regional and Western influences. Juxtaposing and comparing these case studies draws attention to similarities born of a shared geopolitical place in the world while simultaneously providing a heuristic that helps to reveal the fundamental role of local contexts, interests, and meanings.

Without positing some pan-Southeast Asian experience, taken together the chapters do begin to suggest historical patterns and historiographic approaches to the circulation and exchange of ideas and practices regarding health, disease, healing, and medicine across the region. In the case studies presented, language played a particularly significant role, as historical actors have often debated in which language to provide medical education, and changes in the language of medicine often reflect broader political changes. Travel also looms large—both the role of travel in the professional formation of medical practitioners and the selective way in which medical ideas, models, epistemological commitments, and practices moved.[13] The cultural, economic, and political interests that informed medical and health education initiatives also emerge as a persistent theme, with focused local studies showing, for example, how medical education served the larger aims of nationalism, modernization, development, and international diplomacy.

Language was a persistent challenge for Southeast Asian medical education programs, both as a practical matter of access and as an important ideological marker of social, cultural, and political alignments and commitments.[14] Colonial powers promoted medical instruction in Dutch, French, Spanish, or English more often than in the vernacular. Even in initiatives that sought to bring about wider access to health information by using local languages, linguistic issues often led to problems. In an example that Liesbeth Hesselink explores, Malay was the vernacular adopted in Dr. Nel Stokvis-Cohen Stuart's training program for young Javanese women. Yet, subtle communication remained difficult because, as Stokvis-Cohen Stuart noted, "Malay is neither for them nor for us our native tongue." Postcolonial vernacularization often altered the language of instruction without fully resolving the problem. In the 1950s, with the shift from the Dutch to the American model of medical instruction in newly independent Indonesia, Bahasa Indonesia replaced Dutch as the language in which lectures were given, but textbooks were mainly in English or German, languages that could be difficult for most of the students to follow. Many decolonizing nations in Southeast Asia commenced teaching medicine in their own language, which required sustained efforts by an older generation of physicians to write textbooks and to find vernacular equivalents for Western medical concepts.

Cold War geopolitical realignments brought complicated rearrangements in the goals and languages of medical education and professional communication, as Michitake Aso shows in his examination of the generation of Vietnamese physicians trained between 1950 and 1957 at Hanoi Medical University. Educated in the medical school recently opened by the Vietnamese Communist Party, this generation was the first to receive their education in Vietnamese. Their teachers, however, had been taught in French medical schools, spoke French fluently, and were part of a French international network of physicians.[15] After 1955, medical students primarily spoke Vietnamese, with Chinese and Russian as second languages. The move to Vietnamese was driven by practical reasons such as the fact that after 1945, a diminishing number of medical students spoke French well enough to follow medical instruction in that language. It also sustained the anti-colonial impulse of the Communist government to conduct all aspects of life in oral and written Vietnamese. Medical education provided in Vietnamese not only helped to reinforce Vietnamese independence, but also helped to transform medicine into a prime tool of Communist nation-building. Shifts in language both reflected and were constitutive of the social and political realignments that often informed the replacement of one model of medical education with another, shaping the identity of students and forming their particular sense of community within the cacophony of voices that characterized the professional world of Southeast Asian medicine.[16]

We know from other contexts how crucially important travel and study abroad were in the cross-cultural transmission of medical models. French, Dutch, British, Spanish, and American physicians travelling to Southeast Asia brought with them not only medical techniques and theories but also convictions about how medical education was best accomplished. At the same time, indigenous students and practitioners who traveled from the colonies to the medical institutions of the imperial metropolis returned not only with medical ideas, techniques, and epistemological convictions, but also with educational and at times political ideals, as did postcolonial medical travelers from newly independent nations who made the journey to the Soviet Union, China, or the United States. Study abroad was often a fundamentally transformative catalyst in the formation of professional identity, an integral ingredient in the ways returning medical migrants hoped to reshape the Southeast Asian medical world. Equally, though, such medical travelers were nearly always extraordinarily selective in what out of everything they had witnessed abroad, they sought to transplant to their native soil and what they deemed better left behind. Good medical models, like medical knowledge, do not simply travel to where they are in short supply: their dissemination or stasis depends upon cultural appraisals made by their potential couriers, whose agency is critical.[17] Vivek Neelakantan shows, for example, that Indonesian medical students who traveled to the United States for postgraduate training in the 1960s reported disappointment with the experience after their return because they found that much of their American medical education was unsuited to the realities of teaching and practice in Indonesia. Transmission was selective, and what medical students and doctors sought to try to transplant to their home countries was not an inevitable consequence of studying abroad, but rather the expression of active choices and purposeful actions that historians need to analyze and explain.

After the turn of the twentieth century, the colonial powers in Southeast Asia became interested in the health of the indigenous population as they started to see themselves as engaging in a civilizing mission instead of merely exploiting their colonies for monetary gain.[18] Western medical care in the colonies had previously only been provided to soldiers, traders, and administrators, the pillars of the colonial administration. Aside from the vaccination campaigns and quarantine regulations, which were designed to protect Westerners resident in the colonies, the indigenous population had been left to look after itself.[19] Often, the only hospitals available for the indigenous populations were established and run by missionaries. Providing medical care to the indigenous population in the colonies fitted the newly adopted civilizing mission of the major colonial powers. Not only would Western medicine demonstrate the superiority of Western science, it would also impart a belief in the benevolence of colonial powers.[20] At the same time, the economy of most Southeast Asian colonies increasingly shifted from trade to the production of tobacco, rubber, coffee, sugar, and other export staples, on plantations that required a large indigenous labor force. Medicine became an essential element in maintaining and improving this colonial workforce—ideal colonial subjects were healthy and hardworking. After colonies gained independence, the new states of Southeast Asia adopted a very similar stance to medicine and health care as their leaders aspired to develop their economies.

Beyond the pedagogic aim of changing belief and behavior, colonial and most especially postcolonial programs for medical education also encouraged the populace to reconceptualize its own identity in matters of health and health care and to fashion a new sense of health citizenship. A key ingredient in the health education programs conducted by states and by international agencies was to instill in the populace not only a new sense of rights and entitlements in matters of health but also responsibilities and obligations that came with political citizenship. Just as people were encouraged to think differently about their own bodies, their health, and their access to health care, so too they were enjoined to see engagement with educational programs, self-education, and self-transformation in matters of health as a duty. Linking health and citizenship in programs for the medical education of the public implied entitlements, but at the same time imposed the expectation that each individual would be a willing participant in programs for public health and medical change that served such larger ends as economic productivity, modernization, and nationalism. During the Cold War, health and medicine acquired additional political significance as assistance with medical programs became prime bargaining tools used by the great powers to win the hearts and minds of the populations in developing nations. As the contributions to this book begin to show, the global move after World War II to recast medical care as a human right, together with the political and social processes of decolonization, fostered a widespread rethinking about the relationship between health and citizenship in newly independent Asian nations.[21]

## Shaping Medical Practitioners

In the historiography of European and American medicine, the education of medical practitioners is at once the most conventional and one of the most densely studied topics. Long the focus of doctors and nurses intent on tracing their own lineage—often in commemorative histories designed to establish lineage and celebrate progress—since the 1970s it has captured the critical attention of historians and historical sociologists interested in professionalization, the construction of expertise and authority, and the shaping of professional values; of social historians studying midwives, nurses, medical auxiliaries, and the variety of healers who populated the medical marketplace; and scholars in medical history, health policy, medical anthropology, and medical ethics seeking to understand the ethical failings of modern medicine, health disparities, and the shortcomings of modern health care delivery systems. Studies have, in particular, shown how medical education involves not only the acquisition of knowledge but also the formation of professional identity and the training of emotional dispositions.[22]

Like scholars of the history of education more broadly, the contributors to this volume tend to focus on programs of educational reform, precisely because such deliberate efforts to bring about change prompted our historical actors to spell out what otherwise often went unarticulated about what education was designed to do: Who should (and should not) be trained as physicians, nurses, or midwives? How should they be trained? What constitutes a "good" education? What are the larger social, economic, and political purposes that educational programs are designed to serve? What metrics should be enlisted in gauging pedagogic success or failure? And what should the end point—the properly educated practitioner—look like?

The first seven contributions to this volume focus on European- and North American-style medical education in Southeast Asia, ranging from improvised and ad-hoc initiatives in clinics and hospitals to formalized training provided in educational institutions set up by Western powers. Such formal initiatives commenced after the middle of the nineteenth century. In the Philippines, the Spanish colonial administration established the Faculties of Medicine and Pharmacy in 1871 at the University of Santo Tomas. The Philippine Medical School was founded in 1907 by the American colonial government; three years later it was incorporated into the University of the Philippines.[23] In 1851, the colonial administration of the Dutch East Indies opened a school for vaccinators in Batavia; by the turn of the twentieth century, this school had become a full-fledged medical school.[24] The first medical school in French Indochina was established in Hanoi in 1902,[25] while in 1905, the Straits Settlement and Federated Malay States Government Medical School

opened in Singapore.[26] Educational initiatives received a strong induce-
ment around the turn of the twentieth century, after a number of path-
breaking demonstrations (such as the role of microorganisms and insect
vectors in the transmission of malaria, yellow fever, sleeping sickness,
and the plague) provided new perspectives on the diseases that affected
colonizer and colonized alike.[27] Colonial public health initiatives in the
late nineteenth and early twentieth centuries had been largely limited
to enforced, and often resisted, vaccination campaigns and quarantine
regulations.[28] However, the new discoveries in parasitology suggested
ways in which the prevalence of those diseases that most affected colonial populations could be addressed through preventive measures. It was
mostly through the initiatives of the Rockefeller Foundation, starting in
the early 1920s, that colonial health officers started to experiment with
methods of public health education, thereby repeating similar initiatives
that were undertaken in Europe after the bacteriological revolution of
the 1870s and 1880s.[29]

Late-colonial and postcolonial Southeast Asia was awash in a sea
of models for educating medical practitioners, auxiliary health personnel,
and conducting public health education campaigns, models that often
coexisted, competed with, and sometimes supplanted one another. At
times, certain Southeast Asian countries accepted initiatives from different and often competing Western sources, which underscores the fact
that Western medicine was far from monolithic. During the late-colonial
period, such models for educational policy, education reform, and medical school curricula more often than not were selectively adapted from
the dominant imperial powers. In postcolonial nations, however, and
more especially within the context of the Cold War, French, British,
American, Soviet, and Chinese models often vied with one another—
emulated, transformed, or rejected outright in specific local contexts. At
the same time, the World Health Organization (WHO) offered various
forms of assistance for expanding medical research and training in
developing nations. In the charged atmosphere of the Cold War, such
choices had important political ramifications.[30]

Before the turn of the twentieth century, education in Southeast
Asia in Western medicine generally relied on apprenticeship and instruction that was provided outside the confines of conventional schools.
Some colonial physicians cobbled together their own programs for
training auxiliary health workers, as in the instance Hesselink recounts
in her chapter on Stokvis-Cohen Stuart's endeavors on Java. From 1908
to 1920, when she lived and practiced medicine in Semarang, Stokvis-

Cohen Stuart, a Dutch-educated pediatrician who was politically well connected, started a training program in nursing and midwifery for young Javanese women because she felt that the initiatives of the colonial government in this area fell short. Working through an outpatient clinic she had set up in the local hospital, her students worked in turns in the hospital and as district nurses in the kampongs, practicing and proselytizing for Western approaches to maternal and neonatal health care. In Stokvis-Cohen Stuart's view, the task to be taken up by European physicians, nurses, and midwives was "not to just keep on doing ourselves but to train, to transmit, to make others competent enough to take over our work."[31] Indeed, the model at the core of her training program was the example set by the European nurses. Pursued at the margins of colonial society by a politically savvy woman physician, this kind of educational model has received scant historical attention precisely because it was conducted outside official channels. Nonetheless, it can be expected that such local and at times ad-hoc initiatives were far more numerous than their formal counterparts.

Nursing education in Southeast Asia was often the stage for international rivalry between different educational models. Rosemary Wall and Anne Marie Rafferty map out the battle lines in the Federated Malay States and the Straits Settlements and reveal how competing educational models were lightning rods for divergent conceptions of what constituted a good nurse in the Malayan context. Both American and British approaches shared a commitment to training local nurses and to the feminization of the local nursing workforce. The British approach emphasized character as one of the most important elements in well-trained nurses and, in particular, in nursing leaders. In the 1920s and 1930s, British nurses stationed in Malaya were training a growing number of Malay, Eurasian, Chinese, and Indian women. Because these Asian nurses were subordinated to those from Britain, local nurses were not able to fully use their skills and management experience, even at times when hospitals were short of nurses, resulting, in the 1950s and the coming of independence, in a staffing crisis.

In contrast, the American model, for which the Rockefeller Foundation proselytized during the same decades, downplayed matters of character and social status, and instead favored a techno-scientific approach, emphasizing the importance of developing leadership among locally trained Asian nurses. Malaya had been one of the Rockefeller Foundation International Health Commission's first areas for attention in 1913–15, and during the 1920s it was the Rockefeller Foundation, rather than the British, that took the initiative in training public health nurses. The Rockefeller Foundation sought to further promote the American style of nursing education by arranging for British nurses in Malaya to receive advanced training in public health nursing in the United States, a plan that met with limited success. Wall and Rafferty further underscore the contrast between British and American models by pointing to the Americanization of nursing in the Philippines, which from early in the century encouraged the promotion of locally-trained Asian nurses, prioritizing capacity-building and training nursing leaders. The colonial philosophy emphasizing Britishness and character in nursing in Malaya, they conclude, was not as well calculated as the American model to produce an enduring nursing legacy, and after independence from Britain, resulted in a call for help by Malaysia to the World Health Organization (WHO) to assist in building postcolonial nursing leadership.

Debates about the organization of medical education and the indigenization of the health care workforce locally trained in Western medicine were not limited to initiatives in caring for human beings. As Annick Guénel shows, French veterinarians trained Indochinese auxiliary-veterinarians to teach local farmers about hygiene, rational breeding methods, treatment, and animal health. Owing to their knowledge of local language and customs, a French veterinarian commented in 1923, "the auxiliary-veterinarians are the best suited intermediaries" between the "imported scientific methods" of the French veterinarians and the "ignorant" colonized peasants, "and therefore have to play a highly important role as educators. Better enlightened by them, the local farmer will apply all requirements relating to hygiene, treatment, and animal health."[32] Like indigenous nurses and midwives, these veterinary students were educated to practice medicine, but were primarily functioning as go-betweens, intermediaries, or cultural brokers in the wider hygienic education of the populace. These intermediaries translated into indigenous languages and vernacular practices Western ideas and techniques pertaining to animal bodies and the diseases that could potentially limit their productivity with the aim of improving animal health. When these intermediaries were successful, they provided a link between the Western world of science and medicine and indigenous practices. Yet, like locally trained physicians who were often considered auxiliaries positioned below their European counterparts, intermediaries occupied ambiguous and paradoxical positions, as frequently they were not respected as full colleagues by Western physicians and were sometimes regarded as outlandish by the indigenous population.

Embedded in all of the educational models discussed in this volume are assumptions about what kind of individuals were best suited to be recruited as students. This question loomed large for those who spear-headed educational initiatives, shaped policy, and designed programs for reform. Key to Stokvis-Cohen Stuart's plan, for example, was drawing her student nurses from the Javanese elite, in particular young women of noble birth who had already received some education. Hesselink shows how their social status, class, and potential as role models for the general population were essential ingredients in Stokvis-Cohen Stuart's overarching aspiration to see her graduates compete successfully with the greatly respected *dukun bayi*, the traditional birth attendant. In many ways, the education of the former in modern medical methods had to compete with the age, experience, and established social position of the latter. In colonial Malaya, ethnicity and religion also figured prominently in nursing programs in much the same way that class did in the Dutch East Indies. As Wall and Rafferty show, British nursing educators per-sistently tried to recruit Malay women as students, in part because of the challenges they encountered in trying to impose Western structures on a largely Muslim country. However, often they were frustrated by the extent to which they had to resort instead to Eurasian applicants. The case of British Malaya stands in sharp contrast to that of the Philippines, where from the early decades of the American occupation nursing educators successfully promoted the training of nurses from the local population.[33] As Kathryn Sweet notes in her chapter on maternal and child health, the situation in French colonial Laos resembled condi-tions in Malaya rather than those in the Philippines, as recruiting Lao women to nursing and midwifery training programs was a persistent aim and repeated failure. Throughout the colonial period, nearly all hospital staff in Laos were Vietnamese men. Colonial physicians were acutely aware of the difficulties involved in attracting Lao patients to French medical services. They hoped that increasing the number of Lao nurses and midwives would help attract Lao patients, especially women, and in the 1920s deliberately set out to recruit Lao students. This proved difficult, though, not least of all because of the expectation of a primary education and basic literacy in French language.

After Southeast Asian colonies gained independence, they aimed to reconfigure medical education to suit the needs of their newly inde-pendent nations. Neelakantan shows how in Indonesia during the 1950s, leading medical educators sought to replace the Dutch colonial model for training physicians with an American model at the two leading medical schools in Jakarta and Surabaya. Indonesia had inherited the Dutch academic approach to medical education, which in turn was patterned after the German model, an academic approach that emphasized individual "free" study, which allowed students to take their examinations whenever they felt adequately prepared and to sit multiple times for their examination. This approach to medical education emphasized engagement with research and graduated a small number of highly qualified researchers; at the same time, it had astronomical attrition rates. Medical education in the Dutch East Indies had been organized this way since 1927. After 1950, the Faculty of Medicine at the University of Indonesia, which still followed this model, graduated about two dozen highly qualified physicians a year. The model consequently failed to address the acute shortage of physicians in Indonesia, which had, in 1950, about 1,200 physicians for a population of 70 million. Nor did it provide sufficient medical personnel to address pressing public health problems, such as maternal mortality, infant malnutrition, nutritional disorders, resurgent epidemic diseases such as smallpox and cholera, and endemic diseases like malaria and yaws. Starting in 1952, proposals were made to address these problems by remodeling the medical curriculum on the American model, in which classes of medical students moved as a cohort stepwise through the educational program, taking both classes and exams together. To help implement this reform, the medical schools of the University of Indonesia in Jakarta (in 1955) and of Airlangga University in Surabaya (in 1959) affiliated themselves with the University of California's school of medicine in San Francisco.

The attempt to supplant one educational model with another one in the instance of Indonesia was in part an international aid initiative, with funding provided by the Technical Cooperation administration of the United States government and the China Medical Board in New York.[34] For these American funding agencies, the shift from a Dutch to an American model was part of a larger Cold War project to win the confidence and loyalty of emerging nation states. Yet, as in other decolonized Southeast Asian countries, Indonesian politicians were suspicious of such international aid initiatives because they potentially constituted infringements on Indonesia's hard-won political sovereignty. They were wary that the educational alliance between two Indonesian and one American medical schools would enable the United States to exert undue influence on Indonesian politics. The remodeling of medical training at Jakarta's University of Indonesia succeeded, but in 1969 the medical school in Surabaya reverted to the Dutch model. The American version had not turned out to be as successful as its promoters had hoped, in part because of a shortage of qualified instructors, lack of equipment for laboratory classes, and language problems. While medical educators endorsed the ideals of the American model of medical education, they did not have the resources to implement it.

After independence, the new nations in Southeast Asia were able to pick and choose from a whole host of educational models that were available on the international medical market, choices that were shaped and constrained by local health care priorities as well as Cold War geopolitics. In Cambodia, for example, Soviet mentorship and medical aid was part of a larger effort to counter the influence of the United States and Western Europe, and it was in this context during the 1960s that the Soviet Union became the first country to rival the French in setting the model for Cambodian medicine. As Jenna Grant shows, the Soviet Union supplanted colonial French approaches to medical education. Cambodian Prince Sihanouk embraced the Soviet model prioritizing high-tech urban hospitals for state-of-the-art training, care, and knowledge dissemination and cast Soviet-style biomedicine as an instrument of decolonization. The bricks-and-mortar embodiment of this model was the Khmer-Soviet Friendship Hospital, which was built in 1960 in Phnom Penh with funds from the Soviet Union and was, at the time, the largest hospital in Southeast Asia. At this hospital, physicians provided medical training programs and published a Khmer-Soviet medical journal, which clearly expressed Khmer aspirations to a particular kind of cosmopolitan modernity that embraced an ideal of high-tech, hospital-based biomedicine. Equally revealing, though, are the models for medical education that Cambodia rejected. In 1965, for example, Cambodian leaders refused China's offer to build an institute for training barefoot doctors, a distinct counterpoint to the Soviet biomedical model that would have charted a very different path for Cambodia's postcolonial medical education and national identity.[35]

## Public Health Education and the Fashioning of Health Citizenship

Imposition and the use of force rather than persuasion and education characterized most public health campaigns in colonial Southeast Asia before the turn of the twentieth century. Medical and public health interventions alike were often authoritarian—a matter of domination rather than hegemony—exercising the kind of police powers that since the eighteenth century had grown common in the European imperial states.[36] Compulsory vaccination, mandatory quarantines, and the intrusions of the public health apparatus into private spaces and intimate routines exemplified the involuntary nature of much of colonial health care provision, in which compliance was compelled rather than belief remolded or demand created. The use of force was often justified by referring to the low level of development of the indigenous population and the "primitive" beliefs to which they adhered. Colonial administrators were convinced that it was not worth their while trying to convince colonial subjects of the benevolent nature of medical interventions.

Yet, the prominence of teaching in the daily medical practice of doctors, nurses, and midwives in Southeast Asia—particularly in the labors of local, indigenous health care workers—calls attention to the extent to which even in the colonial period, the aim often was not merely to impose, but to persuade. In the lived world of workaday interactions, health care workers educated in Western medicine often found themselves wedged in an ambiguous position between Western physicians and indigenous populations. They also found themselves in competition with a whole host of other indigenous practitioners who relied on healing knowledge that was part and parcel of indigenous epistemologies and held its own social, cultural, and political meanings.[37] They were promoting health products and ideas, practices and practitioners, in pluralistic medical marketplaces. Essential to inculcating new ideas about health and illness was fitting into indigenous society and existing social roles. At times this meant cooperating with traditional healers, incorporating indigenous healing practices, and recasting Western precepts into local frameworks, yet all the while with an aspiration to instill a new medical cosmology. The educational task at hand was not merely to exhort the populace to take up particular health behaviors, but more fundamentally to persuade them to embrace new interpretations, explanations, and expectations—that is, to *convert* them to a new medical belief system.

Sites such as outpatient clinics, hospitals, and infant welfare centers, in addition to providing health care, also functioned as educational institutions. There were also organized initiatives explicitly devoted to promoting Western medical ideas to indigenous populations, such as the Division of Medical-Hygienic Propaganda that the Dutch East Indies Department of Public Health set up in 1925 with funding provided by the Rockefeller Foundation.[38] The most expansively staged and intensively organized educational initiatives were public health campaigns.

Such educational programs were based on the premise that making colonial empires healthy could only be achieved by modifying individual hygiene habits and the conduct of domestic and civic life, which in turn depended on a populace that heeded the lessons of the new public health developed around the turn of the twentieth century in Europe and North America. Educational projects launched by the Rockefeller Foundation, preaching the "gospel of germs," included demonstration projects on how to combat sleeping sickness, the erection of sanitary privies, and the use of movies and slide shows to make the indigenous population familiar with parasites and methods of disease transmission.[39] In the 1920s and 1930s, this educational impulse was vividly displayed by the Rockefeller Foundation's anti-hookworm campaigns, which in places like British Malaya and the American-occupied Philippines, just as in Latin America and the southern United States, carefully sought to cast its lessons about pathology, prevention, and cure in cultural forms that would resonate with the particular population they hoped to reach.[40] Yet, at other times, indigenous physicians embraced activities such as hygienic reform and public health education as forms of protest against the occupying powers and as activities that supported the building of independent societies.[41]

Health initiatives and education programs often failed, sometimes stymied by resentment and resistance to colonial power. As Francis A. Gealogo shows, for example, American colonial authorities in the Philippines viewed the 1918 influenza pandemic as a sterling opportunity to mount a public health education campaign that would not only help check the spread of the disease but also catalyze a more lasting change in Filipino hygienic belief and behavior. Yet, instead of being welcomed as signs of American biomedical expertise and benevolence, the colonial government's health education campaigns were widely regarded as one of the main causes of the suffering of the people. Drawing on popular literature that circulated at the height of the epidemic, Gealogo traces the propagation of alternative interpretations of the influenza epidemic, which related its severity to the poverty of the indigenous population. Filipinos revived the satirical prayers that had been popular during earlier cholera epidemics and transformed them into petitions for deliverance equally from disease and from abusive American oppression. American hygienic instruction had limited purchase in a political context in which most Filipinos held the American colonial occupation and its instruments, including biomedicine, responsible for Filipino suffering.

Medical go-betweens were one vehicle for conveying health lessons to the populace, but there were others, and the chapters in this volume provide glimpses into the sheer variety of media that were enlisted in educational programs. Laurence Monnais, for example, points to how, in French Indochina during the interwar decades, the *Assistance Médicale Indigène* used elementary schools, public conferences, and pamphlets to teach children and adults about hygiene. Guénel, in her exploration of animal health during the same period, calls attention to how leaflets in local languages were distributed to village heads, how school farms supplemented the practical education they conveyed to young Cambodians through courses and films, and how French veterinarians used fairs, agricultural shows, and lectures as vehicles for reaching Indochinese peasants. And Grant notes how, in postcolonial Cambodia, newsreels and films were used to hold up a particular vision of high-tech biomedicine as a model for national aspirations. Local manufacturers of alternative medicines often used newspapers for publishing advertisements and disseminating health information.[42] In the West, where modern medicine and the modern mass media co-developed from the late-nineteenth century into two of the most successful industries of the twentieth century, advertising, newspapers, magazines, exhibitions, radio, film, television, and later the Internet all played critical roles in the communication of health information to the public as well as in forming expectations of medical power and health citizenship. The tantalizing hints in these chapters about the place the media occupied in the wider health education of the Southeast Asian populace suggest the promise of further exploration—as in Gealogo's account of the leaflets and flyers on influenza control that the Bureau of Public Health circulated to Filipino school children, shop-workers, laborers, and householders, and in Monnais' close analysis of the Vietnamese popular press and a health magazine published by a private French pharmacy as a platform for advertising in the 1920s and 1930s, and the role they played in disseminating knowledge about health, prevention, and self-care.

Indeed, Monnais' analysis of the dynamic medical marketplace in which these media circulated enables her to discern important and widely generalizable patterns of popular health care demand and colonial patient agency. The promotion of Western medical practices often met with a recalcitrant populace, something Monnais demonstrates with the examples of Indochinese rejection of vaccines and refusal of quinine. Sometime around World War I, however, there was an intriguing shift among the Vietnamese from rejecting Western medicines to wholeheartedly embracing some Western cures. Looking closely at drug advertisements, packaging, the marketing of medications through newspapers, and at pharmacies themselves, along with the ways that remedies were assimilated into existing local cultural configurations, Monnais reveals the selective process through which some pharmaceuticals were enthusiastically taken up. Demand for certain Western therapies, combined with enduring popular insistence on medical pluralism, in turn encouraged some traditional Sino-Vietnamese practitioners to appropriate biomedical treatments in order to meet their clients' demands. By the late 1930s, instead of simply condemning popular rejection of colonial medicines, some colonial doctors seemed ready to accept therapeutic pluralism as a necessary platform for achieving their wider educational and professional aims.[43] Understanding this "education from below," Monnais concludes, not only underscores the active agency of colonial subjects in the process of medicalization, but also reveals an early form "therapeutic citizenship" in a colonial context.

After World War II, public health education campaigns intensified, and language about civilizing missions gave way to a growing discourse on development. The medical ideas that, during colonial times, had been imported by Western physicians and had often been imposed on indigenous populations were now advocated by indigenous physicians and public health administrators. The international agencies that took an interest in public health education increased sharply, often representing public health as a depoliticized field but—for prospective funders in Western Europe and the United States—simultaneously responding to the fear that poor health was a breeding ground for communism. Organizations like the WHO funded programs of public health nursing in Malaya and rural midwifery in Laos, forms of technical assistance with a strong educational component.

## The Invention of "Traditional Medicine"

While highlighting the plethora of Western models for medical education in Southeast Asia, the essays in this book also point to the deliberate creation of explicitly Asian counter-models. From the colonial era to the present, the graduates of medical schools patterned after Western models to teach Western medicine coexisted and competed with indigenous healers, sometimes trained in formally organized schools but most often by apprenticeship to practicing healers. However, with the intensification of nationalism and broader cultural revivalist movements, such as Ayurveda-Unani Tibb in India, Traditional Chinese Medicine in China, and Kampo in Japan, the politics of medical indigeneity also informed the rise of new kinds of systematic, institutionalized, and increasingly commodified training programs in what came to be styled as "traditional" forms of Southeast Asian medicine.[44] Organized training programs in explicitly alternative forms of medicine and the establishment of organizations of practitioners mirrored the ways in which Western physicians had set up medical education and the medical profession. In Southeast Asia, such programs and associations were set up in response to the incursions of Western medicine.

Junko Iida offers a lucid analysis of the construction of "traditional" Thai medicine and Thai massage at the end of the nineteenth century. Conventional Thai medical knowledge and practice came to be called "traditional" only after Western medicine was introduced in a hospital setting after 1887, and became increasingly marginalized after the Westernization of medical education intensified with support of the Rockefeller Foundation in 1922 and as people came more and more to accept Western medical ways.[45] The collection of texts regarded as canonical today were compiled only in the 1870s, while the first textbooks in Thai traditional medicine were assembled only early in the twentieth century.[46] Buddhist temples started to provide instruction in "traditional" medicine and a number of leading graduates established traditional medical organizations. In the face of anxieties about communism in the 1950s, practitioners of Thai medicine integrated their allegiance to the monarchy and their Buddhist beliefs by forging a link between, on the one hand, teaching, learning, and practicing traditional medicine and, on the other hand, a larger national revivalist project.[47] They established institutions like the School and Association of Traditional Medicine in Thailand in 1957 at Wat Pho in Bangkok and the Old Medical Hospital School in Chiang Mai in the 1960s (which C. Pierce Salguero explores in his chapter). These institutions emerged as prominent centers for educating practitioners of traditional Thai medicine. When in 1978 the WHO started to promote indigenous medicine as part of its global primary health care initiative, Traditional Thai Medicine (TTM) began to gain support from the Thai government, which took an increasingly active role not only in its promotion and standardization but also in the regulation of its training, curriculum, and licensing standards.[48] The government move to institutional TTM in the 1990s established a formalized model for training not only "traditional" practitioners, but also for training biomedical professionals in TTM and providing the expanding tourist industry with commercialized courses.

The creation, perpetuation, and meaning of collective identity is a theme that pervades the contributions to this book, explored in contexts ranging from professional associations of colonial nurses and midwives in Indonesia, Malaysia, and the Philippines, to the imagined community of biomedical physicians in postcolonial Cambodia, to the transitional generation of biomedical doctors medically trained for the first time in Vietnamese in ways that allied them as a group with the political goals of the Viet Minh. It is especially clear in Salguero's analysis of an elaborate version of the annual ceremony for "paying respect to the teachers" celebrated in 2012 at a TTM school in Chiang Mai. Both Iida and Salguero describe the periodic *wai khru* ritual performed by TTM practitioners to honor both their living teachers and the extended lineage of predecessors from whom they have acquired their knowledge and identity, a rite deemed essential to their success as healers. Salguero goes on to show how the ceremony not only links students and staff at the medical school to their mentors and spiritual guides, but also constructs and maintains a sense of tradition and lineage. More than this, it serves to unite a community of practitioners—students, graduates, and a wider network of TTM schools in the region. Here as elsewhere, medical education binds students together in a common lineage, establishing their claim to shared beliefs, practices, and values that defines collective identity, confers a sense of social and cultural belonging, and provides a guiding framework for conduct in the world.

## The Multiple Meanings of Medical Education

While educational models, policy, and programs for reform continue to garner the lion's share of attention in the historiography of medical education, the contributions to this book begin to offer insight into some of the workaday realities of educational practice, including the material culture of pedagogy—classrooms, equipment, laboratories, and bodies. More often than not these drew comments from policy-makers and reformers only when they were targets for change, while the routine, the undisputed, and the stable passed as quite literally unremarkable. But there are particularly intriguing references in the chapters that invite close historical investigation. For example, Hesselink notes that in Stokvis-Cohen Stuart's training program for Javanese nurses in the 1910s, the pupils not only were taught anatomy two to three times a week by a *dokter djawa* but also attended autopsies. Western medicine relied fundamentally on experiential learning through the bodies of teaching subjects, living and dead, and access was often a function of class, race, and ethnicity. And pedagogic access to bodies has often been shown to be a particularly revealing site for identifying differing national sensibilities in medical education and for getting at fundamental issues of ethics.[49] That these Javanese nursing students were able to learn not only by examining the bodies of the sick in the outpatient clinic but also from witnessing dissected bodies at autopsy raises all sorts of questions for further investigation: In Indonesia and elsewhere, for example, where did the bodies come from? Whose bodies were they? Was there a shift in colonial to postcolonial access to human teaching material?

Physician, nurse, and midwife were far from stable categories in Southeast Asia, varying over time and place, and the essays in this collection begin to reveal the multiplicity of envisioned products of various educational models, as well as the larger medical, social, and political work particular educational initiatives were designed to serve. The medically educated graduate was almost always expected to practice as a health care worker, and sometimes as a medical researcher or public health official. Yet, that seldom exhausted the larger work these practitioners were expected to perform in the world—what they were to do, and to be. Accordingly, the contributors to this volume pose the questions: Education for what? What were the students being trained to become? What precisely was their work expected to accomplish? Which social spaces in colonial or postcolonial society were these graduates supposed to occupy? Sometimes the task of the envisioned graduate was quite specific. The Vietnamese doctors Aso examines who started their training in 1950, at the height of the military conflict with France, and who, as students, regularly traveled to the war front to treat the wounded, were educated almost exclusively to meet immediate military needs. In Indonesia during the same decade, the shift from a Dutch to American model was partly designed to replace the education of students to be medical researchers with an orientation towards producing practitioners of medicine and public health. Whereas in Cambodia in the 1960s and Indonesia late in the century, the ideal doctor portrayed in a medium, such as the Khmer-Soviet medical journal Grant examines, was to be an embodiment of biomedical expertise and exemplar of modernity. What counted as a good doctor in one context was not necessarily the same in other contexts.

The most persistent role beyond healer envisioned for the graduates of late-colonial and early-postcolonial Southeast Asian educational programs, though, was that of teacher. And such medical teachers of the public prominently populate nearly all of the contributions to this book. Within the framework of a "civilizing mission"—the Ethical Policy of the Dutch, "white man's burden" of the English, and "mission civilisatrice" of the French—the leading ills they were being educated to cure were those one Dutch East Indies medical educator described as "public prejudice rooted in superstition, ignorance, and customs,"[50] pathologies in which hygienic, aesthetic, and moral symptoms were often intertwined. To this extent, they were being trained to be on-the-ground agents of what might later be described as "hygienic modernity."[51] Through their daily work, medical practitioners functioned as cultural conduits for infusing Western medical ways into the larger society.

This was especially the case with the education of indigenous nurses and midwives of the sort Stokvis-Cohen Stuart trained not only to provide health care, but also to be vehicles for educating the population—to, in her words, "open their eyes to Western ideas about hygiene." At the heart of her program for introducing Western medical convictions and hygienic practices into the kampong was winning over Javanese women through the culture-savvy efforts of women medical practitioner-teachers. As she put it succinctly, "In my view, we can only improve hygiene and sick-care if we reach the women, and the Javanese woman is not easy to reach. Her trust is easiest gained through women, [for] they understand the psyche of the patients much better, and surmount the difficulties much more easily."[52] Pointing to a pattern discernible across Southeast Asia, Hesselink shows how gender, ethnicity, social status, and sometimes even age were as important as any formal training or certification in enabling these nurses and midwives to fit into indigenous society and existing social roles, providing a platform for teaching that was less available to European medical practitioners. They were to be what Stokvis-Cohen Stuart tellingly called "go-betweens."[53] What is especially revealing is how she insisted that even if her graduates married and left the profession, it was no loss to her larger mission, because they would continue to spread the knowledge they had gained about hygiene and nursing to other Javanese women in their community. So too with other kinds of auxiliary medical workers and the indigenization of the health care force locally trained in Western medicine.

One interest that all the contributions to this book share is the way in which they demonstrate in specific local contexts how education is a political act. Exemplified, not least of all, by the ways that Western medical knowledge was promoted in Southeast Asia, both medical and ideological criteria took part in determining what—out of all the available kinds of medical knowledge—was included in the curricula of schools and what was left out, reinforcing prevailing patterns of dominance and subordination.[54] What counts as authoritative medical knowledge, where and how is it best transmitted, and who gets to make these decisions? At the same time, the aims that medical education was designed to serve in particular times and places often embodied quintessentially political commitments and aspirations, evident equally in the colonial project and in programs of decolonization, modernization, international diplomacy, and nation-building. In many ways, physicians of the newly decolonized nations of Southeast Asia transformed medicine from a tool of empire into an instrument of nation-building. Continuities over time in medical initiatives acquired new meanings through discontinuities in political organization.

The overt instrumental aim of keeping people healthy and restoring the ill to health had its own political purposes, which also changed over time. During the colonial period, the shift from guarding the health of civil servants and soldiers to a wider civilizing mission was often bound up with the premise that a healthy populace was important to an economically productive colony. Training medical doctors could also contribute to anti-colonial projects, as Aso notes of the way in which medicine helped the Viet Minh gain legitimacy among the people in their fight against the French. Still later, for the new nations of the region, health and disease—especially epidemics—were one indicator of governmental success or failure, an index of economic well-being and of the state's ability to care for its citizens.[55] The medical education of doctors, nurses, midwives, and citizens alike aimed at reducing the burden of illness on the population while simultaneously guarding the health of the body politic. Modernization was the most pervasive framework for delineating the larger meaning of medical education to postcolonial Southeast Asian societies. Teaching biomedicine to health care professionals and inculcating hygienic modernity in the populace both served the aim of creating new epistemological communities defined most fundamentally by shared trust in the authority and promise of techno-scientific expertise.

Education for health could also be a form of international diplomacy, intensifying during the Cold War as international agencies engaged with medicine proliferated, sponsoring myriad development aid projects. And yet, shifting development priorities and tunnel vision could also work at cross purposes with the power of education to bring about durable change. Sweet, for example, taking the case of Laos, inserts the important caveat that sometimes the complex patchwork of overlapping programs, and the ruptures that came with changes in regime, health policy, or the donors providing international development assistance, were a source of remarkable unsustainability. Focusing on maternal health care, midwifery, and family planning, she finds that among the explanations for poor health outcomes is the repeated failure of the Lao government and international development agencies to critically examine the achievements and shortcomings of previous approaches to women's health. In this instance, she shows, an ahistorical approach to medical education has taken a toll on Lao women's health, underscoring the importance of educating the developers about history.

In the context of postcolonial and Cold War geopolitics, medical education also figured in nation-building. What is particularly intriguing is the strikingly divergent pathways this process could follow, reflecting what, at first glance, might seem like contradictory cultural choices. Grant, for example, by exploring how biomedicine was held up as an emblem of Cambodian nation-building in the 1960s, demonstrates how such medical practices as constructing high-tech hospitals, training professionals, and publishing medical texts all played a role in crafting a very specific model for national medical identity. The first Cambodian medical journal, published between 1961 and 1971 by the Khmer-Soviet Friendship Hospital, itself a vehicle of education, held up a particular model of biomedical rigor and excellence for emulation. For most Cambodian doctors, this Soviet model was an ideal to be aspired to, not a reachable goal, but it invited them to share in a collective national identity that would serve both modernization and nation-building. Tellingly, indigenous medical traditions, robustly cultivated in the community, were all but invisible in the journal's pages, marginalized in the modernist vision of the new Cambodian nation.

In stark contrast is the cultivation of indigenous medical tradition that Iida portrays as part of Thai nation-building. In Thailand, too, indigenous medicine—which began to be called "traditional medicine" only in the late nineteenth century—was marginalized as acceptance of Western medicine increased. Early in the twentieth century, the first publications on "traditional medicine" were compiled as part of the monarch's larger project of reviving the political, social, and cultural aspects of Thai tradition. But it was in the 1950s, when the Thai government was challenged by communism, that the revivalist project intensified. It was within this context, as Iida shows, that the teaching and practice of TTM emerged, celebrated as a distinctively Thai counterpoint to biomedicine. Standardization and institutionalization during the ensuing decades sometimes was modeled after biomedicine, but the TTM revivalist movement remained rooted in a nation-state ideology promoting a Thai national identity.

Medical education, like education in general, is meant to be transformative, intended to provide not only new knowledge and technical skills but also new values, responsibilities, and obligations. One pervasive aim shared by medical educators is to confer a new identity— sometimes tied to larger projects for remolding regional and national identities such as modernization, decolonization, and nation-building. Interwoven in the contributions to this book are fundamental questions about the relationship between medical education and the shaping of individual and collective identities, both those implicated in health citizenship and others fostered by training programs for medical practitioners. Translating the body went hand in hand with fashioning identity. How, for example, did graduates of medical, nursing, or midwifery programs come to see themselves, individually and collectively? How did they conceptualize their place vis-à-vis other healers, their medical, social, and cultural role, and their competitive niche in the medical marketplace? To what extent did they derive their identity and authority from what they were not? So too, how were the practitioners who acquired their identities from various educational plans seen by prospective patients? When did people turn to a biomedically-trained doctor, and when to an indigenous healer? How were their choices informed by programs of medical education aimed at fashioning health citizenship? And how was that education enacted in everyday practice? Medical education initiated students into particular traditions of ideas, practices, and values. How did they display that shared transformative experience once they were out in practice—in, for example, networks or associations among those whose education had conferred the claim to a common lineage?

Taken together, the chapters in this collection, beyond beginning to map out the history of medical education in Southeast Asia, seek to suggest how medical education offers Southeast Asianists a historiographically strategic framework for understanding health and medicine in the region and for getting at wider questions about social, cultural, and political change and choice. A historicized understanding of medical education, we contend, also represents an important resource for guiding health policy and development work in the present. Finally, this collection seeks to help integrate Southeast Asia into a wider understanding of medicine and societies by historians who are not experts in the region but who are working to shape a vision of what a global history of medicine can and should look like and what difference it stands to make to the local studies we all pursue. Ideas of health, disease, and the body went hand in hand with shaping individual identities and building modern nations. Translating the body was, and continues to be, part and parcel of the formation of the global world.

To Southeast Asianists, many of whom might consider history of medicine to be an arcane sub-discipline, the contributions to this volume argue for the larger historiographic promise of exploring how modern understandings of the body have been shaped, as well as the ways in which medicine, health, and health care offer a platform for analyzing larger social, political, economic, and cultural issues. To historians of medicine, whose collective focus until recently tended to be on other parts of the world, the exploration of medical education in Southeast Asia not only suggestively enriches our understanding of European and American contexts but also makes a formidable contribution to the ongoing process of globalizing the history of medicine. To historians interested in the genealogy of the global world, the case studies presented in this book illustrate how international medical initiatives created networks that were among the first connecting different parts of the world together, providing precursors to the appearance of the global world.[56] Together, the essays in this collection constitute a call for Southeast Asianists, historians of the global world, and historians of medicine, health, and health care to consider what the history of medical education in Southeast Asia is and should be, and the wider interpretive work it can do.

## Notes

1.　Gyan Prakash, *Another Reason: Science and the Imagination of Modern India* (Princeton: Princeton University Press, 1999), 5–6.

2.　Vicente L. Rafael, "Betraying Empire: Translation and the Ideology of Conquest," *Translation Studies* 8, no. 1 (2015): 82–93; and see also Rafael's "The War of Translation: Colonial Education, American English, and Tagalog Slang in the Philippines," *Journal of Asian Studies* 74, no. 2 (2015): 283–302, and *Motherless Tongues: The Insurgency of Language amid Wars of Translation* (Durham, NC: Duke University Press, 2016).

3.　This applies not only to the translation of European medical insights into Southeast Asian vernaculars, but also to the transmission of medical knowledge between cultural domains in general. See, for example, C. Pierce Salguero, *Translating Buddhist Medicine in Medieval China* (Philadelphia: University of Pennsylvania Press, 2014).

4.　Sanford Budick, "Crises of Alterity: Cultural Untranslatability and the Experience of Secondary Otherness," in Sanford Budick and Wolfgang Iser, *The Translatability of Cultures: Figurations of the Space Between* (Stanford: Stanford University Press, 1996), 1–22, quote on 11. Eclectic but helpful starting points into the massive literature on translation theory have been Eric Cheyfitz, *The Poetics of Imperialism: Translation and Colonization from* The Tempest *to* Tarzan (New York: Oxford University Press, 1991); Lydia H. Liu, *Translingual Practice: Literature, National Culture, and Translated Modernity—China, 1900–1937* (Stanford: Stanford University Press, 1995); Saliha Paker, *Translations: (Re)Shaping of Literature and Culture* (Istanbul: Boğaziçi University Press, 2002); Hortensia Pârlog, Pia Brînzeu, and Aba-Carina Pârlog, *Translating the Body* (Munich: Lincom Europa, 2007); and especially George Steiner, *After Babel: Aspects of Language and Translation*, 3rd ed. (Oxford: Oxford University Press, 1998).

5.　Particularly helpful here is Michael D. Gordin, *Scientific Babel: How Science Was Done Before and After Global English* (Chicago and London: University of Chicago Press, 2015). The kind of cultural translation at work in medical education should be distinguished in both agency and intent from "the translation of cultures" that since the 1950s has been held up as the distinctive task of social anthropology; see Talal Asad, "The Concept of Cultural Translation in British Social Anthropology," in *Writing Culture: The Poetics and Politics of Ethnography*, ed. James D. Clifford and George E. Marcus (Berkeley, Los Angeles, and London: University of California Press, 1986), 141–64.

6.　A helpful historical exploration of the relationship between health and citizenship in the West is Harry Oosterhuis and Frank Huisman, "The Politics of Health and Citizenship: Historical and Contemporary Perspectives," in

*Health and Citizenship: Political Cultures of Health in Modern Europe*, ed. Huisman and Oosterhuis (London: Pickering and Chatto, 2014), 1–40.

7. George Basalla, "The Spread of Western Science," *Science* 156, no. 3775 (1967): 611–22.

8. David Arnold, *Colonizing the Body: State Medicine and Epidemic Disease in Nineteenth-Century India* (Berkeley: University of California Press, 1993); David Arnold, ed., *Warm Climates and Western Medicine: The Emergence of Tropical Medicine, 1500–1900* (Amsterdam: Rodopi, 1996); Andrew Cunningham and Bridie Andrews, eds, *Western Medicine as Contested Knowledge* (Manchester: Manchester University Press, 1997); Mary P. Sutphen and Bridie Andrews, eds, *Medicine and Colonial Identity* (London: Routledge, 2003); Norman G. Owen, ed., *Death and Disease in Southeast Asia: Explorations in Social Medicine and Demographic History* (Singapore: Oxford University Press, 1987); Ming-Cheng Lo, *Doctors within Borders: Profession, Ethnicity, and Modernity in Colonial Taiwan* (Berkeley: University of California Press, 2002); Steven Palmer, *Launching Global Health: The Caribbean Odyssey of the Rockefeller Foundation* (Ann Arbor: University of Michigan Press, 2010).

9. John R. Pierce, *Yellow Jack: How Yellow Fever Ravaged America and Walter Reed Discovered Its Deadly Secrets* (Hoboken, NJ: Wiley, 2005). For a recent and strong historiographic counterpoint, see Mariola Espinosa, *Epidemic Invasions: Yellow Fever and the Limits of Cuban Independence, 1878–1930* (Chicago: University of Chicago Press, 2009).

10. Ronald Ross Archives, London School of Hygiene and Tropical Medicine, "Letter to William C. Gorgas, March 23, 1914," quoted in R. Patterson, "Dr. William Gorgas and his War with the Mosquito," *Canadian Medical Association Journal* 141, no. 6 (1989): 599.

11. Roy MacLeod and Milton Lewis, "Preface," in *Disease, Medicine, and Empire: Perspectives on Western Medicine and the Experience of European Expansion*, ed. Roy MacLeod and Milton Lewis (London: Routledge, 1988), x.

12. Arnold, *Colonizing the Body*; Cristiana Bastos, "Teaching European Medicine in 19th Century Goa: Local and Colonial Agendas," in *Contesting Colonial Authority: Medicine and Indigenous Responses in Nineteenth- and Twentieth-century India*, ed. Poonam Bala (New York: Lexington Books, 2012); Marcos Cueto and Steven Palmer, *Medicine and Public Health in Latin America: A History* (New York: Cambridge University Press, 2015); Annick Guénel, "La lutte antivariolique en Extrême-Orient: Ruptures et continuité," in *L'Aventure de la Vaccination*, ed. Anne-Marie Moulin (Geneva: Fayard, 1996); Ann Janetta, *The Vaccinators: Smallpox, Medical Knowledge, and the Opening of Japan* (Stanford: Stanford University Press, 2007); C. Michele Thompson, *Vietnamese Traditional Medicine: A Social History* (Singapore: NUS Press, 2015); Megan Vaughan, *Curing*

*Their Ills: Colonial Power and African Illness* (Stanford, CA: Stanford University Press, 1991).

13.   Laurence Monnais and David Wright, eds, *Doctors beyond Borders: The Transnational Migration of Physicians in the Twentieth Century* (Toronto: University of Toronto Press, 2016).

14.   The well-studied East Asian case of hyper-colonized Taiwan—with German, Japanese, Chinese, and English all at play in the medical world— is suggestive here; see in particular Lo, *Doctors within Borders*.

15.   Laurence Monnais-Rousselot, *Médecine et colonisation: L'aventure indo-chinoise, 1860–1939* (Paris: CNRS Editions, 1999). For a historically-grounded discussion of language and linguistic policy in education as an exercise of colonial power, see Johannes Fabian, *Language and Colonial Power: The Appropriation of Swahili in the Former Belgian Congo, 1880–1938* (Cambridge: Cambridge University Press, 1986); and see Prakash, "Translation and Power," in *Another Reason*, 49–85.

16.   On the relationship of physicians to nationalist movements and the process of decolonization, see Warwick Anderson and Hans Pols, "Scientific Patriotism: Medical Science and National Self-Fashioning in Southeast Asia," *Comparative Studies in Society and History* 54, no. 1 (2012): 93–113, and Lo, *Doctors within Borders*.

17.   See, for example, Hsiu-Jane Chen, *"Eine strenge Prüfung deutscher Art": Der Alltag der Japanischen Medizinausbildung im Zeitalter der Reform von 1868 bis 1914* (Husum: Matthiesen Verlag, 2010); John Harley Warner, *Against the Spirit of System: The French Impulse in Nineteenth-Century American Medicine* (Princeton: Princeton University Press, 1998); and John Harley Warner, "The Selective Transport of Medical Knowledge: Antebellum American Physicians and Parisian Medical Therapeutics," *Bulletin of the History of Medicine*, 59 (1985): 213–31.

18.   The American colonial period in the Philippines is an excellent example of this, see Warwick Anderson, *Colonial Pathologies: American Tropical Medicine, Race, and Hygiene in the Philippines* (Durham, NC: Duke University Press, 2006).

19.   Arnold, *Colonizing the Body*.

20.   This was also true for the introduction of other forms of Western science. See Lewis Pyenson, *Civilizing Mission: Exact Sciences and French Overseas Expansion, 1830–1940* (Baltimore: The Johns Hopkins University Press, 1993).

21.   See Hoang Bau Chau, "The Revival and Development of Vietnamese Traditional Medicine: Towards Keeping the Nation in Good Health," in *Southern Medicine*, ed. Monnais, Thompson, and Wahlberg, 133–52. On the larger trajectory in the West of the relationship between health and citizenship, see Oosterhuis and Huisman, "The Politics of Health and Citizenship."

22. Robert K. Merton, George G. Reader, and Patricia L. Kendall, *The Student-Physician: Introductory Studies in the Sociology of Medical Education* (Cambridge: Harvard University Press for the Commonwealth Fund, 1957); Renée C. Fox, *The Sociology of Medicine: A Participant Observer's View* (Englewood Cliffs, NJ: Prentice Hall, 1957); Renée C. Fox, *Experiment Perilous: Physicians and Patients Facing the Unknown* (New York: Free Press, 1959); Renée C. Fox, *Essays in Medical Sociology: Journeys into the Field* (New York: Wiley, 1979). See also Byron J. Good and Mary-Jo DelVecchio Good, "'Learning Medicine': The Constructing of Medical Knowledge at Harvard Medical School," in *Knowledge, Power, and Practice: The Anthropology of Medicine and Everyday Life*, ed. Shirley Lindenbaum and Margaret Lock (Berkeley: University of California Press, 1993), 81–107. Claire Wendland, in her study on medical education in Malawi, has provided one of the only sustained sociological and anthropological analyses of medical education in a non-Western setting: Claire Wendland, *A Heart for the Work: Journeys through an African Medical School* (Chicago: University of Chicago Press, 2010).

23. Warwick Anderson, "Science in the Philippines," *Philippine Studies* 55, no. 3 (2007): 287–318, 289, 298.

24. Liesbeth Hesselink, *Healers on the Colonial Market: Native Doctors and Midwives in the Dutch East Indies* (Leiden: KITLV Press, 2011).

25. Monnais-Rousselot, *Médecine et colonisation.*

26. Lenore Manderson, *Sickness and the State: Health and Illness in Colonial Malaya, 1870–1940* (Cambridge: Cambridge University Press, 1996), 15.

27. For an overview of the development of medicine in colonial empires, see Laurence Monnais and Hans Pols, "Health and Disease in the Colonies: Medicine in the Age of Empire," in *The Routledge History of Western Empires*, ed. Robert Aldrich and Kirsten McKenzie (London: Routledge, 2014), 270–84. See also Arnold, ed., *Warm Climates and Western Medicine*; Roy MacLeod and Milton Lewis, eds, *Disease, Medicine, and Empire: Perspectives on Western Medicine and the Experience of European Expansion* (London: Routledge, 1988); and Michael A. Osborne, *The Emergence of Tropical Medicine in France* (Chicago: University of Chicago Press, 2014).

28. Arnold, *Colonizing the Body*; Guénel, "La lutte antivariolique."

29. Liew Kai Khiun, "Wats and Worms: The Activities of the Rockefeller Foundation's International Health Board in Southeast Asia (1913–1940)," in *Global Movements, Local Concerns: Medicine and Health in Southeast Asia*, ed. Laurence Monnais and Harold J. Cook (Singapore: NUS Press, 2012), 43–61, and Sunil S. Amrith, *Decolonizing International Health: India and Southeast Asia, 1930–1965* (Houndmills, Basingstoke, Hampshire: Palgrave Macmillan, 2006). For an analysis of initiatives in public health education in the United States, see Nancy Tomes, *The Gospel of*

*Germs: Men, Women, and the Microbe in American Life* (Cambridge: Harvard University Press, 1998).

30.   For an overview of health activities on an international scale, see Anne-Emanuelle Birn, Yogan Pillay, and Timothy H. Holtz, "The Historical Origins of Modern Public Health," in *Textbook of International Health: Global Health in a Dynamic World* (New York: Oxford University Press, 2009), 17–60; and Paul Weindling, *International Health Organisations and Movements, 1918–1939* (Cambridge: Cambridge University Press, 1995). See also John Farley, *Brock Chisholm, the World Health Organization, and the Cold War* (Vancouver: University of British Columbia Press, 2008), and Javed Siddiqi, *World Health and World Politics: The World Health Organization and the UN System* (Columbus, SC: University of South Carolina Press, 1995).

31.   Liesbeth Hesselink, "Nel Stokvis-Cohen Stuart (1881–1964) and Her Role in Educating Female Nurses and Midwives in the Dutch East Indies," in this volume, 38–66.

32.   Annick Guénel, "Cattle for the Colony: Veterinary Science and Animal Breeding in Colonial Indochina," in this volume, 95–115.

33.   After World War II, a great number of nurses from the Philippines migrated to the developed world to find employment. See Barbara L. Brush and Julie Sochalski, "International Nurse Migration: Lessons from the Philippines," *Policy, Politics, & Nursing Practice* 8, no. 1 (2007): 37–46. See also Anderson, *Colonial Pathologies*, 201–5.

34.   For an overview of the activities of the China Medical Board in China, see Jennifer Ryan, Lincoln C. Chen, and Anthony J. Saich, eds, *Philanthropy for Health in China* (Bloomington: Indiana University Press, 2014).

35.   A recent investigation of the Chinese barefoot doctors characterizes them as pioneers for introducing Western medicine to the Chinese countryside: Xiaoping Fang, *Barefoot Doctors and Western Medicine in China* (Rochester, NY: Rochester University Press, 2012). See also Jan Ovesen and Ing-Britt Trankell, *Cambodians and Their Doctors: A Medical Anthropology of Colonial and Post-Colonial Cambodia* (Copenhagen: NIAS Press, 2010).

36.   Arnold, *Colonizing the Body*. See also Alison Bashford, *Imperial Hygiene: A Critical History of Colonialism, Nationalism and Public Health* (Basingstoke and New York: Palgrave Macmillan, 2004), and Michael G. Vann, "Hanoi in the Time of Cholera: Epidemic Disease and Racial Power in the Colonial City," in *Global Movements,* ed. Monnais and Cook, 150–70.

37.   See Shaun Kingsley Malarney, "Germ Theory, Hygiene and the Transcendence of 'Backwardness' in Revolutionary Vietnam (1954–60)," in *Southern Medicine for Southern People: Vietnamese Medicine in the Making,* ed. Laurence Monnais, C. Michele Thompson, and Ayo Wahlberg (Newcastle upon Tyne: Cambridge Scholars Publishing, 2012). See also Sokhieng Au, *Mixed Medicines: Health and Culture in French Colonial Cambodia* (Chicago: University of Chicago Press, 2011).

38. See also Eric Andrew Stein, "Hygiene and Decolonization: The Rockefeller Foundation and Indonesian Nationalism, 1933–1958," in *Science, Public Health, and the State in Modern Asia*, ed. Liping Bu, Darwin H. Stapleton, and Ka-Che Yip (New York: Routledge, 2012), 51–70.

39. We take the apt phrase "gospel of germs" from Tomes, *Gospel of Germs*. See Milton Lewis and Kerrie L. MacPherson, *Public Health in Asia and the Pacific: Historical and Comparative Perspectives* (New York: Routledge, 2007). For the Dutch East Indies, see Eric Andrew Stein, "Colonial Theatres of Proof: Representation and Laughter in 1930s Rockefeller Foundation Hygiene Cinema in Java," *Health and History* 8, no. 2 (2006): 14–44, and Liew Kai Khiun, "Wats and Worms." The work of Rockefeller representative John L. Hydrick on Java came to represent this form of intensive public health education. The manual he wrote for the 1937 Intergovernmental Conference on Rural Hygiene was widely disseminated: John L. Hydrick, *Intensive Rural Hygiene Work and Public Health Education of the Public Health Service of Netherlands India* (Batavia: Author, 1937). See also: Amrith, *Decolonizing Public Health*.

40. See, for example, John Ettling, *Germ of Laziness: Rockefeller Philanthropy and Public Health in the New South* (Cambridge, MA: Harvard University Press, 1981); John Farley, *To Cast Out Disease: A History of the International Health Division of the Rockefeller Foundation (1913–1951)* (New York: Oxford University Press, 2004); Steven Palmer, *From Popular Medicine to Medical Populism: Doctors, Healers, and Public Power in Costa Rica, 1800–1940* (Durham, NC: Duke University Press, 2003); and Palmer, *Launching Global Health*.

41. Annick Guénel, "The 1937 Bandung Conference on Rural Hygiene: Toward a New Vision of Healthcare?," in *Global Movements, Local Concerns,* ed. Monnais and Cook, 62–80. See also Malarney, "Germ Theory"; and Robert D. Whitehurst, "Đặng Thùy Trâm and Her Family, Lives in Medicine," in *Southern Medicine*, ed. Monnais, Thompson, and Wahlberg, 85–106.

42. Sherman Cochran, *Chinese Medicine Men: Consumer Culture in China and Southeast Asia* (Cambridge: Harvard University Press, 2006).

43. See also Laurence Monnais, "Traditional, Complementary and Perhaps Scientific? Professional Views of Vietnamese Medicine in the Age of French Colonialism," in *Southern Medicine*, ed. Monnais, Thompson, and Wahlberg, 61–84.

44. See, for example, the essays in Hoang Bao Chau, ed., *Vietnamese Traditional Medicine* (Hanoi: The Gioi, 1999); Ayo Wahlberg, "A Revolutionary Movement to Bring Traditional Medicine Back to the Grassroots Level: On the Biopoliticization of Herbal Medicine in Vietnam," in *Global Movements,* ed. Monnais and Cook, 207–25; and Guy Attewell, *Refiguring Unani Tibb: Plural Healing in Late Colonial India* (New Delhi: Orient Longman, 2007).

45. For the international activities of the Rockefeller Foundation, see William H. Schneider, *Rockefeller Philanthropy and Modern Biomedicine: International Initiatives from World War I to the Cold War* (Bloomington: Indiana University Press, 2002); John Farley, *To Cast Out Disease: A History of the International Health Division of the Rockefeller Foundation (1913–1951)* (New York: Oxford University Press, 2004); Liew Kai Khun "Wats and Worms"; and Palmer, *Launching Global Health.*

46. For an overview of both health matters in Siam in the early twentieth century, see Executive Committee of the Eighth Congress of the Far Eastern Association of Tropical Medicine, *Siam in 1930: General and Medical Features* (reprint) (Bangkok: White Lotus, 2000).

47. For an overview of Thai worries about communism in Asia and the relationship between the Thai monarchy and the Thai Buddhist sangha, see Charles F. Keyes, *Thailand: Buddhist Kingdom as Modern Nation State* (Boulder, CO: Westview, 1987).

48. For WHO initiatives promoting indigenous medicine, see Socrates Litsios, "The Long and Difficult Road to Alma Ata: A Personal Reflection," *International Journal of Health Services* 32 (2002): 709–32. See also, for example, R. Kusumanto Setyonegoro and W.R. Roan, *Traditional Healing Practices: Proceedings, ASEAN Mental Health Teaching Seminar on Traditional Healing, Jakarta, Indonesia, Dec. 3–9, 1979* (Jakarta: Ministry of Health, 1983).

49. See Ruth Richardson, *Death, Dissection, and the Destitute*, 2nd edition with a new afterword (Chicago: University of Chicago, 2000); Helen MacDonald, *Human Remains: Dissection and Its Histories* (New Haven: Yale University Press, 2006); Michael Sappol, *A Traffic of Dead Bodies: Anatomy and Embodied Social Identity in Nineteenth-Century America* (Princeton: Princeton University Press, 2002); and John Harley Warner and James E. Edmonson, *Dissection: Photographs of a Rite of Passage in American Medicine, 1880–1930* (New York: Blast Books, 2009).

50. Geerlof Wassink, quoted in Hesselink, *Healers on the Colonial Market*, 139.

51. We use Ruth Rogaski's term in the expansive sense she develops in *Hygienic Modernity: Meanings of Health and Disease in Treaty-Port China* (Berkeley: University of California Press, 2004).

52. Liesbeth Hesselink, "Nel Stokvis-Cohen Stuart (1881–1964) and Her Role in Educating Female Nurses and Midwives in the Dutch East Indies," in this volume, 38–66.

53. Helpful here is Simon Schaffer, Lissa Roberts, Kapil Raj, and James Delbourgo, eds, *The Brokered World: Go-Betweens and Global Intelligence, 1770–1820* (Sagamore Beach, MA: Science History Publications, 2009).

54. Helpful here are Michael W. Apple, *Ideology and Curriculum* (London: Routledge & Kegan Paul, 1979), and Michael W. Apple and Kristen L.

Buras, eds, *The Subaltern Speak: Curriculum, Power, and Educational Struggles* (New York: Routledge, 2006).

55. Hoang Bau Chau, "Revival and Development."

56. See, for example, David Arnold, "Tropical Governance: Managing Health in Monsoon Asia, 1908–1938," ARI *Working Paper*, no. 116 (2009), http://www.nus.ari.edu.sg/pub/wps.htmm; see also Deborah Neill, *Networks in Tropical Medicine: Internationalism, Colonialism, and the Rise of a Medical Specialty, 1890–1930* (Stanford: Stanford University Press, 2012), and Amrith, *Decolonizing International Health.*

CHAPTER 1

# Nel Stokvis-Cohen Stuart (1881–1964) and Her Role in Educating Female Nurses and Midwives in the Dutch East Indies

*Liesbeth Hesselink*

Studies on the education of medical personnel in the former Dutch colonies have focused on teaching programs and medical schools. Yet many physicians took more or less informal initiatives at local hospitals because of the great need for support staff. The initiative by European physician Nel Stokvis-Cohen Stuart was one of the most extensive in the Dutch East Indies. She can be seen as a pioneer in the education of Indonesian nurses and midwives. Colonial health services initially focused on the health of civil servants and soldiers, all male. However, Stokvis-Cohen Stuart opted from the very start of her career to work among the indigenous population and to focus her work on women: "Naturally, I have dedicated myself in particular to practice among women and children."[1] It was also while training nurses that she set her heart on educating young women. Because of her idealism, devotion, strategic approach, and feel for publicity, she played a crucial role in the establishment of the nursing and midwifery school in Semarang and the district nursing service there.

## Hospitals on Java

Around the turn of the twentieth century, hospitals were not popular with the indigenous population, nor with the European residents of the

Netherlands and in the Indies. This is very understandable in view of the situation in the governmental hospitals of those days: "Gloomy walls of tarred bamboo, mouldy in parts, ravaged by insects, without light, with hard wooden beds, on which lay grimy yellowish brown mats, hard leather rolls for pillows, dirt floors, with red marks here and there from spitting *sirih* [a well-known plum]."[2] Bad hygiene combined with unreliable, incompetent personnel gave the governmental hospitals a bad reputation. Moreover, the indigenous population labored under the misconception that all physicians did in the governmental hospital was '*potong*,' literally 'cut,' that is, operate, in this context.[3]

Due to many developments in the medical sciences, the hospital evolved into a medical treatment institute where one would go to get better. This led to a demand for a more professional way of nursing. The first municipal physician of Semarang, W.Th. de Vogel, stated in his annual report for 1901: "Because the nursing staff is in short supply as well as unreliable, the nursing of the sick leaves much to be desired in governmental hospitals. This could be remedied through a course in sick-nursing among the Natives, but, above all, this ought to be combined with improving the position of the orderlies."[4] In 1904, the head of the Civil Medical Service (CMS), J. Haga, did not have anything good to say about the nursing staff either: "With coolies picked up from the street and *babus* [female servants][5] stealing from the Government and both merely staying in their job until they can get a better position, it is impossible to look after sick and injured patients properly."[6] At the same time, H.F.P. Maasland, who had worked as a health officer in the Indies for some years, also pointed out that the nursing in the Indies' government institutions for the sick generally stood at a "distressingly low level" and that its improvement constituted a prerequisite for any change in the medical field. Only the employment of nurses who had taken exams could bring an improvement of "the dismal situation.... While civilised countries have now universally come to recognize that nursing is a proper profession and that well-trained personnel is a prerequisite, our colony assists its sick by means of folk who often, intellectually and morally, belong to the mire of Indies' society."[7] As of 1900 a number of Dutch nurses came to the Indies, including Johanna Kuyper, the daughter of Prime Minister Abraham Kuyper, and her friend Cornélie Rutgers, the daughter of Professor F.L. Rutgers, two young ladies from the Dutch Reformed elite. However, their number was wholly insufficient to meet the colony's increased demand for competent nursing staff. This is why European physicians themselves started training individuals indigenous to the Indies on their own initiative. Thus, N.F. Lim, second municipal physician in Semarang, began to train young native men,[8] while his colleague Nel Stokvis-Cohen Stuart started training young women.

## Nel Stokvis-Cohen Stuart

Nel (Cornelia J.J.) Stokvis-Cohen Stuart was born in Semarang (Central Java) in 1881. Her father was a high-ranking civil servant in the Indies. Near the end of her secondary school education she was sent to the Netherlands for further education. After finishing secondary school in 1898 she enrolled in medicine at Leiden University. During her student years, she already displayed a pioneering spirit. With two other female students she took the initiative to set up an association for female students in 1901. In those days only a few women attended university; this association aimed to bring them together and provide them with some company. In 1907, just after qualifying as a physician she married Jacques (Zadok) Stokvis (1878–1947).[9] Through self-study and with scholarship support he had studied Dutch and Russian at Leiden University. Shortly after their wedding the young couple received a visit from mission doctor H. Bervoets and his wife, who spoke inspiringly about their work in the mission hospital in Mojowarno (East Java), where they had been working since 1895. This visit strengthened the young couple's resolve to go to the Indies.[10] There they settled in Semarang, where he found a job as a teacher at a secondary school and she set up a private practice.

## Physician in Semarang

The couple fitted in well with the colonial politics of the times. Although the Dutch had been present in the Indonesian archipelago since the early seventeenth century, a fully-fledged colonial state only developed in the nineteenth and early twentieth century. Technical and economic changes as well as feelings of both Western superiority and social concerns about the welfare of the indigenous population resulted in the formulation of a "civilising mission" and a more active colonial policy. Named the Ethical Policy, it was the Dutch version of the British "white man's burden" or the French "mission civilisatrice."[11] According to this policy, the Netherlands "as a Christian power" was obliged "to imbue government policy with the understanding that the Netherlands has to fulfil

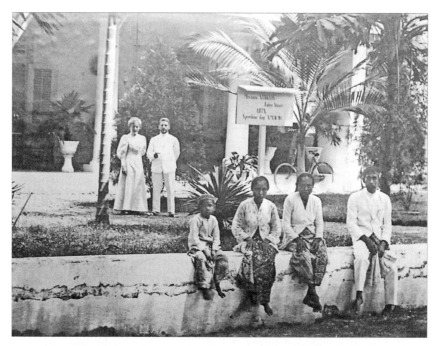

**Figure 1.** The young couple in front of their house in Semarang; on the sign her office hours for private patients (Photograph from the Collectie Cohen-Stuart, Centraal Bureau voor Genealogie, The Hague, inv. no 479).

a moral mission towards the population of these territories."[12] Rather than viewing the colonies as an area to be exploited as a profitable cash cow, the Ethical Policy indicated a novel dedication on the part of the Dutch colonial administration to develop schools and medical services, transportation, and other infrastructural improvements for the indigenous population. The architects of the Ethical Policy aimed at the development of both the land and its people and had in mind a form of (limited) self-government under Dutch leadership following the Western model.

Following similar ethical ideas, Stokvis-Cohen Stuart aimed to improve the health of the indigenous population. "When I arrived in the Indies seven years ago," she told her audience in a lecture at a Red Cross meeting in 1915, "I firmly intended to find employment among the Natives."[13] The director of the Semarang hospital, W.Th. de Vogel, gave her permission—although she was not a government employee— to operate an outpatient clinic for native women and children in the government hospital in the morning. In addition, he agreed to let her continue treating her patients if they had to be admitted to the hospital, instead of them being treated, as the rules dictated, by a male *dokter djawa* (a Western-trained Indonesian physician).[14] The outpatient clinic was attended by poor women only; better-off women stayed away, probably because of the hospital's bad reputation. When Stokvis-Cohen Stuart set up her outpatient clinic from her home, well-to-do women appeared after all and continued coming even when the outpatient clinic was transferred back to the hospital. In addition, she also tended to births in the kampong on her own initiative to build confidence: "If at all possible, I did the delivery in such cases on the spot, with God's grace, and fortunately, things usually worked out fine after all."[15] During her work Stokvis-Cohen Stuart also felt the lack of good helpers.[16] This is how she described the abominable situation in the hospital in the above-mentioned Red Cross lecture:

> Those nurses! They were just *babus*, and not of the best kind, either. They were dressed in their own unsavoury togs, with a white apron on top by way of 'official' uniform. They could neither read nor write; they only knew the numbers from 0 to 9 and on the basis of that they managed to read the thermometer and write down the temperature. They simply had to remember the instructions as to food and medication.[17]

## The First Step is the Hardest One

Stokvis-Cohen Stuart's initial endeavors to train young Javanese women to become nurses were disappointing. Her first student was the daughter of her *babu*, and Stokvis Cohen-Stuart had paid her tuition so that she could learn reading and writing. A great beauty, she had no lack of admirers, and in fact, Stokvis-Cohen Stuart was glad when she got married. The second was a nine-year-old girl who went to school at Stokvis-Cohen Stuart's expense. When she was 13, she stole Stokvis-Cohen Stuart's fountain pen to write short letters to young admirers in the kampong. The third girl died suddenly. The fourth got married when she was 11, after she had attended a mere 3 reading and writing lessons. The fifth girl stayed on for two years until Stokvis-Cohen Stuart sent her away because of her laziness. Next, Stokvis-Cohen Stuart tried to train slightly older young women (17 and 18 years old) to become midwives; both could read and write. But when Stokvis-Cohen Stuart found out that they had boyfriends in the kampong she disapproved of,

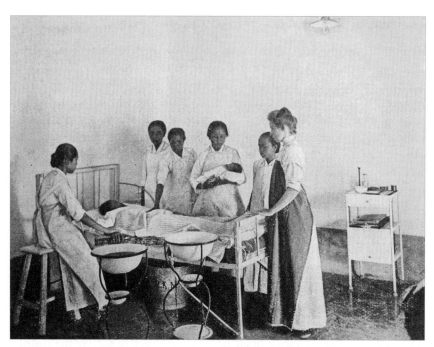

**Figure 2.** A delivery in the hospital supervised by Stokvis-Cohen Stuart; her first pupil Mien holds the newborn baby [Photograph from N. Stokvis-Cohen Stuart, *De Inlandsche Ziekenverpleging te Semarang* (Semarang: H.A. Benjamins, 1916), 19].

she dismissed them. Following these failures, she temporarily disconti-nued trying to educate young indigenous women. At one point, the village head from outside Semarang approached Stokvis-Cohen Stuart together with his 14-year-old daughter, Soetarmijah, or Mien. The young woman very much wished to train as a nurse. Mindful of the fiascos of the past three years, Stokvis-Cohen Stuart was hesitant, but he managed to persuade her that his daughter was in no hurry to get married and was anxious to continue her studies. He rented a small house in the kampong for Mien and a younger sister who was to attend school in Semarang. At first Mien was given theory lessons by Stokvis-Cohen Stuart at the latter's home. To gain hands-on experience she had to work in the clinic. N.F. Lim, by now the director of the hospital, did not object to her presence in the women's ward, but initially did not want to admit her to the lessons he gave to the male students as he did not have enough confidence in the study plans of young Javanese women. Eventually, he changed his mind and let her take part in the lessons.[18]

## Position of Young Women in Javanese Society

The problems Stokvis-Cohen Stuart encountered in training young Javanese women were related to the position they occupied in Javanese
society. Before they could train as nurses, these young women were
required to have received some basic education. In principle, young
women from poor families did not attend school, unlike those from the
middle and upper classes. However, it was considered culturally im-
proper for upper-class girls—the ones who could afford to study—to
live outside their parents' home when they were of marriageable age
(that is, 14 to 16 years old). Further, the bad reputation of the government hospitals made them suitable workplaces only for lower-class
women and women with dubious reputations.[19] According to Stokvis-
Cohen Stuart, the problems with recruiting students were caused "by
an aversion to the hospital."[20] Hospitals were definitely not places for
young women of noble birth.

A related problem pertained to the importance of descent in Javanese society. Most students belonged to the elite—of the 28 students
following the nursing course in 1916, 21 were of noble birth.[21] "It is
quite a job to drum into the students that they have to follow the instructions from the doctors, even when the person concerned is a *Raden Ayu*
(title of a married lady of noble birth) or someone else from the aris-
tocracy."[22] Descent likewise played a role in the students' relationship
with patients, as Stokvis-Cohen Stuart explained in a memorandum to
the Governor-General:

> Our girls do actually distinguish between patients. A 'higher-class'
> patient will be given more attention, more delicacy is brought to
> the care provided. And where appropriate, a wish or a refusal from
> such a 'higher' patient weighs decidedly more heavily than the
> doctor's instruction. This kind of submission to people of a higher
> class, of course, greatly harms the nursing. Conversely, the students'
> conduct towards the ordinary patients frequently leaves much to be
> desired. Unwillingness, especially as to the less pleasant chores of
> nursing, coarse answers, unfortunately, we often catch the girls doing
> so, if we unexpectedly walk into the ward.[23]

## Training for Female Nurses

In 1912 the position of *mantri* nurse was officially established.[24] Government regulations were now put in place for the nursing courses. Students

received an allowance for housing, clothing and food; a maximum of 100 students across the entire archipelago were eligible for this. The trainers received a bonus of *f*500 for each student who graduated,[25] but this was subsequently abolished.[26] Lim was given 20 young men to teach, who were placed in the men's wards to replace the old orderlies.[27] The two young women educated by Stokvis-Cohen Stuart, the above-mentioned Mien and a friend, also fell under the new government regulations.[28]

To be admitted to the training course the following requirements had to be met: applicants had to be at least 16 years old, be of good health and be recipients of a proper primary school education (second-class Native school). When many of the young women registering for the training appeared very thin and gaunt, a minimum height was imposed by way of an additional admission requirement. Young women fulfilling these conditions were given a two-month probation period during which both parties could judge whether it would be useful to continue.[29]

Once the students were admitted, the three-year training course started with a combination of theory and practical lessons. In their first year, the students were instructed in the fundamentals of anatomy two to three times a week by the *dokter djawa*. In addition, Lim taught two one-hour classes a week in pathology, anatomy, infectious diseases, and hygiene to the young men and women. Stokvis-Cohen Stuart taught obstetrics for one hour a week in every study year and took third-year students in pairs to witness deliveries in the kampong or in the hospital. Students were initiated by a European female nurse into the secrets of sick-nursing, infant care and such practical matters as transferring and bathing seriously ill patients. In the morning the students received practical instruction in how to assess and treat leg wounds as often and as long as ward duties allowed. They assisted with operations, attended autopsies and learned to prepare simple prescriptions in the pharmacy. In the evening the students were expected to expand on their theory lessons. Malay was the language of instruction.[30] This sometimes gave rise to problems when, for instance, students were corrected about their conduct towards patients: "it is difficult to discuss such sensitive matters with the students since Malay is neither for them nor for us our mother tongue."[31] The young women were embarrassed when they were reprimanded. They even planned to go on strike on one occasion because the European female nurse "had grumbled too much."[32]

What greatly contributed to the eventual success was the fact that during their training, the students were housed in a kind of boarding

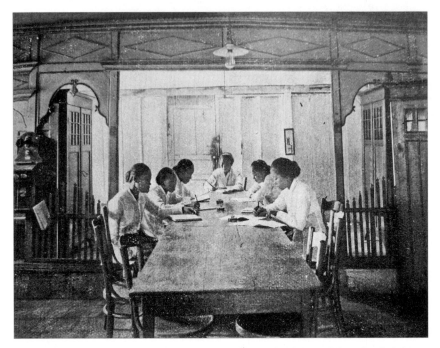

**Figure 3.** The students at work in the boarding school (*pondok moerid*) (Photograph from Stokvis-Cohen Stuart, *Inlandsche Ziekenverpleging Semarang*, 11).

school (*pondok moerid*), although this is a rather grand term for the housing in question. I mentioned before that the father of one of the students had rented a little house in the kampong for his daughter with an old and trusted servant supervising her. As the number of students increased, a second house was rented as well, followed shortly afterwards by a third one; altogether 40 students could be accommodated. Supervision was provided by W.A. Lim-Bergsma, who had been a nurse in Holland before her marriage to Lim.[33]

The hospital numbered 3 European female nurses who supervised about 40 male and female students.[34] They taught them the odd jobs of nursing and checked on their work; according to Stokvis-Cohen Stuart, indigenous female nurses required constant supervision.[35] In her lectures, she emphasized that European nurses played a particularly important part as role models:

> In all this, European female nurses are necessary, the best, but it is not easy to get good European nurses in the Indies, in particular for the job of nursing sick Natives. They really ought to be the best

because they have to serve as an example to our students. And the standing of female nurses should be brought to such high regard in Indies society, by means of the high demands of innate refinement that we set, that it will be considered an *honour* for the Native girls and their environment to be approved of for our service![36]

Stokvis-Cohen Stuart expected a great deal from the influence of European female nurses: "I have placed all my hope in the good example of European nurses."[37]

In 1915 the colonial government started to require an exam in sick-nursing.[38] To be awarded a diploma, candidates had to be at least 20 years of age and were required to produce a certificate of good moral conduct. The examination requirements stated that the students, besides being able to complete common tasks such as making beds, preparing for operations, providing care after operations, and applying different kinds of bandages, also needed to be capable of getting patients out of a vehicle or train compartment, shaving with a knife and trimming hair using clippers, as well as carrying out simple laboratory work such as examining faeces and blood samples. Besides, students had to be knowledgeable about the principles of anatomy, physiology, hygiene, and general and specialist sick-nursing.[39]

## Midwifery Training

Having acquired the diploma of *mantri* nurse, the graduates could—if found suitable—do a follow-up course to obtain the so-called *mantri* nurse diploma first class. After practicing for two years, during which time they were also taught how to do laboratory and pharmacy work, they could take the exam. Then they were authorized to treat the most common diseases, to administer first aid in case of diseases or accidents, and to be in charge of a ward or branch of a hospital, more or less independently.[40] This category of care workers fitted in much better with the policy of the CMS, which prioritized prevention rather than cure and thus provided care that was not hospital-based. In other words, the CMS required nurses, male or female, who were able to staff outpatient departments.

After they had obtained their nursing diploma, female graduates could do a follow-up course for midwives. Stokvis-Cohen Stuart had noticed that most parents found midwifery training more attractive for their daughters than nurse training, because the latter profession was

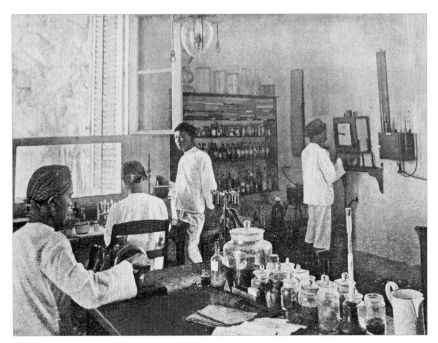

**Figure 4.** A *mantri* nurse (near the window) with some male nursing students (Photograph from Stokvis-Cohen Stuart, *Inlandsche Ziekenverpleging Semarang*, 17).

unknown in Javanese society. Being a midwife was a more appealing alternative because of the financial advantages and better position.[41] She commented that:

> And knowing from experience how desirable the midwifery diploma is generally held to be, and how unpopular the unknown *mantri* nurse diploma still was, I have thought it wise to speed up the process by promising those girls wanting to train for the *mantri* exam the midwifery course, too, by way of a private bonus.[42]

It is likely that the fact that midwives, in contrast to nurses, dealt exclusively with female patients increased the profession's appeal. And, sure enough, almost all the female graduates wanted to train as student-midwives after their nurse exam. Those who showed aptitude and ability were admitted; only a few were not accepted.[43]

The midwifery training consisted of a two-year trajectory in which the student-midwives worked in turns in one of the hospitals and took shifts as district nurses. When they had passed the exam[44] they took the oath: Muslim graduates before the *penghulu* (religious civil servant, cleric), the others before the examination board.[45] Next the graduates just sworn in were awarded certificates stating that they now had the same powers and obligations as European midwives.[46] The graduates were employed by the colonial administration and received a leather bag containing medicines and obstetric instruments such as forceps,[47] which is remarkable as midwives were normally supposed to assist at natural births only.[48] In general they were allotted a post close to their family; if they were not, this often constituted a reason for them to leave the service of the colonial government.[49] If graduates did not accept employment with the colonial government or left within five years, the subsidy had to be paid back.[50] In her memorandum to the Governor-General, Stokvis-Cohen Stuart argued against this governmental stipulation: *"Just as unnecessarily generous as the physician in charge of the midwifery training was remembered, ...just as illogical is the subsidy granted to female (and male) nurses, and just as unreasonable is the requirement that the girls are employed for a five-year period."*[51] This stipulation was a great hindrance to young women. There was a distinct chance that they would get married within five years and leave the civil service. Following a petition submitted by Stokvis-Cohen Stuart, the stipulation concerning the five years of employment was retracted.[52]

## District Nursing

In a letter to her ex-colleague W.Th. de Vogel, who had meanwhile become the head of the CMS, Stokvis-Cohen Stuart expounded her ideas about a district nursing service:

> Yet I would...like to start preparing our 'district service', which, for Semarang, I thought should also be an educational service. Educational for our students, and educational for the population. It could work for the students since they would be put to work more or less independently in an outpatient clinic and would have to perform more or less independently in the kampongs....Educational for the population our district service would have to be because of what I would like to introduce here: no help without payment. How best to arrange this, I do not quite know yet but of course I would want to consult with a few Javanese individuals. I have been pondering this, how we could organize it, in particular so we stand a chance of being granted a subsidy.[53]

With de Vogel's encouragement,[54] Stokvis-Cohen Stuart subsequently wrote a memorandum to the Governor-General about this issue: a district nursing service would have to be set up in association with the nurse and midwifery training, which would consist of one or more outpatient clinics in community centres as well as a home nursing service in the kampong. The district service constituted a useful addition to the training in the hospital. After all, graduates would mainly work in the kampong where they would have to show a high level of independence, because doctors and hospitals would be far away. Moreover, these *mantri* nurses had to be taught how to manage when conditions, particularly as to hygiene, were less favorable than in the hospital. House visits were useful because they might induce more Javanese women to seek medical attention in a timely manner. Moreover, these nurses could help find foci of infection and thereby help combat infectious diseases in the kampong.[55] The positive attitude of de Vogel as head of the CMS made it likely that her ideas might be implemented and the subsidy granted.

However, Stokvis-Cohen Stuart did not await formal approval from the colonial administration and in February 1917 the first outpatient clinic was set up in a small rented house;[56] at the end of that year it moved to a stone building named Mardi Waloejo (The Road to Recovery). Working in the clinic were—apart from a number of Javanese nurses and student-midwives—a European nurse, "a dedicated nurse with sympathy for the Javanese people, and with a good knowledge of district nursing." However, it was not the knowledge of this European nurse that was important but "especially her character, *the good example* she set in coaching our pupils."[57] In other words, European nurses played an important part as role models here as well. The European nurse's salary ($f200$ a month) was subsidized by the colonial government,[58] which implied the official recognition of the district nursing service.[59] On principle, the care administered was not free. In her memorandum to the Govenor-General Stokvis-Cohen Stuart stated that she wished to familiarize the indigenous population with the idea that Western medical help had to be paid for: "It is my personal experience that many Javanese individuals are happy to do something in return for help received; …*The fee of course has to be such that care is accessible for everybody*, including the needy."[60] The fees for the outpatient clinic, house visits, obstetric assistance, and medication were low and progressive.[61]

To ensure that the care provided in the district outpatient clinic was of the same high quality as that given in the hospital, Stokvis-Cohen

Stuart held consultations in the community centre a few times a week. The *mantris* assisted, for example, with treating leg ulcers, chronic eye diseases, and chronic ear infections more or less independently. They examined urine and faeces. If necessary, they referred patients to the hospital. But examining pregnant women and providing infant care was their main priority.[62]

## Strategy

Stokvis-Cohen Stuart set to work very strategically to achieve her aim: to improve health care among the indigenous population by introducing Western medical assistance. In a memorandum to the Governor-General, she expounded on the fundamental position women played in this endeavour:

> In my view, we can only improve hygiene and care for the sick if we reach the women, and the Javanese woman is not easy to reach. Her trust is easiest gained through women. That is why as much female medical help as is possible should be brought to the indigenous hospitals and homes. Of course there will be male physicians who succeed in winning the trust of female patients through their personality.... But the most natural situation is that of a woman seeking medical help from a woman, and I could give plenty of examples of female patients who would much rather go to a female physician with their complaints.... But medical help without trained nurses is powerless. Therefore, if the health care for Javanese women is to be improved, emphasis should be on training nurses.[63]

In order to win over young women and/or their parents and to have them opt for a nursing course, Stokvis-Cohen Stuart emphasized the combined training program she offered: in addition to grounding in nursing, students could enroll, as a bonus, in a follow-up course in the more popular profession of midwifery. To attract students, it was important that the training provided led to a profession with a certain status. Within the Javanese community, graduates had to gain a certain standing to compete with the greatly respected *dukun bayi*, the traditional birth attendant (TBA). Stokvis-Cohen Stuart purposefully picked her students from among the higher classes of society: "I have been busy for a year now consistently propagandizing among the *priyayi* [Javanese nobilities] and other educated Javanese to get girls from their own set as my student-nurses."[64] Apparently, she succeeded in training and holding on to young women from noble families; among the *mantri* midwives we notice two *Raden Ajeng*, unmarried noble ladies.[65] It was common knowledge that her student-nurses were the daughters of *priyayi*.[66]

In Europe, descent played a role in the evolution of the nursing profession as well. Florence Nightingale (1820–1910), the icon of nursing in England, came from a distinguished family. After her work during the Crimean War she took it upon herself to make nursing an accepted profession—rather than a vocation—with proper training and rewards.[67] In the Netherlands, Lady Jeltje de Bosch Kemper (1836–1916) devoted herself to turning sick-nursing into a profession for civilized women. Nursing would become one of the few opportunities for unmarried women and girls from well-to-do families to enter a profession. Nurses were expected to bring a civilizing influence to grubby hospital wards.[68]

A great obstacle for Stokvis-Cohen Stuart to achieve her goals was "the deep distrust in the Native society of our medicine and its practitioners. It is especially because of the latter that we need native male and female nurses, to act as go-betweens."[69] In fact, Stokvis-Cohen Stuart deployed the nurses and midwives as intermediaries to spread Western medicine among the indigenous population. In a lecture for midwives in the Netherlands she set forth her views as follows:

> They understand the psyche of the patients much better, and surmount the difficulties much more easily, especially when they are somewhat older and married. What they should learn from us, except of course the knowledge and techniques that go with the profession, that is empathy, that is *social feeling*, that is the power to persevere and to help bring better notions of hygiene and health care to the uneducated population.[70]

In order to fulfil this role of intermediary, graduates should not provide care to pregnant women among the Chinese, Indo-European, and European communities. "For us, another point we should take into consideration very seriously concerns how we may retain the qualified girls for the *Javanese* population. After all, our main complaint has always been that, over time, many certified midwives choose to work for European and Chinese practices rather than the Native ones for the sake of higher earnings." To avoid this risk, the students were only brought into contact with Javanese patients during their training.[71] Stokvis-Cohen Stuart was not the only one who experienced this problem. The fact that European, Indo-European, and Chinese patients offered better remuneration has always been a problem in training health workers in the Dutch East

Indies, in particular because the salaries offered by the colonial administration were very low. Therefore, it was very difficult to retain trained
workers in their government positions.

The fact that the professional careers of women were almost always
interrupted by marriage and motherhood was often considered to impact
negatively their career prospects. As much happened this time: "So
often the argument is hurled at us that the girls will get married once
they have finished their studies. But that does not mean they are lost to
society!…Rather, married women and mothers can every day spread the
knowledge among their own."[72] In Stokvis-Cohen Stuart's eyes, these
nurses and midwives remained useful as intermediaries of Western health
care, even if they had left the profession because of marriage. Investing
in the training was not a "waste of time and money…since the knowledge gained about hygiene and sick-nursing will not be lost. In her
environment every well-trained nurse or midwife will—in small or great
matters—be a blessing and a help."[73] Stokvis-Cohen Stuart thus did not
belong to the group of ethicists who wanted to hold up the Western
nuclear family with its wage-earning husband and child-rearing wife as

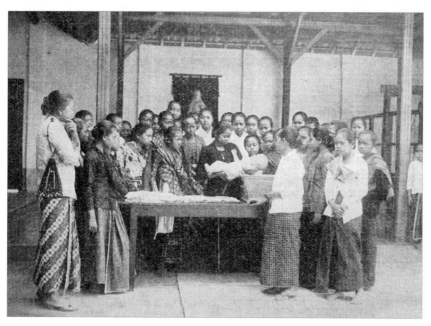

**Figure 5.** The midwife-nurse Raden Ajeng Soelastri opens a course for mothers
in Yogyakarta [Photograph from N. Stokvis-Cohen Stuart, *Leven en Werken in
Indië* (Amsterdam: De Bussy, 1931), 38].

an example. On the contrary: "We should establish a tradition that not every married woman immediately abandons her work, but continues to practice as much as possible what she has learnt."[74]

Educating young women and reaching future mothers has always been emphasized in public health work. Also in Stokvis-Cohen Stuart's strategy, women were not merely important as helpers—as nurses or midwives—but also constituted her target group: "In my view we can only improve hygiene and sick-care by reaching the women."[75] "Hygienic emancipation of the Native population is impossible without the cooperation of the Native woman."[76] Stokvis-Cohen Stuart regarded housewives and mothers as central figures whose cooperation was absolutely necessary for achieving and effecting improvements in the field of health care and hygiene. In one of her lectures she told the audience: "And truly, it is not out of feminist considerations that I have reached this conclusion—*it is the women, the mothers that we depend on!*"[77] Javanese women had to be persuaded to use Western medical assistance, not only through the deployment of female caregivers but also by means of little presents. If Javanese women gave birth in hospital, the young mothers received a small parcel with clothes as a gift.[78] "In the beginning we did everything for free [at the outpatient clinic], we even gave away nappies and baby clothes by way of propaganda. This was also to propagandize good baby clothes because usually there was no special baby wear."[79] Infant care offered an entrance into the world of mothers: "And via a one-year-old infant, we got to treat the woman during her pregnancy of next year's child!"[80] "And time and time again we found the great power of propaganda that emanates from such infant welfare centres, or, as you wish, outpatient clinics."[81]

Another prong of her strategy involved establishing the Society for the Promotion of Native Nursing Practices (Vereeniging tot Bevordering van de Inlandsche Ziekenverpleging) whose aim was to promote the interests of indigenous nursing in the broadest sense.[82] At its outset the Society was especially orientated towards providing training by funding the girls' and, later, also, the boys'[83] accommodation and the first outpatient clinic.[84] Stokvis-Cohen Stuart wished to broaden the scope of the Society: "We could try to make our Society known across the Native society; we could seek the cooperation of more educated Javanese."[85] Thus, the Society was used to garner support among the population by inviting them to the board and admitting them as members. Nearly all members, both in the Indies and in the Netherlands, belonged to the upper classes. The board deliberately consisted of both European and

Javanese individuals, mostly *priyayi*. As an example, Raden Ayu Poerbo-hadiningrat and Raden Ayu Sosrohadikoesoemo,[86] two noble ladies, sat on the board. Its secretary was an assistant district head (*wedono*), Mas Soedjono.[87] Since he was also the chairman of the Semarang branch of the Sarekat Islam (Islamic Union), a nationalist organization, the Society also received support from that quarter.[88] The Society organized lectures: "By means of lectures to Natives, we may endeavour to open their eyes to the Western ideas of hygiene, in other words, contribute to the promotion of public health."[89] The lectures, often accompanied by slides, were given by Stokvis-Cohen Stuart or by one of the Javanese board members.[90] Occasionally, a lecture was published in the form of a leaflet or article.

The Society was also important because it took care of all ex-penses, sometimes in advance of the subsidy from the colonial govern-ment. Stokvis-Cohen Stuart was frequently impatient and could not always wait for the colonial government to provide subsidies; in such cases, the Society would pay for activities instead. Apart from govern-ment subsidies, the Society's activities were funded by members' contri-butions and the proceeds of the lectures given by Stokvis-Cohen Stuart. When she returned to the Indies from overseas leave in 1915, she car-ried a nicely filled money bag with her, thanks to recommendations by Prince Henry, Queen Wilhelmina's husband, and by the former Minister of Colonial Affairs J.T. Cremer.[91] These funds provided the Society's starting capital. During her next leave (early 1916) she replenished the Society's coffers by giving lectures to the Red Cross and at the request of the wife of Minister for Colonial Affairs Th.B. Pleyte. The proceeds of both lectures amounted to ƒ17,000, an enormous amount (current value €150,000). The great interest shown in the Netherlands in the work of the Society led Stokvis-Cohen Stuart to appoint a local repre-sentative of the Society.[92] She allocated this task to her own mother.

## In Practice

The indigenous population continued to be averse to Western medicine, even if care was offered by women. Stokvis-Cohen Stuart experienced this in person: "yet it has even happened to me a few times that a patient already lying in the examination chair jumped out and went home before anything had been done because she did not wish to be examined, not even by a woman."[93] However, the main cause lay in the fact that Javanese women, when pregnant, remained loyal to the *dukun bayi*. *Dukuns bayi* derived their reputation from their advanced age, which meant that not only had they assisted many deliveries, they were also mothers who had had several children themselves and knew the intimate details of childbirth. The student-midwives were distrusted because of their young age and their unmarried status.[94] "It is greatly disappointing for the girls to find that despite their diploma all kinds of patients consider their youth and unmarried status as shortcomings."[95]

The competition from the *dukun* was constantly felt. Stokvis-Cohen Stuart was quite aware of the fact that graduates working in remote areas, "the interior," would occasionally have to provide help in "a field that is most definitely not hers." Even so, in her memorandum to the Governor-General, Stokvis-Cohen Stuart expressed the hope that they "would be of more benefit and cause less damage than the *dukuns* have thus far."[96] As they worked shifts in the kampong the midwives would encounter resistance not only from housemates and family members but also from *dukuns*.[97] Concepts from *adat* (indigenous customs and law) concerning pregnancy and delivery were especially deep-rooted and they were, as a matter of course, observed by the *dukun bayi*. The *adat* determined that the umbilical cord could only be cut after the placenta was delivered because the baby and its afterbirth were siblings. In a number of cases this had caused the death of the mother, the child or both. Since such mishaps were easily remedied in the eyes of Western physicians, they fulminated against the incompetence of the *dukun bayi*. Remarkably, Stokvis-Cohen Stuart mentioned this *adat* rule just once.[98] Did she not feel very strongly about this matter because she thought that these traditional customs would disappear with the introduction of Western medicine? Or should we interpret her silence on this issue as a form of fatalism, a 'you can't change such an internalized custom anyhow' attitude?

There are indications that *dukuns* regarded Western-trained midwives as their rivals and tried to put them in a bad light. According to Stokvis-Cohen Stuart, the *dukuns* spread "the usual tales about 'cutting', steep bills, etc....[to] try to create distrust of the midwife."[99] Further, *dukuns* attempted to imitate Western-trained midwives. They were often present incognito when Stokvis-Cohen Stuart or one of her students assisted with a delivery and would witness them performing internal examinations or removing placentas. *Dukuns* then started to do these things themselves, but with unwashed hands. Incidentally, Stokvis-Cohen Stuart could muster some sympathy for the fact that in some circumstances *dukuns* might well be of use, if only because they gave moral support to the woman in labor or when, as it sometimes happened, no one else was available.[100] She dared charge for the services of the graduates since the Javanese population was used to paying a *dukun bayi*.[101] She suspected that *dukun*s were often a lot more expensive.[102] Not everybody in the colony advocated levying a charge for Western medical help. In fact, a prominent medical committee rejected the idea: "If the Natives are to be won over to European medicine, you can hardly start by asking them for money for medicines."[103]

In practice, the number of patients fell short of expectations, even though it did show a slight increase over time: in 1915, the first year of midwifery training, 75 women were given obstetric help while in 1929, 1,400 women received this help (200 in the clinic and 1,200 in the kampong).[104] The training for *mantri* nurses (male and female) soon became enormously popular: in 1914 there were merely 90 students,[105] while 7 years later, in 1921, there were 787 of them;[106] unfortunately, how these numbers were divided over the sexes is only known for the year 1924, when 325 young men and 228 young women received training.[107] Meanwhile, the colonial government had increased the total

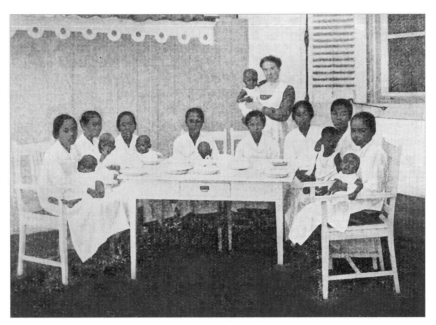

**Figure 6.** The students and a European nurse with babies in the garden of the Semarang hospital (Photograph from Stokvis-Cohen Stuart, *Leven en Werken in Indië*, 21).

number of young individuals whose training was subsidized to 500.[108] Not surprisingly, there were more graduates: in 1924, 41 female *and* 306 male *mantri* nurses finished the course.[109] A few years earlier, in 1918, there had been only 102 male and female *mantri* graduates.[110] The number of student-midwives was, in comparison, low (18) in 1918,[111] and in 1922 they only numbered 43.[112] These numbers contradict the remarks by Stokvis-Cohen Stuart that midwifery training was more popular and that almost all qualified nurses wanted to continue their studies to become midwives. Yet experience had shown that training midwives was an uphill struggle. As a result, the old regulation whereby physicians could train young women to become midwives in two years at home was abolished for lack of interest—on the part of both trainers and students.[113]

With her suggestion to propagandize Western medicine through the district nursing service, Stokvis-Cohen Stuart fitted in very well with the health policies of the day. In a lecture delivered in Amsterdam in 1915, W.Th. de Vogel, head of the CMS since 1913, emphasized that a special task of his organization was to promulgate Western medicine among the indigenous population, which continued to hold on to its own folk medicine. To instil trust in Western medicine, it was important to use propaganda among the population prudently.[114] A separate department of Medical-Hygienic Propaganda was set up within the CMS in 1925 for this purpose.[115]

## Conclusion

Stokvis-Cohen Stuart was unusual in several ways. Both from a medical and a social perspective her interventions are interesting. However, the plans that Stokvis-Cohen Stuart implemented—nurse and midwifery training, and outpatient clinics—were hardly new. As early as 1906 de Vogel had advocated establishing model hospitals in the three major cities, where indigenous male and female staff, including nurses, were to be trained. The nurses would gradually replace the *dukuns* in the kampongs. The best nurses were to be trained as midwives after they had worked in hospitals for at least two years.[116] Stokvis-Cohen Stuart's combined training was her own idea. She may not have been aware of earlier proposals because they had not received much attention. Regardless, the fact remains that she contributed district nursing services as a new element in the colonial health service. Stokvis-Cohen Stuart occupies a unique position as she put these ideas into actual practice.

She could only do so because of her perseverance, strategic insight, and idealism. Long after her return to the Netherlands, she kept fighting for her ideals. For example, she called on female physicians to go to the Indies: "A fine task awaits female physicians in the Indies: contributing to the *training of Native girls to become nurses and midwives*."[117] She also wrote several articles about working in the Indies in a journal on nursing to prepare nurses who wanted to go to the colony.[118] In the end she even organized a course on nursing in the tropics for them.[119] Apart from carrying out her duties as a physician and an educator, she also wrote memorandums, twice to the Governor-General of the Dutch East Indies. A third element in her success was the Society for the Promotion of Native Nursing Practices and her lectures, which created support among the Europeans and Javanese. The quotations from her lectures and her articles are wonderfully vivid as my quotations illustrate. Her presentations were a necessary part of her strategy because they were the means for her cause and her ideals. Stokvis-Cohen Stuart deployed the graduates of her courses as agents of Western medicine, but she herself was a change agent as she helped build and institutionalize the nursing profession. Within a relatively short time—from 1908 until her move to Bogor in 1920—she managed to put her ideals into practice. In part, her ideas fitted in with the spirit of the age, the Ethical Policy, as with her commitment to the welfare of the indigenous population; but she was also ahead of her time, given her focus on women and the transfer of knowledge to Javanese women. In her view, the task facing European physicians, nurses, and midwives was "not to just *keep on doing ourselves but to train*, to transmit, to make others competent enough to take over our work."[120]

In those days it was highly unusual for a married woman to work outside the home: in 1930 a mere 5.5 per cent of married European women in the colony did so.[121] Her being a physician made her exceptional: apart from her, there were only two other female physicians in the colony in 1908.[122] In 1908 she set up a private practice,[123] but most of her time was spent on the outpatient clinic and providing training activities that did not bring in any earnings. Stokvis-Cohen Stuart could afford to engage in these activities because her husband had a well-paying job and because the couple had remained childless.

It goes without saying that Stokvis-Cohen Stuart did not achieve all this all by herself. She was inspired by the mission. She admired missionary-physician H. Bervoets and his wife, a nurse.[124] She even worked a few months in a missionary hospital in Yogyakarta to learn how the mission educated Javanese women to become nurses and mid-wives. Further, she could not but have been greatly inspired by her uncle J.H. Abendanon, the personification of the Ethical Policy (he was director of the Department of Education, Religion and Industry from 1900 to 1905). Her husband, too, supported her in her work. As a member of the People's Council (Volksraad, the proto-parliament in the Dutch Indies), he was a staunch advocate of building a new hospital in Semarang, which was important for the nursing training courses. Together with others, he managed to double the amount budgeted for this purpose: from 200,000 to 400,000 guilders.[125] She received a great deal of practical help from her colleague N.F. Lim and his wife W.A. Lim-Bergsma; the book on sick-nursing that she published in 1928 was dedicated to Lim.[126] Of similar importance was the support of W.Th. de Vogel, first in his position as director of the hospital in Semarang and later as head of the CMS. In turn, de Vogel showed appreciation for her work: "In Semarang the sustained efforts on the part of Dr. Lim and Mrs. Stokvis-Cohen Stuart have been successful in persuading Native women and men from the upper classes to devote themselves to sick-nursing and to train as qualified nurses. Once they return to their Native society, they will be the true propagators of Western medicine among the people."[127] It was also helpful that she already spoke the language and had a good social network (she called Governor-General Idenburg "uncle")[128] when she arrived in Semarang. Naturally, she also met with opposition, among others, from Lim's successor.[129]

Ultimately, her work can be characterized as an intervention in indigenous patterns of birthing and mothering. Fundamental to such interventions were attacks on indigenous modes of birthing and nurturing as well as on TBAs. Stokvis-Cohen Stuart hardly ever mentioned *adat* when she introduced Western approaches to birthing and infant care. At the same time, her policy of giving away free baby clothes is reminiscent of a kind of civilizing mission: "Through this system [of free baby clothes instead of clothes made from old sarongs] we sought to have the people break with the old custom, but, even more so, to teach the mothers, once everything had ended well, the enjoyment of taking proper care of their baby, of making him or her look smart."[130] Yet we have seen that Javanese women did not simply succumb to the message of "enlightenment" through maternal improvement, but variously rejected or embraced such advice, or accommodated it selectively. Many clung to the intimate practices of confinement and labor, traditional sexual and dietary taboos during and after pregnancy, breast-feeding, and early infant care. They rejected modernity in the form of hygienic injunctions, and antenatal and postnatal checks.[131] Around 1920 the CMS was pleased to note that the annual reports of the physicians of the colonial government across various parts of the archipelago increasingly mentioned the rapprochement of the indigenous population with European medicine, yet that this was found to be less the case for obstetric help. Even today, *dukun bayis* have a strong position. They are still responsible for around 35 per cent of all deliveries, even though the Indonesian government stipulated in 2000 that only qualified midwives should be responsible for deliveries.[132]

## Archives Consulted

Collectie W.Th. de Vogel, KITLV (Royal Institute for Carribean and Southeast Asian Studies), Leiden, The Netherlands, inv. no. H 214.
Collectie Cohen-Stuart, Centraal Bureau voor Genealogie, The Hague, The Netherlands, inv. no. 479.

## Notes

1.  N. Stokvis-Cohen Stuart, "Nota betreffende de noodzakelijkheid van verbetering van de ziekenzorg voor Javaansche vrouwen," *Bulletin van den Bond van Geneesheeren in Ned.-Indië* 97 (1914): 1.
2.  O. Degeller, "Inlandsche Ziekenverpleging," Part 1, *Bulletin van den Bond van Geneesheeren in Ned.-Indië* 19 (1910): 1. Government hospitals were called *stadsverband*. As this article deals only with government hospitals, I have simply termed them hospitals.
3.  N. Stokvis-Cohen Stuart, "Plan tot instelling eener wijkverpleging," *Bulletin van den Bond van Geneesheeren in Ned.-Indië* 25 (1916): 8.
4.  W.Th de Vogel, Concept-geneeskundig Jaarverslag Semarang over 1901, Collectie W.Th. de Vogel, no. 5.
5.  Indonesian does not have separate forms to indicate plurals; nonetheless for this article English plurals will be used for Indonesian words such as *babu, mantri, dukun*.
6.  J. Bijker, *Rapport der Commissie tot Voorbereiding eener Reorganisatie van den Burgerlijken Geneeskundigen Dienst* (Batavia: Landsdrukkerij, 1908), 96.
7.  H.F.P. Maasland, "Ziekenverpleging door Vrouwen" (paper presented at the conference to discuss the work done by women in various societal areas in our Indies possessions, Amsterdam, August 22, 1898), 1, 5.
8.  N. Stokvis-Cohen Stuart, "Over Inlandsche Ziekenverpleging in Nederlandsch-Indië," *De Indische Gids* 37 (1915): 795 (paper presented at a meeting at the Red Cross, The Hague, April 14, 1915).

9.  Her family was of Jewish descent but converted to Christianity at the beginning of the eighteenth century.

10. N. Stokvis-Cohen Stuart, "Medisch-sociaal Werk in Indië," *Leven en Werken* 16 (1931): 471–2; N. Stokvis-Cohen Stuart, "Leven en Werken in Indië," part I, *Tijdschrift voor Ziekenverpleging* 41 (1931): 142 ("I myself was attracted to this work through the enthusiasm of the well-known missionary doctor Bervoets."). Jacques Stokvis too relates the visit from the Bervoets to their departure for the Indies, *Autobiography Jacques Stokvis*, 1945, Collectie Cohen Stuart, no. 309.

11. Elsbeth Locher-Scholten, *Women and the Colonial State: Essays on Gender and Modernity in the Netherlands Indies 1900–1942* (Amsterdam: Amsterdam University Press, 2000), 16.

12. H.W. van den Doel, *Het Rijk van Insulinde: Opkomst en Ondergang van een Nederlandse Kolonie* (Amsterdam: Prometheus, 1996), 157.

13. Stokvis-Cohen Stuart, "Over Inlandsche Ziekenverpleging," 793.

14. Ibid.

15. N. Stokvis-Cohen Stuart, "Vroedvrouw-opleiding in Indië en Verloskundig Werk onder de Inlandsche Bevolking," *Tijdschrift voor Sociale Hygiëne* 33 (1931): 84.

16. Stokvis-Cohen Stuart, "Over Inlandsche Ziekenverpleging," 791.

17. Ibid., 794.

18. Ibid., 797–800.

19. N. Stokvis-Cohen Stuart, "De huidige koers ten aanzien van de gezondheidszorg in Indië," *Indisch Genootschap, Verslagen der Vergaderingen over de Jaren 1926–1930*, 1930: 19–22.

20. Stokvis-Cohen Stuart, *Inlandsche Ziekenverpleging Semarang*, 3–5.

21. *Jaarverslag der Vereeniging tot Bevordering der Inlandsche Ziekenverpleging*, vol. 2 (Semarang: H.A. Benjamins, 1916), 24.

22. Stokvis-Cohen Stuart, *Inlandsche Ziekenverpleging Semarang*, 12–14.

23. Stokvis-Cohen Stuart, "Plan Wijkverpleging," 5–6.

24. *Staatsblad van Nederlandsch-Indië* 1912, no. 87. *Mantri* refers to a lower civil servant; the word is used to form all manner of compound nouns. Here, *mantri* nurse is used to distinguish from those who carried out unqualified nursing work. Wherever the connection is clear, *mantri* may also be used on its own, in other words, *mantri* can mean "nurse" in this article.

25. GB dated 6-8-1911 no. 31, *Jaarverslag Vereeniging* 2 (1916): 17.

26. GB dated 19-3-1917 no. 20, *Bijblad op het Staatsblad van Nederlandsch-Indië*, no. 8727.

27. Stokvis-Cohen Stuart, "Over Inlandsche Ziekenverpleging," 797.

28. *Koloniaal Verslag* 1914, Appendix U mentions only one midwife-student with a private female physician in Semarang; these must have been Stokvis-Cohen Stuart and her first student Mien.

29. Stokvis-Cohen Stuart, *Inlandsche Ziekenverpleging Semarang*, 10–11.

30. *Jaarverslag Vereeniging* 2 (1916): 7–9.
31. Stokvis-Cohen Stuart, *Inlandsche Ziekenverpleging Semarang*, 12–14.
32. Ibid., 12.
33. *Jaarverslag Vereeniging* 2 (1916): 10.
34. Stokvis-Cohen Stuart, "Over Inlandsche Ziekenverpleging," 803. In 1914 the CMS was authorized to appoint three European sisters on a temporary basis; two out of the three came to work in Semarang (*Koloniaal Verslag* 1915, 134), probably because of the nurse training.
35. Stokvis-Cohen Stuart, "Over Inlandsche Ziekenverpleging," 803.
36. Stokvis-Cohen Stuart, *Inlandsche Ziekenverpleging Semarang*, 21; italics by Stokvis-Cohen Stuart.
37. Stokvis-Cohen Stuart, *Inlandsche Ziekenverpleging Semarang*, 15.
38. *Staatsblad van Nederlandsch-Indië* 1915, no. 514.
39. *Bijblad op het Staatsblad van Nederlandsch-Indië*, no. 8378.
40. *Staatsblad van Nederlandsch-Indië*, no. 438.
41. Stokvis-Cohen Stuart, "Over Inlandsche Ziekenverpleging," 801.
42. Stokvis-Cohen Stuart, *Inlandsche Ziekenverpleging Semarang*, 8.
43. *Jaarverslag Vereeniging* 9 (1923): 13.
44. Examination requirements were laid down in *Bijblad op het Staatsblad van Nederlandsch-Indië*, no. 8251.
45. *Jaarverslag Vereeniging* 5 (1919): 8.
46. *Bijblad op het Staatsblad van Nederlandsch-Indië*, no. 8055.
47. Liesbeth Hesselink, *Healers on the Colonial Market: Native Doctors and Midwives in the Dutch East Indies* (Leiden: KITLV Press, 2011), 147.
48. The committee to reorganize the CMS advocated an absolute ban on using instruments. Bijker, *Rapport Reorganisatiecommissie*, 95.
49. *Jaarverslag Vereeniging* 9 (1923): 8.
50. *Jaarverslag Vereeniging* 2 (1916): 5.
51. Stokvis-Cohen Stuart, "Nota Ziekenzorg Javaansche Vrouwen," 9; italics by Stokvis-Cohen Stuart.
52. *Jaarverslag Vereeniging* 2 (1916): 7. The petition was formally submitted by the Society but it is most likely that Stokvis-Cohen Stuart, being in the chair, was the driving force; in her 1914 memorandum to the Governor-General she already fulminated against this regulation.
53. Letter from Stokvis-Cohen Stuart dated 9-3-1916 to de Vogel, Collectie W.Th. de Vogel, no. 4.
54. Ibid.
55. Stokvis-Cohen Stuart, "Plan Wijkverpleging," 1, 3–4, 6, 7. The memorandum was formally sent on behalf of the Society but its author was, in fact, Stokvis-Cohen Stuart, the chair; in several instances in the memorandum she writes in the first person.
56. *Jaarverslag Vereeniging* 4 (1918): 7–8.

57. Stokvis-Cohen Stuart, "Plan Wijkverpleging," 14–15; italics by Stokvis-Cohen Stuart.

58. *Jaarverslag Vereeniging* 4 (1918): 9.

59. *Koloniaal Verslag* 1919, 171; *Staatsblad van Nederlandsch-Indië* 1918, no. 466.

60. Stokvis-Cohen Stuart, "Plan Wijkverpleging," 9–10; italics by Stokvis-Cohen Stuart.

61. Stokvis-Cohen Stuart, "Plan Wijkverpleging," 16; *Jaarverslag Vereeniging* 4 (1918): 13.

62. Stokvis-Cohen Stuart, "Plan Wijkverpleging," 11–12.

63. Stokvis-Cohen Stuart, "Nota Ziekenzorg Javaansche Vrouwen," 2.

64. Ibid.

65. In December 1918 Raden Ajeng Soelastri was in charge of a branch of the outpatient clinic and worked as a teacher at the training, while Raden Ajeng Roebiah was in charge of laboratory research and a book of photographs. See Collectie Cohen Stuart, no. 1174.

66. G.J. Dreckmeier, "Zendingsarts op Java," in *En nog steeds hebben wij twee Vaderlanden": Op Avontuur in Nederlands-Indië*, ed. Carolijn Visser and Sasza Malko (Amsterdam: Meulenhoff, 2001), 145.

67. A.P.M. van der Meij-de Leur, *Van olie en Wijn: Geschiedenis van Verpleegkunde, Geneeskunde en Sociale Zorg* (Amsterdam/Brussel: Agon Elsevier, 1974), 168.

68. Nanny Wiegman, "'De Verpleegster zij in de eerste plaats Vrouw van Karakter': Ziekenverpleging als Vrouwenzaak (1898–1998)," in *Gezond en Wel: Vrouwen en de Zorg voor Gezondheid in de 20ᵉ Eeuw*, ed. Rineke van Daalen and Marijke Gijswijt-Hofstra (Amsterdam: Amsterdam University Press, 1998), 129–30.

69. Stokvis-Cohen Stuart, *Inlandsche Ziekenverpleging Semarang*, 3–5.

70. Stokvis-Cohen Stuart, "Vroedvrouw-opleiding in Indië," 80–1; italics by Stokvis-Cohen Stuart.

71. Stokvis-Cohen Stuart, *Inlandsche Ziekenverpleging Semarang*, 20–1; italics by Stokvis-Cohen Stuart.

72. Stokvis-Cohen Stuart, *Inlandsche Ziekenverpleging Semarang*, 19.

73. Stokvis-Cohen Stuart, "Nota Ziekenzorg Javaansche Vrouwen," 13.

74. Letter from Stokvis-Cohen Stuart dated 9-3-1916 to de Vogel, Collectie W.Th. de Vogel, no. 4.

75. Stokvis-Cohen Stuart, "Nota Ziekenzorg Javaansche Vrouwen," 2.

76. Stokvis-Cohen Stuart, "Vrouwelijke Artsen voor Indië," *Nederlands Tijdschrift voor Geneeskunde* 74 (1930): 1269.

77. Stokvis-Cohen Stuart, *Inlandsche Ziekenverpleging Semarang*, 21–3; italics by Stokvis-Cohen Stuart.

78. *Jaarverslag Vereeniging* 2 (1916): 13–14.

79. Stokvis-Cohen Stuart, "Vroedvrouw-opleiding," 91.
80. Ibid., 89.
81. Ibid., 92.
82. Approved by order of the colonial government no. 42 dated 21-1-1915. However, the Society was already in existence as the statutes had been submitted to the Governor-General for approval in August 1914, *Jaarverslag Vereeniging* 2 (1916): 18.
83. Stokvis-Cohen Stuart, *Inlandsche Ziekenverpleging Semarang*, 10–11.
84. *Jaarverslag Vereeniging* 4 (1918): 7–8.
85. Stokvis-Cohen Stuart, *Inlandsche Ziekenverpleging Semarang*, 19, 21–2.
86. Soematri, a sister of the Indonesian national heroine Kartini.
87. He was a stepson of Roekmini, another sister of Kartini. Mas is the title of the lowest noble rank.
88. Stokvis-Cohen Stuart, "Over Inlandsche Ziekenverpleging," 801.
89. Stokvis-Cohen Stuart, *Inlandsche Ziekenverpleging Semarang*, 19.
90. *Jaarverslag Vereeniging* 2 (1916): 12–13; Stokvis-Cohen Stuart, *Inlandsche Ziekenverpleging Semarang*, 24.
91. Autobiography Jacques Stokvis.
92. *Jaarverslag Vereeniging* 2 (1916): 3–5.
93. Stokvis-Cohen Stuart, "Vrouwelijke Artsen," 1269.
94. Ibid.
95. *Jaarverslag Vereeniging* 4 (1918): 23.
96. Stokvis-Cohen Stuart, "Plan Wijkverpleging," 1–2.
97. Ibid., 6.
98. Stokvis-Cohen Stuart, "Vroedvrouw-opleiding," 77.
99. *Jaarverslag Vereeniging* 5 (1919): 19.
100. Stokvis-Cohen Stuart, "Vroedvrouw-opleiding," 81.
101. Stokvis-Cohen Stuart, "Plan Wijkverpleging," 16.
102. Stokvis-Cohen Stuart, "Vroedvrouw-opleiding," 92.
103. Bijker, *Rapport Reorganisatiecommissie*, 53. Lower civil servants, poor Indo-Europeans and poor natives—according to the definition of the government, 95 per cent of the native population was poor—were entitled to free medical care. See W.Th. de Vogel, "De Taak van den Burgerlijken Geneeskundigen Dienst in Nederlandsch-Indië," *Mededeeling Koloniaal Instituut Amsterdam* 8, no. 4 (1917): 22.
104. Stokvis-Cohen Stuart, "Vroedvrouw-opleiding," 90.
105. *Koloniaal Verslag* 1915, 134.
106. *Koloniaal Verslag* 1922, 213.
107. "Jaarverslag van den Burgerlijken Geneeskundigen Dienst in Nederlandsch-Indië over 1924," *Mededeelingen van den Dienst der Volksgezondheid in Nederlandsch-Indië* 1927: 206, 239.
108. *Koloniaal Verslag* 1919, 170.
109. "Jaarverslag Burgerlijken Geneeskundigen Dienst 1924," 206, 239.

110. *Beknopt Verslag over den Burgerlijken Geneeskundigen Dienst van 1911 t/m 1918* (Weltevreden: Albrecht, 1920), 38.
111. *Koloniaal Verslag* 1919, 171.
112. *Koloniaal Verslag* 1923, 119.
113. Hesselink, *Healers on the Colonial Market*, 232; *Staatsblad van Nederlandsch-Indië* 1920, no. 602.
114. De Vogel, "De Taak Burgerlijken Geneeskundigen Dienst," 9.
115. J.A. Verdoorn, *Verloskundige Hulp voor de Inheemsche Bevolking van Nederlandsch-Indië* ('s-Gravenhage: Boekencentrum, 1941), 263.
116. W.Th. de Vogel, "Memorie betreffende den Burgerlijken Geneeskundigen Dienst," *Bulletin van den Bond van Geneesheeren in Ned.-Indië* 14 (1906): 39–40.
117. Stokvis-Cohen Stuart, "Vrouwelijke Artsen," 1269; italics by Stokvis-Cohen Stuart.
118. Stokvis-Cohen Stuart, *Leven en Werken in Indië.*
119. N. Stokvis-Cohen Stuart, "Tropenleergang voor Verplegenden", *Tijdschrift voor Ziekenverpleging* 41 (1931): 43–5; 388–90; 511–14; 651–2; 42 (1932): 20–1.
120. Stokvis-Cohen Stuart, "Vroedvrouw-opleiding," 81; italics by Stokvis-Cohen Stuart.
121. Elsbeth Locher-Scholten, "Door een gekleurde bril: Koloniale bronnen over Vrouwenarbeid op Java in de negentiende en twintigste Eeuw," in *Vrouwen in de Nederlandse Koloniën, 7ᵉ Jaarboek voor Vrouwengeschiedenis*, ed. Jeske Reijs et al. (Nijmegen: SUN, 1986), 48.
122. P. Pet-van Wijngaarden, a private doctor in Surabaya, and A. Pijsel, a missionary doctor in Mojowarno. In total, European physicians in the entire archipelago then numbered 329.
123. Later she became locum physician for the colonial government with the CMS, *Javasche Courant*, February 1, 1916, no. 9.
124. *Jaarverslag Vereeniging* 5 (1919): 8.
125. Ibid.: 6–7.
126. N. Stokvis-Cohen Stuart, *Ilmoe pembĕla orang sakit* (Groningen: Wolters, 1928); with several later reprints.
127. De Vogel, "Taak Burgerlijken Geneeskundigen Dienst," 18.
128. Autobiography Jacques Stokvis and book of photographs, Collectie Cohen Stuart, no. 523.
129. Autobiography Jacques Stokvis; Dreckmeier, "Zendingsarts op Java," 145 writes: "she met with opposition from the physicians and the hospitals, the whole lot in Semarang."
130. Stokvis-Cohen Stuart, "Vroedvrouw-opleiding," 91.
131. *Koloniaal Verslag*, 1918, 129.
132. Deborah Hennessy, Carolyn Hick, and Harni Koesno, "The Training and Development of Needs of Midwives in Indonesia," *Human Resources for Health* 4 (2006): 9.

## CHAPTER 2

# Trouble with "Status": Competing Models of British and North American Public Health Nursing Education and Practice in British Malaya

*Rosemary Wall and Anne Marie Rafferty*

Two distinct nursing styles fought for dominance within the nursing world in the interwar period and British Malaya provides a historical laboratory with which to study the varied goals of British and North American nursing. Where the British approach in the field relied upon the notion of "character," the North American model favored a more techno-scientific approach emphasizing the importance of leadership. The "organic" British approach appears to contrast with that of American colonial policy and that of the American Rockefeller Foundation (RF) in the Philippines, where there was a concerted attempt to lay down a legacy and create "lighthouses" of leadership.[1] Yet, British and North American attitudes were initially similar in two respects: training of local nurses and the feminization of the local nursing workforce. However, the focus of this chapter is the collaboration and conflict between American and British nursing styles in British Malaya in the 1920s and 1930s. The title of this chapter refers to the experience of a nurse, Elizabeth Darville, who was trained in Britain, recruited by the Overseas Nursing Association (ONA), and was inspired by further training in North America before working in Malaya where she experienced a clash of attitudes. The challenges which Darville faced reveal that "Western" nursing and medical leadership styles were not homogenous in colonial contexts.[2] The chapter concludes by considering how lethargic British nursing was in laying down a clear legacy of leadership throughout the period of British rule.

In this chapter, Darville's experience of working with the American Rockefeller Foundation's Straits Settlement Rural Sanitation Campaign (SSRSC) is situated within an analysis of the history of colonial nursing policy in British Malaya from the 1890s to the 1950s. Independence of Malaya and Singapore from 1957 and 1959 resulted in dependence upon the World Health Organization (WHO) for assistance with training. We explore the twists and turns that shaped nursing in Malaya before independence from the United Kingdom. The themes of integration and inhibition are used to explore the processes at work that drove the supply and demand factors for female British and Asian nurses in British Malaya in the early to mid-twentieth century.

Between 1896 and 1966 the Colonial Nursing Association (CNA) recruited and sent 8,450 nurses to areas overseas. The Association was run by volunteers, but quickly came to serve the Colonial Office, with this relationship finally formalized in 1940.[3] The CNA changed its name to the ONA in 1918, in recognition of the fact that it not only served the colonies but other areas with British populations.[4] From the 1920s on, Malaya hosted the most British colonial nurses, only overtaken by the East African colonies in the late 1950s, after Malaya gained independence in 1957.[5] Figure 1 illustrates the concentration of these nurses in Malaya during the years that this chapter largely focuses upon: 1925–35. The graph illustrates the number of nurses in the six most common destinations during that period. Malaya was able to employ so many nurses because the colonies of East and Southeast Asia were amongst the richest in the British Empire.[6] Before World War II, services within colonies were funded internally.[7] Therefore the Eastern colonies of Malaya, Hong Kong, and Ceylon, and the international concession in Shanghai were in an economic position to employ British nurses. India does not feature in this graph as a separate organization supplied most of its British nurses, Lady Minto's Indian Nursing Association. Despite this concentration of nurses in the area, British Malaya has been largely neglected by historians of nursing. The most extensive works on nursing in Southeast Asia have focused on the US experience in the Philippines.[8]

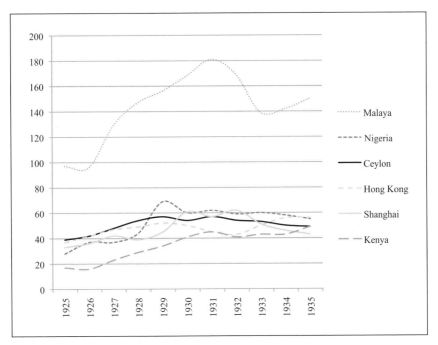

**Figure 1.** Number of nurses in territories with the highest number of Overseas Nursing Association nurses, 1925–35 (Source: Colonial/Overseas Nursing Association, *Annual Reports*, 1925–35, box 131, MSS Brit Emp s400, Overseas Nursing Association Collection, Commonwealth and African Studies, Bodleian Library, University of Oxford).

## Early Colonial Nursing in British Malaya

The term British Malaya is used to denote the three administrative areas —the Federated Malay States (FMS), Unfederated Malay States (UFMS), and the Straits Settlements—which were further divided into "twelve geopolitical units."[9] European health care began with trade and military medical care in the Straits Settlements in the eighteenth century, organized centrally from the nineteenth century. The FMS were formed in 1895, with little co-ordination of medical provision between the states and no uniformity in provision until 1911.[10] The RF interventions, on which this chapter is centered, took place within the Straits Settlements in the 1920s. In 1932, during the economic depression, the medical and health departments of the Straits Settlements and the FMS were joined in order to cut costs and became the Malayan Medical Services.[11] Following World War II, the Malayan Union was created by the British, with the FMS, UFMS, and Penang and Malacca (formerly in the Straits Settlements), administered separately from Singapore.[12] Not only was British Malaya a complex administrative construct but its population was a complicated ethnic mix as a result of the colonial economy. Muslim Malays, together with the immigrant populations from China and the Indian subcontinent, presented ethnic and gender hierarchies and political policies that needed to be navigated in nurses' work and social lives.[13]

Prior to the arrival of colonial nurses, the FMS medical department was staffed by European surgeons and Chinese or Indian apothecaries, the majority being Chinese or Indian dressers and apprentices; the entire staff was male.[14] Male dressers performed a role similar to that of nurses, but their responsibilities included additional tasks such as microscopy.[15] Therefore, the role of a "dresser" was not equivalent to the role with this title in Britain at that time, which described medical students on surgical placements. This system of using dressers for the care of patients became unpopular with the British doctors and Residents (the term used for the representatives of the British government in each of the states comprising the FMS). In the 1893 Perak report, the Resident commented that patients in hospitals were only being looked after in the daytime and were left without nursing at night, when "many of their lives depend on being fed and attended to every hour."[16] In Negri Sembilan, dressers were learning and being slowly promoted on the job, but the Resident bemoaned the fact that they were "plunged straight away into the mysteries of surgery and medicine and the prescribing of drugs of whose action they know nothing."[17] In Pahang, the Resident was concerned that the Malay community did not generally attend hospitals, as they viewed the Chinese and Indian dressers with suspicion. In 1896, he suggested training Malay dressers to encourage the Malays to attend. However, he noted that the situation was still complicated as Malays wanted to be treated by female family members, and Malay families would not allow women to be treated in hospital.[18]

At this stage, the training of local women as nurses was not considered appropriate. It was not the custom for Malay women to work within the colonial economy.[19] Training of other Asian women was problematic as the British treated the Chinese and Indian populations as transient migrant labor, adopting a laissez-faire attitude towards them until the 1920s, after which Chinese and Indian women were encouraged to migrate, marry, and reproduce. A paternalist attitude, including education, was reserved for the Malays.[20] Treatment by male medical staff, in particular physical exposure of the female patient to the male doctor, was anathema to Muslim Malays. This led to increased provision of Lady Medical Officers in the 1920s. However, female doctors could not devote all of their time to Malays as there was demand in the towns from Chinese and Tamils, and it was a strain to spend day after day visiting rural kampongs.[21] A Malay-only hospital opened in Perak at the beginning of the twentieth century, which had improved attendance, but this experiment was not repeated in the state.[22] Concerns about provision of maternity care resulted in an emphasis on training local women in antiseptic procedures for childbirth, leading to many more locally trained midwives than nurses in the rural areas.[23]

Despite these challenges, as soon as female British nurses arrived, an attempt was made to train a female nursing workforce. Although some colonies, such as Hong Kong, had already begun recruiting British nurses in the 1890s, the Colonial Office's suggestion of employing British nurses made a radical change to nursing in Malaya.[24] In 1898, European nurses were obtained from Britain.[25] Although there are records of a British nurse being sought for Selangor in 1889, and of a nurse being sent from the London Hospital to Perak in 1897, there are no records in the FMS reports that these nurses arrived.[26]

An alternative pattern of nursing care emerged in the Straits Settlements. Although care was initially primarily carried out by male attendants, suggestions of employing British- or Madras-trained nurses were made by the Principal Civil Medical Officer and the Surgeon-in-Charge of the General Hospital in Singapore in the 1880s. However, it was deemed uneconomical to bring nurses from Britain, and nurses from Madras did not want to come to Singapore.[27] The male attendants were replaced with partially trained female nurses of mixed nationalities from Roman Catholic convents in Singapore, Penang, and Malacca.[28] Even though there were benefits to employing the nuns as they were multilingual, cheap to employ, and the convents sent replacements when the nurses were unwell, there were protests as the nuns came from foreign-run convents and could not look at naked bodies. A total of 144 European residents petitioned for recruiting English nurses instead.[29]

In 1896, J. Irvine Rowell, head of the medical services in the Straits Settlements, and William Hoad, who was in charge of medical services in Singapore, wanted to pilot British nursing in the Straits Settlements by starting with "one fully trained nurse, from some good home hospital" who would be paid by the government to start organizing the scheme. This nurse would have to have "marked intelligence, energy, and tact, physically strong, not less than 35 years old, and with, if possible, few home ties." Rowell's and Hoad's initial intention was to employ nurses to teach women in the pauper hospital in order for women of different nationalities to nurse their own "race." They thought that "in the Eurasian community there will be found many members who will gladly lend themselves to a service of this nature, and who would probably be found, in the end, to make excellent nurses for general purposes."[30] However, as Felicia Yap has discussed, Eurasians had a marginal status, with difficulties integrating into colonial and Asian society, with many Europeans perceiving them as the "embodiment of degeneration," a product of a moral lapse as many were illegitimate.[31] Therefore, they may not have been able to fulfil the role which locally trained health care workers could have as "cultural brokers," disseminating Western ideas of health education.[32] Nevertheless, only two British nurses would be brought over as they wished to use the "ample material available in the Colony itself."[33] By November 1900 their ideas had clearly changed as eight British nursing sisters were employed in Singapore.[34]

The introduction of female British nurses who would train women locally was part of a plan to feminize the nursing workforce. Feminization was equated with modernization, whether in the case of British military nursing in the mid-nineteenth century or replacing male dressers in the colonies.[35] This pattern was also followed in the Philippines, where American nurses actively aimed to delineate the male and female spheres, a process which was seen as part of civilizing a race.[36] Yet in contrast to Malaya, where the feminization program persisted, from 1913 on Filipino men were reintegrated into nurse training and some were promoted to senior hospital positions; they were also recognized as valuable for remote public health nursing work.[37] Catherine Choy suggests this reintegration of men may have been accepted as there was a minority of male nurses working in the US.[38]

The process of feminization was complicated as recruitment of local female Asian nurses could be difficult with nursing not always seen as a desirable vocation. This also explains the recruitment of Eurasians. In an oral testimony recorded in the 1980s, one woman recalled that in the 1930s, her parents would not allow her to be a nurse as it was thought that boys and men visited the nurses in their hostels.[39] Even by the early 1960s, an interviewee's mother asked her why she was training to be a nurse, worried that her friends thought that nursing was menial and not respectable.[40] A danger was perceived that the nurses might consider certain duties beneath them. In the early 1940s, a British nurse wrote about an Asian nurse who had only been training for 18 months, yet complained that she was "too senior to be a 'temperature nurse'." Another, who had been told to give an enema, was "found holding the funnel, but she had called the *ayah* to insert the catheter!"[41] Despite these limitations on recruitment, census statistics reveal that the numbers of Malay and other nurses were increasing. In 1921, there were 43 Malay nurses, 48 Eurasian nurses, 34 Chinese nurses, and 22 Indian nurses in British Malaya.[42] As Figure 1 illustrates, by 1930 the number of British nurses in Malaya had increased dramatically to 168. These nurses were training an increasing number of Asian women from Malay, Eurasian, Chinese, and Indian ethnic origins to work in nursing. By 1947, there were 301 Malay women working as midwives, nurses, or mental attendants, though this must have been minuscule compared to the demand.[43] However, much of the emphasis was on midwifery rather than general nursing, with efforts to enhance maternity care by training the existing *bidan* (traditional midwives) and other Asian women beginning in the Straits Settlements in 1905, leading to at least 1,518 trained midwives working in the Straits Settlements by 1936, but far fewer in the FMS and UFMS, where training programs began in 1914 and 1929 respectively.[44] Also, as the following section reveals, Asian nurses were subordinated within the British colonial health care system.

## Critique and Americanization of British Colonial Nursing in Malaya

The health care system that had been established by the British became the subject of critique by the RF from 1915 on. In that year, the International Health Commission (IHC) of the RF surveyed and attempted to influence British policy and practice in Malaya. Although nursing was not a priority for the RF, over 34 years the Foundation assisted with nursing education in 44 countries.[45] When the IHC was established in 1913 the main foci were eradicating hookworm, malaria, and yellow fever, as well as training public health physicians and public health nurses. Malaya was one of the IHC's first areas for attention in 1913–15, along with British Guiana, the British West Indies, Egypt, and Ceylon, illustrating that the IHC was not afraid to intervene in British territories.[46]

Subordination of Asian nurses through limited training and lack of promotion was highlighted in 1915, when a survey of medical education in Malaya was undertaken by Victor Heiser, the IHC's Director for the East. Heiser worried much more about hospital assistants, nurses, pharmacists, and dentists than about doctors. He found nursing more racially divided than medicine, with medical courses primarily attracting Malays, whilst nursing was limited to European and Eurasian applicants. The course attracted only a few students. Heiser also observed that the British nurses in Penang did not wash the patients or apply dressings, leaving this to the locally trained staff. Heiser wanted to provide scholarships for Malayan nurses to train at the American-run nursing school in Manila in the Philippines, as he believed the Malayan patients were not receiving the care they would if they were cared for by nurses trained to American standards.[47] However, Heiser had arrived in Malaya after ten years as Director of Health for the Philippines (1905–15) and was therefore praising his own nursing program.[48]

Heiser noted that training and prospects for Asian nurses were very different in Malaya than in the American Philippines. The American rule of the Philippines was, according to Sunil Amrith, "self-consciously 'progressive'" with more focus on the health of indigenous populations.[49] American colonial rule had a "light bureaucratic presence" administered through a "public-private" nexus, in comparison to European tropical colonies in the early twentieth century.[50] The Philippines were acquired abruptly in 1898 as a result of the Spanish-American War, and the American colonizers initially intended to reform the style of Spanish centralized colonial rule. Yet the Philippines were inherited as nationalism was brewing, which resulted in four years of American pacification, surveillance, and control.[51] Whereas Malaya and Singapore were highly significant for the British in terms of raw materials and trade—hence the protracted struggle to maintain the area as a colony after World War II—the Philippines were valuable to the US as the archipelago was well located for trade and as a military base close to China.[52] Nevertheless the stages of "retention and self-rule" transitioned much more swiftly in the American than the British Empire.[53] Although the American colonizers initially infantilized the Filipinos, as Warwick Anderson has argued with the example of public health policy, in contrast to other colonial powers, the Americans soon moved towards "civilizing" as a "precursor" to the "development" projects organized by other colonial powers from the 1940s.[54]

The legacy of Spanish colonization led to religious differences between the populations in some areas of the Philippines, in comparison to largely Muslim Malaya, which must have made a key difference in the recruitment of nurses for training. The Philippines had been exposed to 300 years of Spanish "clerical colonialism" by the Catholic orders, with hospitals for the poor and universities for the elite, and, from 1806, a vaccination program.[55] Religion and politics also played an important role in terms of greater empowerment in nursing, as from 1905 Christian provinces were granted "partial, local self-government," in contrast to nearly half the territory which was populated by animists (who believe that natural objects have souls and are invested with spirits) and Muslims and which remained under American control. However, American colonists used comparisons between the administrations to justify why this bifurcated system should continue, arguing that this revealed that Christian Filipinos did not have the capacity for full self-government.[56]

William H. Taft, the first civil governor, thought that the Christian Filipinos could be trained for self-government over many generations.[57] His perception of Filipinos as infantilized led him to believe that they could be trained. He developed a "policy of attraction," aiming to show benevolence following the suppression of the people in the Philippine-American War.[58] Adam D. Burns relates this "hearts and minds" strategy to recent US foreign policy.[59] However, in terms of empowerment of nurses, Tafts' policy can be related to the actions of the British colonial government as a reaction to the Malayan Emergency in the 1940s and 1950s, which we have written about in detail elsewhere.[60] American training in the Philippines would have accelerated following anti-imperialist lobbying in the US, which argued that a "subservient empire" was contrary to the nation's ideals; as early as 1907, President Theodore Roosevelt was concerned that the islands should be independent, with legislation passed in 1916 promising future independence.[61] From 1911, Filipino nurses were funded to travel to the US by the RF and other organizations.[62] However, American nurses still led most of the hospital training schools and from the 1920s, more American nurses worked in the Philippines, funded by the RF in an attempt to improve public health.[63] Although Americans had been keen to promote Asian nurses, they exerted cultural dominance in their conviction of the supremacy of American nursing, and as Choy has shown, used racist and patronizing language in discussing Filipino nurses.[64]

In 1925, the RF returned to British Malaya, and continued to question the quality of the training of British public health nurses. The RF established the SSRSC, largely concentrating on hookworm and on implementing American-style public health nursing, a strategy that had been used within RF Health Units in the US.[65] When the Straits Settlements government agreed to cooperate with the RF, Milford Barnes, an RF doctor, doubted that English nurses would initiate activities of the kind American County Health nurses undertook. He worried about convincing the British to accept North American training for the public health nurses who were to be sent to work on the campaign. According to A.L. Hoops, the Principal Civil Medical Officer for Singapore, the British felt a "loss of prestige" in accepting help from Americans.[66]

Politically, this was a difficult period for American intervention. After World War I, Britain remained the country with the largest foreign trade, foreign income, share of international services, and merchant fleet in the world. However, British finances had been weakened by the loss of dollar securities to the US in order to finance the war.[67] Frederick Gates, who helped to establish the RF as the philanthropic arm of John D. Rockefeller's Standard Oil, saw American influence in non-industrialized colonies as an opportunity to increase markets, whereas Dr Howard, who also worked for the RF, directly linked improved health with productivity, happiness, and prosperity.[68] Revealing the perception of British attitudes towards American internationalism in Malaya in 1928, Heiser wrote in his diary, "America is reviled and slandered almost continuously in the press. This seems a strange thing to do to your best customer."[69]

Despite these political tensions, Barnes succeeded in convincing the colonial government that the British nurses required extra American training.[70] The RF provided them with experience in public health nursing in America for three months, with the British government paying the salaries, whilst the RF paid the extra expenses—their board and travel in North America, and the extra expenditure on travel incurred by traveling to Singapore via North America.[71] RF funding for rural health was perhaps welcome at a time of increased Malayan nationalism in the 1920s.[72] This rural campaign may have been seen as valuable for reaching more of the population through Western medicine, seen by historians as accelerating "cultural colonialism" and justification of empire.[73]

In 1926, Elizabeth Darville and Annabella McNeill were recruited by the ONA to lead public health nursing in the Straits Settlements.[74] Darville had worked as a health visitor in England, with four years' school nurse experience, a health visitors' diploma, and work in a sanatorium. McNeill had some specialist training—a Sanitary Science Health Visitors certificate from the University of Liverpool—plus maternity and children's nursing experience.[75] Although they had some experience of training and working in public health, the RF did not view British public health nursing and training highly, as shown in Barnes' letter and a disparaging RF survey of public health nursing in Britain. The RF's criticism targeted a "jumble" of qualifications and the need to build leadership capacity in the field.[76] These findings were a disappointment to the RF as they had hoped to establish demonstration projects in England that could be used across the British Empire.[77] In 1923 an RF survey stated that trained nurses should be carrying out the role of health education. American RF nurse, Elizabeth Crowell, reported back from the UK that fellowships should be awarded for nurses to study in the US, Canada, and France, where superior training facilities for public health nurses were to be found.[78] These concerns were not unfounded. A survey carried out in 1926 showed that 1,974 health visitors had between them 22 different kinds of certificates or varieties of experience, held in 88 combinations, with some holding as many as 5 separate certificates. Health visiting lacked direction and the College of Nursing (now the Royal College of Nursing) was concerned about standards. In 1925 the College was successful in gaining the necessary government approval for a full-time course in health-visiting for nurses.[79]

The RF continued to be exercised about the quality of British public health nurse training in the 1930s.[80] Americans believed that nurses needed a college-based education, in contrast to the apprenticeship-style training within British hospitals.[81] In another example of Anglo-American collaboration in the 1920s, the RF believed that the international courses in public health nursing at King's College for Women and Bedford College, London, in the 1920s, influenced by American vision, and financed and organized through the League of Red Cross Societies, were led by "unimpressive individuals."[82] The North American leaders of nursing education, Annie Goodrich, Dean of the Yale University School of Nursing, and Kathleen Russell, Director of the School of Nursing at the University of Toronto, believed standards at the colleges were low. Hence, the leader of those courses, Olive Baggallay, was provided with an RF fellowship in public health nursing undertaken in the US and a second in Europe accompanied by Goodrich.[83] Additionally, nurses were trained in public health alongside "engineers… statisticians, bacteriologists, chemists, administrators, sociologists and economists" in the US.[84] Although American training in public health was established 50 years later than in the UK, it provided nurses with esteem and was located in centers of prestige in American universities, as exemplified by the training which Darville and McNeill received in North America.

Darville and McNeill's training in the US began with three-and-a-half weeks at the East Harlem Nursing and Health Demonstration in New York. Next, they spent three-and-a-half weeks in rural Alabama, including visits to the Public Health Nurses Annual Conference in Birmingham and the Tuskegee Institute. Then they visited Yale University and Providence, Rhode Island. They attended public health lectures at the Massachusetts Institute of Technology (MIT), where a School for Health Officers had been established in 1913 to train postgraduate sanitary engineers, biologists, and physicians.[85] In Toronto, Canada, they learnt about the chlorination of water and pasteurization of milk, visited schools and clinics, and met with the head of the nursing school at the University of Toronto.[86] This school of nursing had attracted RF attention as it was the only program where nurses were trained in public health as well as hospital nursing. The RF officers also considered the school's director, Russell, to be the best nurse educator in the world.[87] Therefore, Darville and McNeill were treated with corresponding respect, meeting with the leaders in North American nursing education, Goodrich and Russell.[88] Perhaps the experience of this higher status of nursing in North American higher education affected their attitude when they reached Malaya. In contrast, it was not until the 1950s that serious associations between public health nursing and universities occurred in Britain.[89]

Once in the Straits Settlements, the health sisters undertook an enormous amount of work for the RF campaign, which was led by Dr Paul Russell, and they were based in new District Health Centers.[90] These were introduced to provide more rural health care for Malays, adding to the provision of traveling dispensaries which were established in the late nineteenth century, and the Infant Welfare Centers which were introduced as another part of this increased rural service in the 1920s.[91] McNeill was stationed in Singapore and Darville in Penang. In 1927, there were a total of 13,024 home visits by health sisters or nurses in the six district health centers involved in the project. Additionally, there were 5,539 visits to the Health Centers. Darville and McNeill were by now joined by another British public health nurse, an unofficial health visitor, plus their Asian nurse assistants.[92] The functions of the Health Centers went beyond hookworm eradication.[93] The more scientific role of the nurses in the District Health Centers, compared to British nursing, is indicated by the training which Darville and

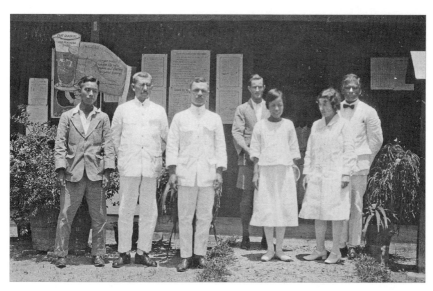

**Figure 2.** Elizabeth Darville in Penang, second from right, with staff of the Government Health Center at Tanjong Tokong, Penang rural area, including a Chinese health nurse, third from right (Source: Straits Settlements Rural Sanitation Campaign, Report for the Third Quarter of 1927, 13, folder 2594, box 210, series 473H, RG 5.3, Rockefeller Foundation records, Rockefeller Archive Center, © Courtesy of Rockefeller Archive Center).

McNeill received at MIT and in Toronto, as well as the laboratory work in these health centers. Significantly, Darville's uniform resembles a laboratory coat rather than a nurse's dress (see Figure 2).

Darville was invited to discuss her work in maternity and child welfare in a lecture to the students of tropical hygiene at the London School of Hygiene and Tropical Medicine (LSHTM). Her early work involved visiting local areas, including visiting girls' schools with Russell where they treated children for hookworm. After establishing the six district centers, Darville attended a different one each day, meeting with the local staff, which consisted of a Chinese, Indian, or Eurasian nurse; a Chinese attendant acting as cleaner and interpreter; and a Chinese or Malay midwife. As requested, the lecture emphasized her role with mothers and infants, but she also listed the other work which took place within the centers: prevention of diseases involving worms, skin, and eyes; breaking down "old traditions, prejudices and superstitions;" and improvement of "domestic sanitation and hygienic living" and Malay attendance at government hospitals. Part of Darville's role was also to provide locally educated health visitors with training in "curative and preventive work," including advice for mothers, but also regarding malaria transmission, insanitary conditions, as well as the importance of "tact and patience and courtesy in dealing with the mixed races."[94]

Heiser was full of praise for McNeill and Darville. In 1927, Heiser wrote to Russell, considering that the two British nurses had benefited greatly from their trip to the US and hoping that they would be an added stimulus for developing public health nursing in Malaya.[95] Heiser went on to commend the importance of Darville in Butterworth, Penang, demonstrated by the reduction in attendance whilst she was on holiday.[96] He gave special mention to Darville and McNeill in his summary of his 1931 trip around the Straits Settlements:

> Another Rockefeller Foundation investment that has produced profitable returns was in having Miss Darville and Miss O'Neill [sic] come to the United States for a brief study tour. Their example has interested others in health center work, and the apprentice system has already produced a considerable number of women, both native and foreign, who are doing acceptable public health nurse work.[97]

The British nurses received great praise in confidential British colonial documentation too.[98] Contrary to Lenore Manderson's argument that RF influence was short-lived in Malaya, with public health nursing the RF fulfilled one of their crucial intentions of creating a sustainable scheme through short-term funding.[99] The British hired another specific public health nurse in 1927 and Darville and McNeill remained working in Singapore into the 1940s.[100] As Heiser noted in 1931, the three public health nurses had already trained a significant number of Asian women.

## Integration or Inhibition?

Although Darville appears to have integrated with the locals in Malaya, demonstrated by the decreased attendance at clinics whilst she was on leave, integration into hierarchical colonial society could be more difficult. Darville confided in Heiser that it was hard to convince local British doctors of her ideas and that she was having "troubles with status."[101] This was exemplified by how she could speak to Heiser about her problems, yet was unable to "call" in this way in England or in "British circles" in Penang.[102] Her life was also unpleasant as another nurse was jealous of her role as a public health nurse because she worked fewer days. She told Heiser she would have resigned but for the "sympathy" of Paul Russell.[103] Stark differences in the hierarchy in the colonial Philippines can be seen by RF nurse Alice Fitzgerald's ability to meet with the Director of the Health Service, and persuade the Governor General to send out a telegram encouraging provincial governors to hire new graduates of public health nursing.[104] Filipino nurses were invited to meet government officials and attend government functions, though Choy suggests this could have been to showcase how Americans had nurtured Filipinos. However, a Filipino nurse interpreted these opportunities as the prestige which Americans bestowed on nursing.[105]

Darville was not the only person to find working amongst the British difficult. American doctors appear to have been marginalized in British colonial society. Heiser described their encounters with the British as a "veritable hell" as they had not been introduced to the Colonial Club or social amenities.[106] They were classed socially among the lowest assistant surgeons, and Barnes even had problems gaining permission to practice medicine.[107] Heiser's diaries cannot be taken at face value. Rather they are judgmental, bloated accounts designed to bolster the reputation of the RF's approach to public health. For example, in the Dutch East Indies, Heiser was also dismissive of the Dutch, dubbing them "stupid or discourteous."[108]

It is unlikely that Darville would have presented difficulties with her British colleagues when she discussed her work at LSHTM, which trained Colonial Medical Officers. Indeed, in 1935 she told students that the Senior Health Officer in Penang "took endless trouble to make things as easy as possible for me.... He has always been most sympathetic and I always feel that I can rely on him to give me any advice or assistance that I may need," and that the other European and Asian staff were very helpful. She also acknowledged the help she received from Paul Russell.[109] Contrary to Heiser's account, she claimed that she was "allowed to organize the work in my own way, which I did as far as possible on the same lines as it was done in Surrey [England]," thus not referring to the American model.[110] Given that Heiser's diary was a report of his trip, submitted to the RF, and that Darville was presenting to potential Colonial Medical Officers, each were probably propagandizing their own national interests. Perhaps the reality of Darville's situation is somewhere in between—she did boldly tell the students that she had difficulties with her salary.[111] With their new colleague, I. Simmons, McNeill complained from 1927 as they were concerned that they were unable to receive promotion like their hospital sister colleagues, arguing for the creation of a public health matron post.[112]

In September 1929, A.L. Hoops, the Medical Officer for Singapore, argued that these nurses needed to know the habits and customs of the various races and that "their work is more responsible and more independent, and they have to be specially trained and selected if they are to succeed."[113] From January 1930 they were provided with an extra $10 per month and the promise of an extra $30 per month if they passed their Malay examination.[114]

Despite the difficulties which British nurses could face in Malaya, Asian nurses were subjected to far more hierarchical subordination, as highlighted by Heiser's survey in 1915. Although there was an early attempt to integrate a black nurse into the ONA in 1903, patients objected and her contract in Sierra Leone was not continued after her six-month probationary period ended.[115] Until the late 1940s, the ONA placed a great deal of importance on the nurses it sent out to the colonies being not only white, but almost always British.[116] There was an impetus for change in the early 1940s, when Asian nurses and doctors ran the health care systems in East and Southeast Asia, as British nurses either left, were interned, or died when the Japanese seized British Malaya.[117] Locally-recruited Malayan Medical Service staff could continue their work, but their job was harder as the Japanese took from the hospitals what they needed to treat their forces, and largely took over from the Malayans in 1943.[118] British control of health care in Malaya was regained in the summer and autumn of 1945. Heiser's concerns about the subordination of Asian nurses were echoed in reports by a Colonial Office doctor after World War II; in 1946, A.G.H. Smart, Medical Adviser to the Secretary of State for the Colonies, visited Malaya. His purview was to recommend actions following the Japanese occupation, but he also critiqued Malayan medical planning prior to World War II.[119] Like Heiser's report of 1915, Smart recommended in his summary that training of local nurses had to be increased, as recommended by the British Rushcliffe Committee on the Training of Nurses in the Colonies (1943–45), which encouraged training equivalent to that in Britain. Smart found that the subordination of local nurses' training and prospects was highlighted by Asians' work during the occupation, and he discussed several nurses and dressers who could be selected for more training and promotion.[120] World War II changed the relationship between Asian health care staff and the British. For example, Chee Kong Tet, a hospital administrator and later a doctor in Singapore, remembered that local people could not tolerate the British sisters who returned, as the locals were put back in their old positions whilst the British took charge again.[121] Indeed, Smart noted that the local staff were "tired out after a period of great stress and exhaustion...[and] are asking for a clear statement as to their future prospects."[122] The push for the feminization of nursing endured with Smart's belief that he could see the difference between hospitals with female nurses compared to those with male nurses.[123] Smart also documented the neglect of rural health relative to urban health in Malaya, and the need for more public health nurses.[124]

There had been some efforts to train local nurses in Singapore since 1913. In 1934 a plan was made for a nursing school with a full-time Tutor Sister for 1935. With a larger settler population in Singapore than elsewhere in Malaya, there were more European and Eurasian children from which to recruit nurses: in the 1920s, 72 per cent of the 12,645 Eurasians in Malaya lived in the Straits Settlements.[125] By 1949, training in Singapore was recognized as equivalent to that of the UK and nurses were given reciprocity with the UK's General Nursing Council.[126]

At the nursing school in Penang, 66 nurses completed their general training in 1949.[127] Gradually, efforts were made to train Asian nurses for more prestigious posts. In 1949, two fully qualified local nurses were given the opportunity to undertake a tutor's course and were subsequently sent to the Royal College of Nursing in London to study for the Sister Tutor's diploma. Two more received training in teaching.[128] In the same year, 28 Asian women worked as health or nursing sisters, positions previously limited to Europeans; this increased to 67 in 1952.[129] In 1952, the training in Penang was deemed to be equivalent to that in Britain with the School gaining reciprocity.[130] By 1953, the School was offering a three-month public health nursing course and was planning an expanded course complying with the Royal Sanitary Institute.[131]

Presumably inspired by the British model of State Enrolled Nurses, established in 1943, an Assistant Nurses scheme began in 1951, with a two-year training course that aimed to improve the "haphazard" work which was carried out by attendants, and to relieve trained nurses from tasks requiring less responsibility.[132] WHO doctor Donald Huggins noted the utility of these assistant nurses in his yaws report, noting that they were drawn from the kampongs and were young and able to approach shy Malay women.[133]

Remedying the under-provision of nurse training, particularly in rural areas, became a goal of international health organizations visiting

Malaya in the 1950s. This came at a particularly difficult time for Malaya. The Malayan Emergency (1948–60) affected nursing recruitment, with staffing still badly affected by World War II.[134] There were 176 British colonial nurses in Malaya in 1942, 48 of whom died during the war. By 1948, 137 colonial nurses were working in Malaya, slowly increasing to 166 by 1955.[135] During the Emergency, large nursing teams from the Red Cross, the Order of St. John, and the Soldier, Sailors, Airmen and Families Association provided care in rural areas of Malaya.[136]

The Cold War led to increased funding for public health, which was seen as a "depoliticized field" of goodwill, particularly as Asian states were not willing to spend large amounts on it themselves.[137] In the 1940s and 1950s, poor health was believed to result in a "breeding ground for communism."[138] With policy and funding being driven by experts in Western biomedicine in the US and Europe, the Cold War climate demanded quick remedies rather than slow economic and social change to improve health and win "hearts and minds."[139] Alongside developments in techno-centric biomedicine, including DDT, antibiotics, and vaccination, the WHO included interventions in public health nursing under the banner of "technical assistance."[140] From 1950, various WHO nurses were appointed in Malaya, mainly in teaching roles.[141] In 1953, the WHO agreed to funding of $47,000 for a Rural Health Center, attaching "unusual importance" to this project of "very considerable potential value," even though there were financial challenges at this time. Between 1950 and 1953 the United Nations Children's Emergency Fund (UNICEF) provided an additional $100,000 for equipment.[142]

Prior to independence, Malayanization of public services resulted in an official policy of the cessation of recruitment of British nurses from the mid-1950s.[143] The Malayanization program and independence from Britain in Malaya (1957) and Singapore (1959) had a drastic effect on the number of British colonial nurses. Between 1955 and 1960 they declined from 90 to 25 in the Federation of Malaya and from 62 to 22 in Singapore.[144] Staff shortages resulted in the WHO being asked to assist again in 1957.[145] Australia also provided assistance through the Colombo Aid Plan for Southeast Asia, providing Australian nurses and training for at least 48 Malay nurses in Australia in the mid-1950s.[146] A consequence of the Malayanization program was the acceptance of male Malayan nursing after half a century of attempting to feminize nursing. In 1954, an unpopular proposal aimed to recruit male nurses and pay both male and female nurses the same rate.[147] In 1955, male practitioners who had formerly been called hospital assistants were able to register as nurses. Men would no longer be recruited as hospital assistants.[148]

## Conclusion

This chapter has explored the role of training and education as a lightning rod for rival models and interpretations of public health nursing. Nurses faced the constraints of conventional British social norms of class and gender in Malaya, contrasted with respect, status, and opportunities from North Americans. Hostility was displayed towards Americans within the Malayan medical services, affecting the way in which the RF-trained British nurses perceived colonial society, following their interaction with their friendlier and more egalitarian cross-Atlantic colleagues. The chapter also reveals how British, American, and international organizations' efforts and funding to improve public health nursing in rural areas coincided with periods of increased nationalism in the 1920s and communism in the late 1940s and early 1950s. In the 1920s, in particular, the RF, rather than the British, drove public health nursing in Malaya, enhancing health care in politically fragile rural areas.

The difficulties of imposing Western structures on a largely Muslim, Asian country have been demonstrated by the failed attempt to feminize Malayan nursing. The misplaced expectation of recruiting enough girls educated to School Certificate standard led to the eventual return to training men as well as women, although men continued to be trained as dressers and hospital assistants.[149] Yet the goal of feminization persisted far longer than in the American Philippines, where men had been reintegrated into nursing 30 years earlier.

Comparisons with American colonial nursing also reveal that the long-term subordination of and lack of career opportunities for Asian nurses in Malaya led to continual nursing shortages in comparison to the Philippines, where locally trained nurses had better career prospects and believed their profession to be prestigious.[150] But the approach adopted by the RF by investing in "lighthouses of leadership" belies deeper tensions within American nurse leadership regarding what an appropriate model for training development should be.[151] This tension reflected differences in philosophy derived from contextual conditions with which American and British nurse leaders had to contend to build capacity.[152] Assistance from the RF, the WHO, and Australia highlights the declining prestige of British nursing and the legacy of under-investment in higher education that would constrain its global competitive edge for decades to come.

## Acknowledgements

Research for this chapter has been supported by two grants from the Wellcome Trust; "Nurses Abroad: The Colonial Nursing Association, 1896–1966" (084990), 2008, and "The Boundaries of Illness" (086071), 2009–15; a Grant-in-Aid from the Rockefeller Archive Center, 2010; as well as a travel award from the University of London, 2010. The authors are grateful for permission from the Rockefeller Archive Center to reproduce Figure 2, and to the National Archives of Singapore for permission to use the Oral History Interviews collection. Many thanks to staff in all of the archives which we have accessed, in particular to Lucy McCann at the University of Oxford for her continued help with our ongoing research. Thank you for helpful comments at seminars at Imperial College London and the University of Oxford in 2011, and a work-in-progress session at Imperial College London in 2012.

## Archives Consulted

Arkib Negara Malaysia, Kuala Lumpur, Malaysia
Colonial Office records, The National Archives, UK (hereafter TNA)
Hong Kong University Library, Special Collections, Hong Kong
Commonwealth and African Studies Collections, Bodleian Libraries, University of Oxford, UK
National Archives of Singapore Oral History Center, National Archives, Singapore
Rockefeller Foundation records, Rockefeller Archive Center, Sleepy Hollow, NY, USA
Royal London Hospital Archive, London, UK

## Government Reports Consulted

*Protected Malay States Reports*, 1890–95
*Reports on the Federated Malay States*, 1896–99
*Annual Report of the Malayan Union*, 1946
*Report of the Medical Department, Malaya*, 1949–52, 1954–56
*Colony of Singapore Medical Report*, 1957

# Notes

1. See John Farley, *To Cast Out Disease: A History of the International Health Division of Rockefeller Foundation, 1913–51* (Oxford: Oxford University Press, 2003), 223–35.
2. Victor Heiser, "Diary, 1927–8," Jan. 25, 1928, box 217, RG 12, Officers' Diaries, Rockefeller Foundation records (hereafter RF), Rockefeller Archive Center.
3. H.P. Dickson, *The Badge of Britannia: The History and Reminiscences of the Queen Elizabeth's Overseas Nursing Service, 1886–1966* (Edinburgh: Pentland Press, 1990), 5 and 21; Overseas Nursing Association, *Annual Report*, 1966, box 131, MSS Brit Emp s400, Overseas Nursing Association Collection (hereafter ONA Collection), Commonwealth and African Studies, Bodleian Libraries (hereafter CASBL), University of Oxford.
4. Dickson, *Badge of Britannia*, 14; ONA, *Annual Reports*, 1897–1919.
5. ONA, *Annual Reports*, 1900–66, ONA Collection.
6. Michael Havinden and David Meredith, *Colonialism and Development: Britain and Its Tropical Colonies, 1850–1960* (London: Routledge, 1996), 63, 92–4, 97, 107–10 and 236–7.
7. See Phua Kai Hong, "The Development of Health Services in Malaya and Singapore, 1867–1960" (PhD diss., London School of Economics, 1987), 7.
8. Catherine Ceniza Choy, *Empire of Care: Nursing and Migration in Filipino American History* (Durham, NC: Duke University Press, 2003); Barbara L. Brush, "The Rockefeller Agenda for American/Philippines Nursing Relations," in Anne Marie Rafferty, Jane Robinson and Ruth Elkan, eds, *Nursing History and the Politics of Welfare* (London: Routledge, 1997), 45–63; Winifred Connerton, "Have Cap, Will Travel: U.S. Nurses Abroad 1898–1917" (PhD diss., University of Pennsylvania, 2010).
9. Lenore Manderson, *Sickness and the State: Health and Illness in Colonial Malaya, 1870–1940* (Cambridge: Cambridge University Press, 1996), 1, 15, 18.
10. Wan Faizah binti Wan Yusoff, "Malay Responses to the Promotion of Western Medicine, with Particular Reference to Women and Child Healthcare in the Federated Malay States, 1920–1939" (PhD diss., University of London, 2010), 48; Manderson, *Sickness and the State*, 1 and 15.
11. Wan Faizah, "Malay Responses," 54.
12. Barbara Andaya and Leonard Andaya, *A History of Malaysia* (Basingstoke: Palgrave, 2001), 266.
13. See Lynn Hollen Lees, "Being British in Malaya," *Journal of British Studies* 48 (2009): 82.
14. *Protected Malay States (PMS) Reports*, 1890–95; *Reports on the Federated Malay States (FMS)*, 1896–99.
15. *Reports on the FMS*, 1899, 55, 74.

16.  *PMS Reports*, 1893, 12–13.

17.  *Reports on the FMS*, 1898, 53.

18.  *Reports on the FMS*, 1896, 69.

19.  Andaya and Andaya, *A History of Malaysia*, 178; Manderson, *Sickness and the State*, 210.

20.  Andaya and Andaya, *A History of Malaysia*, 240–1; Manderson, *Sickness and the State*, 31.

21.  Wan Faizah, "Malay Responses," 105–6.

22.  Ibid., 100.

23.  Manderson, *Sickness and the State*, 206–7; J.E. Nathan, *The Census of British Malaya, 1921* (London: Waterlow and Sons, 1922), 252, 258, 264.

24.  J. Irvine Rowell and William Hoad to Charles Gage Brown, and P.B.C. Ayres to Charles Gage Brown, "Papers on the Subject of Nurses and Training of Nurses, Hong Kong," Jan. 18, 1896, 5–6 and 8–10, HKP 610.73 G78, Hong Kong University Library, Special Collections (hereafter, HKUL); Eva Lückes, "Matron's Annual Letter No. 1," London Hospital, 1894, LH/N/7/1/1; Eva Lückes, "Matron's Annual Letter No. 4," London Hospital, 1897, LH/N.7/1/4, Royal London Hospital Archive (hereafter RLHA).

25.  *Reports on the FMS*, 1899, 23.

26.  Lückes, "Matron's Annual Letter No. 4"; John L. Welch, Residency Surgeon to British Resident, Selangor, July 5, 1889, "Asks to secure the services of a capable European nurse," 1889, Item 7, 1957.0015797, Arkib Negara Malaysia, Kuala Lumpur.

27.  Lee Yong Kiat, "Nursing and the Beginnings of Specialised Nursing in Early Singapore," *Singapore Medical Journal* 46 (2005): 601.

28.  Rowell and Hoad to Gage Brown, "Papers on the Subject of Nurses," 9.

29.  Ibid., 9–10; See also Lee, "Nursing," 602; Lee Yong Kiat, "The Origins of Nursing in Singapore," *Singapore Medical Journal* 26 (1985): 58.

30.  Rowell and Hoad to Gage Brown, "Papers on the Subject of Nurses," 9.

31.  Felicia Yap, "Eurasians in British Asia during the Second World War," *Journal of the Royal Asiatic Society* (Third Series) 21 (2011): 488.

32.  For the term "cultural brokers," see Manderson, *Sickness and the State*, 232.

33.  Rowell and Hoad to Gage Brown, "Papers on the Subject of Nurses," 9.

34.  Lee, "Nursing," 603.

35.  Anne Summers, *Angels and Citizens: British Women as Military Nurses, 1854–1914* (London: Routledge and Kegan Paul, 1988), 23–7; Shula Marks, *Divided Sisterhood: Race, Class and Gender in the South African Nursing Profession* (Basingstoke: Macmillan, 1994), 86–8.

36.  Choy, *Empire of Care*, 26.

37.  Ibid., 48; Brush, "The Rockefeller Agenda," 56.

38.  Choy, *Empire of Care*, 48.

39.  Interview with Chan Keong Poh, Reel 1, 000802, July 27, 1987, National Archives of Singapore Oral History Center (hereafter NASOHC).

40. Interview with Chan Poh Goon, Reel 1, 002063, Oct. 16, 1998, NASOHC.

41. E.M. Fowler Wright, "The Singapore General Hospital," *Nursing Times*, Sept. 20, 1941, 765–6.

42. Nathan, *The Census of British Malaya, 1921*, 269–312.

43. Vincent Del Tufo, *Malaya Comprising the Federation of Malaya and the Colony of Singapore: A Report on the 1947 Census of the Population* (London: Crown Agents for the Colonies, 1949), 481.

44. Manderson, *Sickness and the State*, 206–11.

45. Anne Marie Rafferty, "Internationalising Nursing Education During the Interwar Period," in *International Health Organisations and Movements, 1918–1939*, ed. Paul Weindling (Cambridge: Cambridge University Press, 1995), 267. The IHC became the International Health Board from 1916–27 and the International Health Division from 1927–51. For an early account of some of the ideas presented within this chapter, and for more context regarding the RF records discussed, see Rosemary Wall, "The International Health Division's Views on Nursing Practice, Policy and Education in British Malaya," *Rockefeller Archive Center Research Reports* (2010), http://www.rockarch.org/publications/resrep/wall.pdf, accessed June 27, 2015.

46. Farley, *To Cast Out Disease*, 62–6.

47. Victor G. Heiser, "Memorandum on Medical Education in Malaya, 1915," folder 1, box 1, series 473A, RG 1.1, RF.

48. "Victor George Heiser (1873–1972)," reprint from *Year Book of the American Philosophical Society*, 1972, 194–7, in "Victor Heiser," Biography File, RF.

49. Sunil Amrith, *Decolonising International Health: India and Southeast Asia, 1930–65* (Basingstoke: Palgrave Macmillan, 2006), 9.

50. Alfred W. McCoy, Francisco A. Scarano, and Courtney Johnson, "On the Tropic of Cancer: Transitions and Transformations in the US Imperial State," in *Colonial Crucible: Empire in the Making of the Modern American State*, ed. Alfred W. McCoy and Francisco A. Scarano (Madison: The University of Wisconsin Press, 2009), 7.

51. Ibid., 11–18; Alfred W. McCoy, "Policing the Imperial Periphery: Philippine Pacification and the Rise of the US National Security State," in *Colonial Crucible*, 109.

52. Thomas McCormick, "From Old Empire to New: The Changing Dynamics and Tactics of American Empire," in *Colonial Crucible*, 77.

53. McCoy et al., "On the Tropic of Cancer," 25.

54. Warwick Anderson, "Pacific Crossings: Imperial Logics in United States' Public Health Programs," in *Colonial Crucible*, 279–80.

55. Warwick Anderson, *Colonial Pathologies: American Tropical Medicine, Race, and Hygiene in the Philippines* (Durham, NC: Duke University Press, 2006), 28.

56. Paul A. Kramer, "Race, Empire and Transnational History," in *Colonial Crucible*, 206–8.

57. Anderson, *Colonial Pathologies*, 55, 58.

58. Adam D. Burns, "Winning 'Hearts and Minds': American Imperial Designs of the Early Twentieth and Twenty-First Centuries," History and Policy, http://www.historyandpolicy.org/policy-papers/papers/winning-hearts-and-minds-american-imperial-designs-of-the-early-twentieth-a, accessed June 24, 2015.

59. Ibid.

60. Rosemary Wall and Anne Marie Rafferty, "Nursing and the 'Hearts and Minds' Campaign, 1948–1958: The Malayan Emergency," in *Routledge Handbook on the Global History of Nursing*, ed. Patricia D'Antonio, Julie Fairman, and Jean Whelan (New York: Routledge, 2013), 218–36.

61. Burns, "Winning 'Hearts and Minds'."

62. Brush, "The Rockefeller Agenda," 47. See Choy, *Empire of Care*, 33, for more examples.

63. Brush, "The Rockefeller Agenda," 48–51.

64. Ibid., 49–50; Choy, *Empire of Care*, 35.

65. "Tentative Draft of the Agreement between the Straits Settlements Government and the International Health Board of the Rockefeller Foundation," 1925, folder 2971, box 233, series 1.2, RG 5, RF; Farley, *To Cast Out Disease*, 31–3.

66. M.E. Barnes to Victor Heiser, May 18, 1925, folder 2971, box 233, series 1.2, RG 5, RF.

67. John Darwin, *The Empire Project: The Rise and Fall of the British World-System, 1830–1970* (Cambridge: Cambridge University Press, 2009), 326–7.

68. Soma Hewa, *Colonialism, Tropical Disease and Imperial Medicine: Rockefeller Philanthropy in Sri Lanka* (Lanham, MD: University Press of America, 1995), 68–71.

69. Heiser, "Diary, 1927–29," Feb. 24, 1928.

70. M.E. Barnes to Victor Heiser, May 18, 1925, folder 2971, box 233, series 1.2, RG 5, RF.

71. Victor Heiser to A.L. Hoops, Feb. 5, 1927; H.M. Gillette to the Under Secretary of State, Colonial Office, England, July 28, 1927, folder 3869, box 304, series 1.2, RG 5, RF.

72. Wan Faizah, "Malay Responses," 58.

73. Manderson, *Sickness and the State*, 242; Wan Faizah, "Malay Responses," 49; Mark Harrison, *Public Health in British India: Anglo-Indian Preventive Medicine 1859–1914* (Cambridge: Cambridge University Press, 1994), 60–98.

74. J.E. Shuckburgh to Victor Heiser, Jan. 4, 1927, folder 2869, box 304, series 1.2, RG 5, RF.

75. Mary Beard to Florence Read, Jan. 31, 1927, folder 3869, box 304, series 1.2, RG 5, RF.

76. Elizabeth Crowell, "Memorandum on the Study of Sick Nursing and Health Visiting in England," folder 427, box 401C, series 1.1, RF, iv, cited in Rafferty, "Internationalising Nursing Education," 271. See also Jaime Lapeyre, "'The Idea of Better Nursing': The American Battle for Control over Standards of Nursing Education in Europe, 1918–1925" (PhD diss., University of Toronto, 2013), 139 and 213; and Susan McGann, "Collaboration and Conflict in International Nursing, 1920–39," *Nursing History Review* 16 (2008): 29–57.

77. Rafferty, "Internationalising Nursing Education," 271.

78. McGann, "Collaboration and Conflict," 34 and 38; Lapeyre, "'The Idea of Better Nursing'," 67.

79. Helen Sweet with Rona Dougall, *Community Nursing and Primary Healthcare in Britain in the Twentieth Century* (New York: Routledge, 2008), 37–8.

80. Rafferty, "Internationalising Nursing Education," 276.

81. McGann, "Collaboration and Conflict," 30.

82. Ibid., 43.

83. Ibid., 43–6 and 52; Rafferty, "Internationalising Nursing Education," 275.

84. Elizabeth Fee and Roy M. Acheson, "Introduction," in *A History of Education in Public Health: Health that Mocks the Doctors' Rules*, ed. Elizabeth Fee and Roy M. Acheson (Oxford: Oxford University Press, 1991), 1–3.

85. A.M. McNeill to Mary Beard, Apr. 8, 1927; A.M. McNeill to Florence Read, Apr. 8, 1927, folder 3869, box 304, series 1.2, RG 5, RF; Barbara Rosenkrantz, *Public Health and the State: Changing Views in Massachusetts, 1842–1936* (Cambridge, MA: Harvard University Press, 1972), 169.

86. A.M. McNeill to Miss Beard, Apr. 8, 1927; A.M. McNeill to Miss Read, Apr. 8, 1927, folder 3869, box 304, series 1.2, RG 5, RF.

87. Farley, *To Cast Out Disease*, 230–5.

88. A.M. McNeill to Miss Beard, Apr. 8, 1927; A.M. McNeill to Miss Read, Apr. 8 1927, folder 3869, box 304, series 1.2, RG 5, RF.

89. Susan McGann, Anne Crowther, and Rona Dougall, *A History of the Royal College of Nursing, 1916–90: A Voice for Nurses* (Manchester: Manchester University Press, 2009), 187; Jane Brooks and Anne Marie Rafferty, "Degrees of Ambivalence: Attitudes towards Pre-registration University Education for Nurses in Britain, 1930–1960," *Nurse Education Today* 30, 6 (2010): 579–83.

90. "Straits Settlements Rural Sanitation Campaign Reports," 1927, folder 2595, box 210, series 473H, RG 5.3, RF.

91. Wan Faizah, "Malay Responses," 107; Manderson, *Sickness and the State*, 16.

92. "District Health Centre Statistics, 1927," table 26, folder 2595, box 210, series 473H, RG 5.3, RF.

93. "Straits Settlements Rural Sanitation Campaign Reports," 1927.
94. Elizabeth Darville, "Maternity and Child Welfare Work in Penang," Lecture to students of tropical hygiene at the London School of Hygiene and Tropical Medicine, 1935, Mss. Ind. Ocn. s 134, 2–3 and 25–6, CASBL.
95. Victor Heiser to Paul Russell, July 1, 1927, folder 3871, box 305, series 1.2, RG5, RF.
96. Victor Heiser, "Diary, 1930–1," Feb. 28, 1931, box 217, RG 12, RF.
97. Ibid.
98. A. O'Brien, "Public Health Nursing Sisters in Malaya, 1929–34," Item 4, CO 717/67/15, The National Archives, UK (hereafter TNA).
99. Lenore Manderson, "Race, Colonial Mentality and Public Health in Early Twentieth Century Malaya," in *The Underside of Malaysian History: Pullers, Prostitutes, Plantation Workers*, ed. P.J. Rimmer and L.M. Allen (Singapore: Singapore University Press, 1990), 210.
100. ONA, *Annual Reports*, 1927–49, ONAC.
101. Heiser, "Diary, 1927–28," Jan. 25, 1928.
102. Ibid.
103. Ibid.
104. Brush, "The Rockefeller Agenda," 54–5.
105. Choy, *Empire of Care*, 32.
106. Victor Heiser, "Diary, 1925–26," Dec. 30, 1925, box 216, RG 12, RF.
107. Ibid.
108. Cited in Terence H. Hull, "Conflict and Collaboration in Public Health: The Rockefeller Foundation and the Dutch Colonial Government in Indonesia," in *Public Health in Asia and the Pacific: Historical and Comparative perspectives*, ed. Milton J. Lewis and Kerrie L. MacPherson (London: Routledge, 2008), 143, and see 141.
109. Darville, "Maternity and Child Welfare Work," 2, 9–10.
110. Ibid., 2–3.
111. Ibid., 1–2.
112. Governor's Deputy, Straits Settlements, to L.C.M.S. Amery, Colonial Office, 29 Dec. 1927, "1928 Straits, Infant Welfare Nurses, Salaries of," item 1, CO 273/546/1, TNA; A. O'Brien, "Public Health Nursing Sisters in Malaya."
113. A. O'Brien, "Public Health Nursing Sisters in Malaya."
114. Walter D. Ellis to the Under Secretary of State, Colonial Office, London, Nov. 30, 1929, Item 52, "1913–1964 Straits Settlements," folder 1, box 137, ONAC.
115. ONA, "Minutes of the Nursing Committee," June 8, 1903 and Nov. 18, 1903, MSS B. Emp. S.400/19, ONAC.
116. ONA Executive Committee Minutes, June 5, 1945 and Dec. 4, 1945, vol. 18, ONAC.

117. Dickson, *Badge of Britannia*, 21–2, 100–7.
118. Malayan Union, *Annual Report of the Malayan Union*, 1946, 66–8.
119. R.J.G. Dewar to Mr. Morgan, Apr. 1, 1946, CO 273/679, TNA.
120. A.G.H. Smart, "Report on some aspects of medical planning for Malaya," CO 273/679, TNA.
121. Chee Kong Tet, Reel 12, 000683, June 27, 1986, NASOHC.
122. Smart, "Report on Some Aspects."
123. Ibid.
124. Ibid.
125. R.L. German (compiler), *Handbook to British Malaya* (London: Malayan Civil Service, 1927).
126. Phua, "Development of Health Services," 240.
127. *Report of the Medical Department, Malaya*, 1949, 24.
128. Ibid.
129. *Report of the Medical Department, Malaya*, 1949, 103; 1952, 94.
130. Ibid., 1952, 21.
131. "Plan of Operations for the Establishment of a Rural Health Training Centre at Jitra in Kedah in Malaya, Fourth Draft," CO859/415, TNA.
132. Anne Marie Rafferty, *The Politics of Nursing Knowledge* (London: Routledge, 1996), 169. *Report of the Medical Department, Malaya*, 1951, 16.
133. D.H. Huggins, 'The Yaws Problem in the Federation of Malaya,' 1953, CO859/415, TNA, 20.
134. Wall and Rafferty, "Nursing and the 'Hearts and Minds' Campaign," 218–36.
135. ONA, *Annual Reports*, 1942–55.
136. Wall and Rafferty, "Nursing and the 'Hearts and Minds' Campaign," 226–30.
137. Amrith, *Decolonising International Health*, 84.
138. John Farley, *Brock Chisholm, the World Health Organization, and the Cold War* (Vancouver: University of British Columbia Press, 2008), 83.
139. Amrith, *Decolonising International Health*, 17 and 53–6, 98; Farley, *Brock Chisholm*, 2, 79, 84, 86 and 116–17.
140. Amrith, *Decolonising International Health*, 102.
141. *Report of the Medical Department, Malaya*, 1950, 21.
142. I.C. Fang, Regional Director, Western Pacific, to the Member for Health, Penang, Sept. 2, 1952; "UNICEF Recommendation of the Executive Director for an Apportionment to Malaya," Aug. 25, 1953; I.C. Fang, to the Member for Health, Penang, Jan. 9, 1953, CO 859/415, TNA; Malayan Union, *Report of the Medical Department, Malaya*, 1950, 23.
143. *Report of the Medical Department, Malaya*, 1955, 28.
144. ONA, *Annual Reports*, 1955–60.
145. *Colony of Singapore Medical Report*, 1957, 1–4.

146. *Report of the Medical Department, Malaya*, 1956, 29.
147. Ibid., 1954, 24.
148. Ibid., 1955, 29.
149. Del Tufo, *Malaya*, 481.
150. Choy, *Empire of Care*, 38.
151. Lapeyre, "'The Idea of Better Nursing'."
152. Rafferty, *Politics of Nursing Knowledge*, 7.

CHAPTER 3

# Cattle for the Colony: Veterinary Science and Animal Breeding in Colonial Indochina

*Annick Guénel*

Henri Jacotot, a veterinarian who succeeded Alexandre Yersin as head of the Pasteur Institute in Nha Trang (Central Vietnam), wrote in 1947 in a French scientific publication: "It is no exaggeration to say that in Indochina the exploitation of domestic animals has been conducted methodically since the day settlers and French technicians began to develop the natural productions of the country." This development, Jacotot added, was achieved through a "set of scientific disciplines," previously unknown to local populations, including the elite, as well as through control of the murderous epizootics, against which "the Annamese, Cambodian, Laotian breeders [...] were defenseless."[1]

Scientific resource management, or "*mise en valeur*" in the French terminology, was a key element in colonial policy. This policy often attempted to convince local people to adopt new modes of exploitation of the country's natural resources and to change their relationships with the environment. In this respect, French colonial veterinarians had a particularly important role to play, due to their expertise in various areas. The products of a long tradition of training in veterinary schools in France, they acquired knowledge not only in animal medicine but also in agronomy and other fields together referred to as zootechny. Diana Davis explored the multiple tasks of veterinarians in North African colonies, and stressed their role in the introduction of what she has called "livestock and range management."[2] In contrast, as she also noticed, colonial veterinarians in British India contributed little to this field. Aside from the differences between French and British veterinary

95

education, she raised two dissimilar factors: the animal diseases in each of the colonies, and the respective modes of governance of the two European powers.[3]

Far from the African colonies, in Indochina, French veterinarians were also charged with contributing to domestic animal breeding development. They had a dual role: the protection of livestock and the "popularization and application of animal husbandry methods."[4] Much focus was put on cattle. In 1901, soon after the completion of the conquest of all territories, E. Douarche, then head of the veterinary service, provided a promising report, stating that, "Cattle constitute a large part of the country's wealth and one of the most important factors in its economic future."[5]

Nevertheless, Indochina may be said to resemble more closely India than the Maghreb because of its geographical situation and climate, its wild and domestic animals, the regional epizootics, and, to a lesser extent, its economy and culture, all obstacles to the colonial agenda. Furthermore, unlike Maghreb countries where big land concessions were allocated to Europeans, Indochina was never a settlement colony. Instead, the colonial administration tried to rely on the major Vietnamese ethnic group, the Kinh, living in the plains. In the colonial classification of societies in a scale of 'civilisation,' although the Vietnamese were mostly rice farmers, they were the best placed to be educated in new methods of breeding.

Adaptability or "acclimatization" of colonial policy to the natural and social environment in disciplines such as forestry and human medicine has been postulated.[6] Examining first the social, economic, and geographical realities of colonial Indochina, then the civilizing mission entrusted to the veterinarians, it will be argued here that in some cases this postulate can be challenged.

## Mapping Breeding Areas

French Indochina included five administrative territories. Cochinchina (present-day southern Vietnam) was the first to be conquered and the only colony, while Tonkin and Annam (respectively northern and central Vietnam) as well as Cambodia and Laos were protectorates. Added to the topographic and climatic diversity, were important demographic, economic, and cultural differences between Vietnam and the two other countries, between the north and the south, and between the plains and the highlands.

With the highest population density and the most lands dedicated to intensive rice-growing, the Red River delta was in sharp contrast to the highlands of northern Tonkin, sparsely populated by ethnic minorities practicing slash-and-burn agriculture. Early French observers reported on the good quality of pastures and livestock in the High Region. The importance of water buffalo breeding to some mountain dwellers was particularly emphasized.[7]

At the time of the French annexation of Cochinchina, vast areas were not yet cleared.[8] The colonial administration initially considered converting lands into pastures.[9] This project was dropped not so much because of unfavorable natural and climatic conditions as because the expansion of rice cultivation in the Mekong delta and the rubber plantations contributed much more to the colony's wealth.[10] The grasslands of the Annamese plateaus were more favorable to animal breeding. In 1901, a veterinarian, Schein, reported that he met a village chief at the Lao border who owned 10,000 to 12,000 oxen or cows and 8,000 water buffaloes.[11] Although not all the villages were as rich as the latter, it was recognized that, despite their small size, the oxen were "well-formed" and provided rather good quality beef.[12] Water buffaloes, paddy field animals par excellence, were produced in sufficient quantities to be exported not only to the Indochinese plains, but also to neighboring countries.[13]

However, Cambodia offered the most unique conditions and was soon considered "the supplier of the Far East." Its population density was much lower than that of the neighboring southern Vietnamese provinces,[14] and the country had wide uncultivated areas covered with natural vegetation. Cattle breeding was carried out throughout the territory. Baradat, a French veterinarian, argued that the Cambodian breed of cattle was probably not so different from the other regional breeds;[15] its robustness was due rather to the abundance of food and its variety, the watering facilities for livestock, as well as the care provided by the breeders.[16]

Before colonization, beef and buffalo meat consumption was rare in the three countries outside occasional rituals and sacrifices, or the death of an animal. Milk was totally absent from the local diet. Pierre Gourou, in *L'utilisation du sol en Indochine française*, published in 1940, introduced the idea of a civilization of plants (*la civilisation du végétal*). The use of plants as the primary source of food, Gourou said, was above all characteristic of civilization, and had "important consequences for land use."[17] The importance of agricultural crops left little room for animal breeding.

But oxen and water buffalo had a crucial role in field work and transport. Usually, cattle lived in unfenced spaces and fed on what could be found in their natural surroundings, but because of the scarcity of animal food in intensively cultivated areas, such as in the Red River delta, some peasants bought one or two head of cattle before plowing and sold them thereafter. The coastal plains of Annam were more favored, as the herds could be led to the nearby hillsides during the dry season.[18] There was a long-standing cattle trade with bordering countries, China and Siam, as well as an intense animal trade between and within the Indochinese countries. In the north, the mountain dwellers had provided cattle, especially water buffaloes, to the rice growers of the plains for a long time, as is suggested by the multitude of markets on the trails linking the Red River delta and the High Region.[19] Laos and North Annam also supplied draft animals to Tonkin. In Cochinchina, the importation of cattle increased with the extension of land cultivation. Cattle came mainly from Cambodia, but also from Laos and Southern Annam. Yet, although the high regions of Vietnam constituted a cattle reserve for the plains, it cannot be considered that real pastoral activity was well developed there. The livestock density was lower than that in the plains and the cattle grazed almost totally freely. According to Gourou, only in some Cambodian provinces were there real pastoral activities, due to Indian influence.[20]

Moreover, after European settlement, cattle trade not only concerned draft animals, but also animals delivered to slaughterhouses of the cities occupied by Europeans. Finally, colonization introduced new trade routes to neighboring countries. The Philippines was the first and the most promising foreign market, before cattle were shipped to Singapore and Hong Kong as well.[21]

Control of animal movement was an early concern of the colonial administration. The frequency of cattle diseases, some of which had been endemic in Asia for centuries, had quickly drawn veterinarians' attention. A focus on the prevention of epizootics was also expected to give "immediate and much more demonstrative results to the native than any zootechnical method."[22]

## The Veterinary Service and Training of Local Staff

The development of the Indochinese veterinary service was encouraged by the first research on animal epidemiology. Alexandre Yersin, after his discovery of the human plague bacillus in Hong Kong in 1894, set up a laboratory in Nha Trang (Annam), which rapidly turned its attention to animal diseases.[23] The first investigations focused on rinderpest (commonly called cattle plague). This viral disease proved to be the most murderous disease of bovidae in Indochina. Two veterinarians, Carré and Fraimbault, who identified the disease during an epizootic in Tonkin,[24] succeeded in producing, not a vaccine, but a serum in 1898. One year later, the institute sent 2,000 doses of serum to Tonkin, and from 1904 serotherapy extended to other Indochinese territories.

At the turn of the twentieth century, veterinarians of the Nha Trang Institute were also interested in two other contagious diseases against which serums and vaccines were available. Bovine hemorrhagic septicemia, or bovine pasteurellosis, caused by a coccobacillus, was the second most important cause of cattle mortality after rinderpest. It was sometimes confused with anthrax which was more geographically limited, and which was investigated during outbreaks in two provinces of the High Region of Tonkin.[25]

These scientific achievements were in line with General Governor Paul Doumer's policy. In 1899, he had created the General Directorate of Agriculture, Forests, and Commerce for the rational and scientific use of natural resources of the Empire.[26] Under its supervision, the Veterinary, Zootechnical, and Epizootics Service was reorganized two years later. In each of the five Indochinese territories, a veterinary service reporting to the local administrators was to be set up. The territories were divided into sectors headed by veterinary-inspectors to be recruited from among graduates of veterinary schools in France. It should be noted, however, that in Laos a veterinary service was not created until 1921.[27]

Until its reorganization, the colonial veterinary service comprised exclusively military personnel and was mainly interested in the supply of horses to the army. The recruitment of civilian personnel was problematic from the outset. In 1907, when the services really started working, only 14 out of 23 positions of veterinary-inspectors were filled because of a lack of sufficient candidates.[28] It soon became clear that the veterinary service could not work without local staff.

Initially provided by a single institution, the Ecole de Médecine de Hanoi created in 1904, veterinary and medical education experienced similar limits and vicissitudes. First, the school applicants were more numerous than the small number of student places set by the colonial authorities.[29] The independence of the Veterinary School in 1918 (henceforth attached to the local veterinary service in Tonkin) was a signal of greater attention paid to the profession. Several successive reforms raised the educational level, and with the introduction or strengthening of disciplines, such as prophylaxis of animal diseases and zootechny, the program was extended from three to four years. Yet, the closure of the School between 1935 and 1940 put an end to reforms and the Hanoi Veterinary School never granted diplomas equivalent to the Metropolitan schools. From its creation until 1935, about 150 Indochinese veterinarians graduated from the school.[30]

The Pasteur Institute in Nha Trang also took on an educational role. A practical and theoretical training program on local animal diseases was initially exclusively intended for the colonial veterinarians newly graduated from a French university after their arrival in Indochina. Nevertheless, from the 1920s on, Indochinese veterinarians also received a three-month practical training at the Nha Trang Institute, before their assignment to a position.[31]

But the first and foremost educational task of the Institute was the training of vaccinators. As early as 1899, the Résidents Supérieurs in Annam and Tonkin had sent some young indigenous people to the Nha Trang Institute for training as vaccinators.[32] Selected by their local administrators, they were required to have a primary school certificate and sufficient knowledge of the French language to serve as interpreters for the farmers. The training program, which expanded over the years, included general notions of animal anatomy and physiology, some data on the country's contagious diseases, their causes, their prophylaxis, and related animal health rules. The students also learned how to take blood or tissue samples, and to practice inoculations, microscopic examinations, autopsy, and minor surgery.[33]

As noted in 1927 in a circular from the Agriculture General Inspector addressed to the authorities of the different Indochinese Union's countries and regions, the veterinary-inspectors' function was to supervise and oversee, not to execute. However, in many circumstances, not all the veterinary-inspector posts were filled by French veterinarians, and auxiliary-veterinarians filled vacancies, at least temporarily. Most generally, the workload of the veterinary staff, especially in times of an epizootic, could lead to some responsibilities being delegated to lower-grade staff members. Certainly some auxiliary-veterinarians, and vaccinators as well, acquired skills and efficiency that sometimes earned them very positive assessments from their superiors. Grouped in a professional association, the auxiliary veterinarians started a publication called *Bulletin des vétérinaires auxiliaires de l'Indochine* in 1923. In the first issue, a French veterinarian underlined their educational mission:

Thanks to their in-depth knowledge of the Annamese language and customs, the auxiliary-veterinarians are the best suited intermediaries between the French veterinarians who have imported scientific methods and the Nhà Quê [vietnamese pejorative word for the peasants], totally ignorant, and therefore have to play a highly important role as educators. Better enlightened by them, the local farmer will apply all requirements relating to hygiene, treatment and animal health with a more complete understanding, and thus with more willingness and a better return than those seen to date.

And he concluded rather emphatically: "So, the usefulness and importance of the service to which the auxiliary-veterinarians have the honor of belonging will be visible to everybody."[34]

However, the appropriateness of auxiliaries in higher veterinary education was questioned by some colonial veterinarians, as in other scientific branches such as human medicine.[35] Henri Schein, a "prominent" veterinarian and a Pastorian (graduate of the Pasteur Institute), argued that the training of vaccinators in larger numbers would be better than useless investments in the veterinary school. To support his opinion about the necessity of increasing vaccinators, he pointed out that the auxiliary staff was mostly composed of Vietnamese, even in Laos and Cambodia. He also suggested the training of "healers" among minority groups in the high regions. He considered the veterinary school to be a "toy" school; furthermore he maintained that many auxiliary-veterinarians, as was the rest of the "Annamese" people, were "3,000 years behind us" and easily reverted to their ancestor's beliefs and their superstitions in the performance of their duties.[36]

However, the slow response time of the veterinary service when an epidemic broke out was mostly blamed on the local population. For example, the spread of rinderpest from the Tonkin highlands to the delta in 1907–08 was attributed to several factors. The first was local farmers who did not report the illness in order to move their cattle and those who did not bury the carcasses of sick animals to avoid the required tax. The second was a lack of interest on the part of native authorities in their district. The third was the failure of the native authorities, when warned of an epidemic outbreak, to implement the law on the declaration of infection and the prohibition of free cattle movement. Finally, the purchase of livestock in the contaminated areas and its sale in areas still free of rinderpest also favored the propagation of the disease.[37]

From the 1920s on, leaflets in local languages were distributed to the village heads, or Lý Trưởng, in charge of diffusing information on symptoms of different contagious diseases and requirements of animal health policy to the farmers. A bleak picture of the terrible consequences of animal diseases was drawn in the introduction: spread of epizootics to an entire province, impediments to fieldwork, and finally poverty and starvation. In order to make a stronger impact on the public, this publicity would be followed by details of heavy fines and, in some cases, prison sentences in events of non-compliance with health measures such as rapid reportage of animal diseases to the authorities, burying of carcasses, disinfection, quarantine, and so on.[38]

It is noteworthy that the culling of infected animals and animals suspected of contamination, a measure modeled on the metropolitan law, had to be abolished, given the general endemicity of the animal diseases. Not only would this have resulted in a massive slaughter of Indochinese livestock, but application of the law encountered all kinds of difficulties.[39] Furthermore, there was a broad agreement that, in Indochinese countries, unlike European ones, epizootic control could not be achieved through sanitary measures alone.

Although the list of communicable diseases of domestic animals grew substantially over the years, with documented cases of foot and mouth disease, blackleg, pleuropneumonia, malignant catarrhal fever, and bovine tuberculosis, to name but cattle diseases, rinderpest control remained the biggest challenge. The first immunization method, with a serum produced at the Pasteur Institute, only provided short-term immunity, was not very effective in water buffaloes—which were more sensitive to the disease than oxen—and had several other drawbacks.[40] Longer lasting protection was given by sero-infection, also called serum-simultaneous vaccine, but despite better outcomes, this method was tricky and not without risk of a new epizootic.[41]

At the end of the 1920s, the first successful immunization trials with vaccines developed from rinderpest-infected organ extracts were carried out both at the Nha Trang Institute and in the laboratory of the Veterinary School in Hanoi.[42] Soon after, the veterinary service launched the first vaccination campaigns in Tonkin, then in Cochinchina, where the rinderpest epizootic that broke out in 1929 caused the loss of nearly 30,000 head of cattle.[43] The vaccines did not provide complete protective immunity and had a short shelf life. Nevertheless they were much more likely to win farmers' trust because of their safety and the simplicity of their use, as compared with earlier protective methods. According to Bergeon, head of a laboratory in Hanoi, after only few years of campaigns, "the indigenous farmers are the first to claim immunization of threatened herds; they even offer calves for vaccine production."[44]

The conditions were still far from perfect for practicing systematic immunization among Indochinese livestock. Most of the time, the veterinary service intervened when an outbreak had already occurred.[45] However, a turning point in the history of rinderpest control occurred in the 1930s. Despite the persistence of frequent rinderpest outbreaks all over Indochina, these vaccines led, apparently, to a downward trend in cattle mortality. A new impetus was given to the development of animal husbandry.

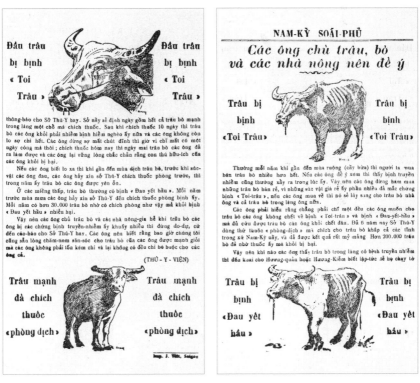

**Figures 1 and 2.** Brochure produced by the veterinary service and distributed by the government of Cochinchina. Its purpose was to urge farmers to report bovine contagious diseases (particularly rinderpest and bovine pasteurellosis) to the local authorities as soon as these occurred in the villages, by informing farmers of the benefits of vaccinations (Source: ANOM: GGI, Services Economiques, 2520 Elevage et services vétérinaires. Correspondances diverses, 1937–43).

## Pursuit of a Colonial Dream: The Livestock Improvement Program

In his comprehensive report on animal production for the international colonial exhibition of 1931 in Paris, the Inspector-General of Veterinary Service in Indochina, Le Louët, wrote:

> It can be said that Indochina does not raise cattle; actually cattle is only a natural production like trees of the forest, a production on which the natives seldom have any influence. We can also say... that Indochina produces bovine, bubaline, porcine, etc. species, but does not create, does not keep, and does not develop breeds in each of these species.[46]

Yet, the improvement of livestock production had been an early concern of the Inspector of Agriculture, and a council for animal husbandry development was established in Annam-Tonkin in 1904.[47] Introduction of "rational farming systems," the Council members agreed, was "the role of the official institutions and of enlightened settlers." They also emphasized that educating the ethnic minority groups, "semi-savage" backward people who lived in the high region where the cattle breeding stock was, would be a very long process. The "Annamese," or lowland Vietnamese people who settled in regions of natural grasslands yet to be exploited outside the deltas, were seen as more likely to adopt new methods of farming.[48]

Not only were calls to both the Europeans and the Vietnamese to start animal farms in favorable areas little heard, but the few new farmers "too often do no better than the savages, when they do no worse," in terms of the lack of breed selection and hay supply, as was reported to the Inspector of agriculture. The risks of cattle loss to breeders, due to epizootics, tigers, and animal theft, required strengthening state intervention, concluded the report. Aside from the necessary increase of veterinary staff and the rigorous application of animal health rules, it also stressed the barriers to free trade that prevented the breeders from investing in animal food supply and adequate equipment.[49]

Actually, the main measure was a ban, enacted in 1911, on the slaughter of cows under the age of nine, following warnings about the risk of Cambodian livestock degeneration due to the acceleration of the cattle trade. This measure caused disagreements between some veterinarians and administrators, the latter arguing that the ban might discourage local farmers who had just found a new source of profitable revenue. The matter was not resolved, as veterinarians pointed out that the development of cattle breeding aimed to allow the Indochinese to purchase low-priced working animals.[50] This notwithstanding, they were equally critical of local breeding methods, stating, in particular, that the Indochinese practiced "reverse selection," that is to say that they kept the males of lowest breeding quality and sold or castrated the best ones. To prevent this practice, rounds of castrations were organized by the veterinary service.[51]

Another measure was the purchase of carefully selected bulls that were made available to breeders who requested for them. So in the 1920s, the issue of cattle breeding development in Cochinchina re-emerged due to its high dependence on draft animals, and the bad quality of beef and milk coming on the city market. At the request of the Colonial Council, the administration acquired 20 bulls on the Cambodian market, some of which were intended for cattle breeders. It seems that this initiative was successful mainly among owners of big rubber tree companies. In any case, the idea of developing pastoral activity in Cochinchina to supply slaughter and draft animals to the colony was finally abandoned. But it was the starting point of a cattle selection program in an experimental farm settled in Tan Son Nhut (a village close to Saigon).[52]

The farm also hosted Indian breeding animals for milk production. While the first crossbreeding attempts between local and European breeds had led to failure, good results were obtained in Cochinchina by the Indian community which introduced Ongole, Bangalore and other Indian breeds. Most of the dairies in Saigon belonged to Indian people.[53] From a survey of these dairies conducted by the veterinary service, their hygiene conditions were very unsatisfactory. However, even the Indian-local crossbred cows were better milk producers than any autochthonous breed.[54] On the basis of these good results, in 1923 the veterinary service started the breeding of Sind-bred animals brought back from India.[55]

From the beginning of 1930s, the studies carried out by the veterinary service in experimental farms expanded. In the rearing unit at Nong-Công (Thanh Hoa province, North Annam), Le Louët intended to demonstrate that extensive farming was possible: the herd composed of carefully selected animals of the local breed, protected against the main cattle diseases, and provided with a minimum of feed, water and shelter at night, and had a fertility index higher than 80 per cent.[56] In the high regions at An Khê and Dankia (Central Annam, at respectively 500 and

1,400 meter altitudes), and at Nước Hai (Tonkin), trials of crossbreeding for the dairy industry, cattle selection programs, and adaptation of fodder plants were conducted. To give new impetus to animal husbandry, bonuses were also proposed for breeders and a new scheme of farming concessions was set up.[57]

The province's residents were encouraged to organize animal competitions, which had the dual objective of "giving the native the wish to have beautiful animals, to expand its livestock and improve it," and of selecting the best breeding animals to lend them to breeders.[58] The competitions also allowed assessing the outcomes of educational measures. According to Evanno, head of the veterinary service in Tonkin, apart from a certain homogenization due to the introduction of the Sind breed, the results were rather disappointing. Pointing out that animal feed was the most important factor in the development of cattle husbandry, he recognized that, although the Vietnamese were "enterprising and hard-working...the low value of livestock did not encourage farmers to undertake cultural improvements" and that the peasants "will never impose methods [in use in experimental farms] on themselves, which would be able to tip the annual account balance on the wrong side."[59] Evanno stressed that European settlers did not contribute more than Vietnamese breeders to changes in breeding practices. They owned no more than 2–3 per cent of the total livestock, and most of them were big planters using cattle for manure production.[60]

In the 1930s, peasant poverty, which was exacerbated by the economic crisis, was even more of an obstacle to change than before. The head of the veterinary service in Annam also noted that "the current farm crisis and the slump in cattle sales prevent any change in traditional livestock rearing" and that, in the inland region where lands were yet to be cleared, to poverty was also added sickness due to endemic malaria.[61]

Baradat, head of the Battambang sector in western Cambodia, gave a slightly more positive report. Although he subscribed to the colonial stereotype of the Cambodian peasant as "reluctant to effort," he was also a good observer of rural life, laying out in great detail the care with which the rice farmers chose their cattle. After a competition organized in order to show the influence of the soil and pasture on cattle size, he noticed that:

> Farmers in the region were quick to point out that the cattle coming
> from siliceous soils and seasonally dry pastures were small and had

a late development, and that, if when still young they were carried to alluvial soils, the same cattle acquire powerful bones and good harmony of muscles.[62]

Baradat proposed following another education model. Using farms in Brazil and Venezuela as examples, he created a project to set up improvement trials of the zootechnic characters of local bovine breeds as well as the acclimatization of various fodder plants in a series of school farms. These school farms would be manned by "young Cambodians having received rudimentary education, intending to take over from their parents in the country," who would be also selected for "their athletic qualities." Baradat proposed that:

> [those recruited] would carry out most of the work. This mainly practical education would be complemented by some courses and film projections. Any ambition they may have to embark on a career of civil servant should be destroyed; [instead,] their peasant life vocation should be encouraged; and, as they finish their schooling, they should be immediately helped in getting back to their villages wherein, among other humble roles, they would demonstrate the efficacy of their work for the cattle of this country. For the sake of the masses' education, the one who practises what one preaches is better than the one who contents himself with advising.[63]

Probably due to schedule problems, this paternalistic program could not be implemented. As the looming war caused fear of meat supply disruption, Jules Brévié, who had been appointed Governor-General of Indochina in 1936, called on an agronomist to reassess the possibility of livestock development in the colony.[64] While recognizing the importance of the role of the veterinarians as hygienists or as "geneticists," he called into question their other functions. Brévié, previously the administrator of French West Africa, nominated Havard-Duclos, who had carried out missions in several French African colonies as well as in the Belgian Congo.[65] Havard-Duclos was also professor of zootechnics at the Institut National d'Agronomie de la France d'Outre-Mer. His mission only lasted from February to November 1939, but gave rise to a long report.

Havard-Duclos was not very flattering about the veterinarian's work in zootechny, emphasizing that the improvement of pasture was a matter for agronomists. In fact, like his predecessors, he pointed out that the main problem facing Indochinese breeding was the locals' failure to understand the need of stocking fodder for the dry season. In turn, he advocated a battery of collective propaganda among peasants: fairs, agricultural shows, and short lectures. He recommended a slow cautious learning process that would not discourage the peasant, on the one hand, and would spare the colonial instructor from "losing face," on the other hand. First of all, he recommended education at school about animal food, care, and housing by means of pictures and observation.

However, Havard-Duclos did not dwell on the local farming systems. At the present time, he concluded, Europeans alone would be able to give an impetus to breeding. The only way to attract new settlers and to provide incentives for European breeding activity, according to him, was to create conditions for large-scale production. Indeed, because of the low value of domestic animals in the colony, this activity would be profitable only above the threshold of 3,000 cattle and 20,000 hectares.[66] Large European breeding centers would enable the *mise en valeur* of high plateaus, such as in Tran-Ninh, Cammon, Kontum, Darlac, and the Plateau des Herbes, for exportation of canned and frozen meat, as well as milk products. Scientific methods used in South Africa, Central Africa, Australia, and South America would regenerate the land spoiled by the "ignorant locals." Last but not least, Havard-Duclos envisioned either putting the ethnic minorities in reservations inside the concessions or "clearing off" the territories in exchange for material compensation to local inhabitants.[67]

Finally, Havard-Duclos devoted some thoughts to a theme that was much debated during the 1930s—the food intake requirements of the natives. He noted an increase, especially in urban areas, in the consumption of beef, the protein content of which is much higher than that of pork, the population's basic meat, and envisaged a constant rise in beef consumption. The army played an important role in his projection, first due to the growth of the troops, and second, as a vehicle for a change in food habits. He also advocated bringing numerous selected animals to propitious areas where they would constitute a food source for a time of self-reliance if such were imposed on the colony.[68]

## Conclusion

Whether or not Havard-Duclos' mission was organized to prepare for war, his report was bitterly received by veterinarians who had long experience of the country and had become familiar with rural life.[69] Jacotot, who had arrived in Indochina in 1922, reacted to Havard-Duclos's report:

The increase in the number of farms and moreover the improvement of domestic animals of Indochina's various regions can be carried out immediately and can continue rather easily if we keep it within measured limits; but, within these limits, the achievements will contribute to the recovery of the Indochinese economy and to the enrichment of the country only if they will concern a progressively increasing proportion of indigenous farms.

The progress achieved will benefit not, as has been the case up to now, the privileged few but will extend to all small farmers, to the mass of peasants. The Technical, Veterinary and Agronomical Services would thus contribute directly, to the improvement of the rural population's condition as well as to increasing the economic potential of French Indochina.[70]

In the 1930s, Jacotot was not the only veterinarian to think both in terms of economic growth and of social progress. During the interwar period, special focus was given to living conditions in the rural areas and to one of the direct consequences of the poverty of inhabitants—malnutrition—which became a growing concern in some colonial political and scientific circles.[71] While estimates of local meat consumption (beef and pork) in Indochina showed a surplus of production, the average protein intake per inhabitant was only about a tenth of the estimated consumption required by a worker. Education on a diet richer in animal protein, especially beef, was envisaged, both as a means of promoting animal breeding with "rational" methods and as a complement to education of the colonized people.[72] However, projections concerning the possible development of the Indochinese herd were rather pessimistic, stating that it would take at least 40 years to attain a beef production level that would satisfy the minimum needs of the population.[73]

This certainly challenged the exporting activity of livestock farming —the overriding colonial purpose—and seriously thwarted the colonial ambition of transforming Indochina into a cattle producer like big countries such as Brazil, South Africa, or Australia. Despite this, the myth of the European settler-farmer reappeared on the eve of World War II, largely due to the competition of a new generation of agronomists who called into question the veterinarian's competence in zootechny. However, as pointed out by Etienne Landais, in French colonial sub-Saharan Africa, veterinarians kept a monopoly on the animal husbandry service at least until independence.[74] We can assume that the situation was rather similar in Indochina, not least because of the economic consequences of animal diseases. Undoubtedly, disease control was the veterinarian's biggest contribution. But the imprint of the wide range of competencies in animal farming, which the French colonial veterinarians claimed, is obvious in the work conducted by their Indochinese students until at least the 1960s.[75]

## Notes

1.   Henri Jacotot, "La situation de l'élevage indochinois au début du siècle et à la fin de la Deuxième Guerre Mondiale," *Revue d'Elevage et de Médecine Vétérinaire des Pays Tropicaux* 1 (1947): 287.

2.   Diana K. Davis, "Prescribing Progress: French Veterinary Medicine in the Service of Empire," *Veterinary Heritage* 29, no. 1 (2006): 1–7. http://www.utexas.edu/depts/grg/davis/PrescProgress.pdf [site no longer available].

3.   Diana K. Davis, "Brutes, Beasts and Empire: Veterinary Medicine and Environmental Policy in French North Africa and British India," *Journal of Historical Geography* 34 (2008): 242–67.

4.   F. Lepinte, "Rapport sur le service vétérinaire, zootechnique et des épizooties," *Bulletin Economique de l'Indochine* 11 (Sept.–Oct. 1908): 461–85.

5.   E. Douarche, "Les bovins d'Indochine," *Bulletin Economique de l'Indochine* 5 (Oct. 1902): 689–705.

6.   For a review on these topics as well as on education, see Robert Aldrich, "Imperial *Mise en Valeur* et *Mise en Scène*: Recent Works on French Colonialism," *The Historical Journal* 15, no. 4 (2002): 925–6.

7.   P. Famin, *Au Tonkin et sur la frontière du Kwang-Si* (Paris: Challamel, 1895); W. Lichtenfelder, "Rapport sur les cultures et l'élevage dans la haute-Région du Tonkin," *Bulletin Economique de l'Indochine* 5 (Nov. 1902): 804–13.

8.   The annexation of the entire territory was achieved in 1862. The occupation of southern lands (part of the country the French named "Cochinchina") by the Viêts was relatively recent. Indeed, from the eleventh century, Vietnam's borders progressively shifted from the north (and the Red River delta) to the south, first incorporating the Champa kingdom in the center, then the former Khmer provinces in the south. This is called the "Nam Tiên," or drive to the south.

9.   In 1872, Condamine, then director of the stud farm in Saigon, was appointed to investigate the current status of animal breeding and the possibilities of land conversion into pastures. National Archives of Vietnam (NAV), Centre no. 2, Goucoch, IA 4/152(1): "Elève du bétail dans la colonie," Rapport de Mr Condamine (directeur du haras), Dec. 2, 1872.

10.   Pierre Brocheux, *Une histoire économique du Viet Nam 1850–2007: la palanche et le camion* (Paris: Les Indes Savantes, 2009), 72–83.

11.   "L'élevage du bétail en Annam", *Bulletin Economique de l'Indochine* 4 (Nov. 1901): 1016–17.

12. Without a hump such as a Zebu (Bos primagenius indicus).

13. L. Gilbert, "Annam, Chapitre II: animaux domestiques et sauvages," *Bulletin Economique de l'Indochine* 28 (1925): 126–7.

14. About demography and cultivated areas, see Pierre Brocheux and Daniel Hémery, *Indochine, la colonisation ambiguë 1858–1954* (Paris: Editions La Découverte, 1995), 245–74.

15. The Indochinese bovine species are described as a mosaic of breeds due to numerous influences from India, Siam, and China. See: G. Le Louët, "La production animale en Indochine," *Revue de Médecine Vétérinaire Exotique* 5 (Apr.–June 1932): 144–56.

16. R. Baradat, "Conditions d'élevage au Cambodge: A., 5e Secteur vétérinaire," *Bulletin Economique de l'Indochine* 40, no. 3 (1937): 547–56.

17. Pierre Gourou, *L'utilisation du sol en Indochine française* (Paris: Hartmann, 1940).

18. "Mouvement des animaux en Indochine: transhumance, marché et commerce du bétail," *Revue de Médecine Vétérinaire Exotique* 2 (Apr.–June 1929): 85.

19. Lucien Choquart, *Les marchés de bestiaux et le commerce du bétail au Tonkin*, thèse de doctorat vétérinaire (Paris, 1928).

20. Gourou, *L'utilisation du sol*, 196–207.

21. Due to the decimation of the archipelago's carabao (water buffalo) from rinderpest in the late 1880s, which was a disaster for the sugar cane planters. See: Ken De Bevoise, *Agents of Apocalypse: Epidemic Disease in the Colonial Philippines* (Princeton: Princeton University Press, 1995). Arleigh Ross D. De la Cruz, "Epizootics and the Colonial Legacies of the United States in Philippine Veterinary Science," *International Review of Environmental History* 2 (2016): 143–72.

22. J. Bauche, "Rapport sur le service vétérinaire, zootechnique et des épizooties de l'Indochine," *Bulletin Economique de l'Indochine* 11 (Nov.–Dec. 1908): 677.

23. The laboratory progressively expanded and was renamed the Pasteur Institute in 1904, as was the Saigon laboratory created by Albert Calmette in 1891.

24. Until the end of the nineteenth century, the nature of the main animal diseases in Indochina were not identified.

25. J. Blin, "Note sur des vaccinations anticharbonneuses et sur le trypanosome des mammifères," *Bulletin Economique de l'Indochine* 5 (Aug. 1902): 585–8; J. Blin and Carougeau, "La septicémie hémorragique aiguë des buffles," *Bulletin Economique de l'Indochine* 6 (Jan. 1903): 60–74; L. Lepinte, E. Douarche, and J. Bauche, "Rapport sur le charbon bactéridien au Tonkin," *Bulletin Economique de l'Indochine* 6 (Sept. 1903): 628–37.

26. Brocheux, *Une histoire économique du Viet Nam 1850–2007*, 72.

27. M.P. Conti, "Note sur les dix premières années de l'action vétérinaire au Laos," *Revue de Médecine Vétérinaire Exotique* 5 (Apr.–June 1932): 80–3.

28.  In 1907, Tonkin was divided into ten sectors, Annam four, Cambodia three, and Cochinchina only two. There were four higher-rank inspectors at the head of Tonkin, Annam, Cochinchina, and Cambodia, but no veterinary position allocated to Laos: L. Lepinte, "Rapport sur le service vétérinaire, zootechnique et des épizooties de 'Indo-Chine'," *Bulletin Economique de l'Indochine* 11 (Sept.–Oct. 1908): 462–85; (Nov.–Dec. 1908): 600–93.

29.  For more details on the Hanoi Medical School, see Laurence Monnais, *Médecine et colonisation: l'aventure indochinoise 1860–1939* (Paris: CNRS Editions, 1999).

30.  R. Jauffret, "L'école vétérinaire de l'Indochine: son but, son organisation, ses résultats, son avenir," *Bulletin Economique de l'Indochine* 46, no. 3 (1943): 351–62.

31.  Anonymous, "Recrutement et formation du personnel vétérinaire indigène en Indochine," *Recueil de Médecine Vétérinaire Exotique* 1 (Oct.–Dec. 1928): 177–8; H.G. Morin, H. Jacotot, and J. Genevray, "Les Instituts Pasteur d'Indochine en 1934," *Archives des Instituts Pasteur d'Indochine*, no. 20 (1934): 492–3. Between 1924 and 1934, 35 French veterinarians, 75 Indochinese veterinarians, and 150 vaccinators were trained at the Nha Trang Institute.

32.  Pasteur Institute Archives, "L'Institut Pasteur de Nha Trang," by Jacotot, Aug. 15, 1930, FR AIP IND-C1; A. Yersin, "Fonctionnement de l'Institut Pasteur de Nha Trang (Annam)," *Annales d'Hygiène et de Médecine Coloniales*, Tome 3 (1900): 506–20.

33.  Ibid.

34.  E.H. Choquart, *Bulletin des vétérinaires auxiliaires de l'Indochine*, no. 1 (1923). Most of the journal articles were from French authors. Between 1923 and 1925, the journal was twice retitled: *Bulletin vétérinaire de l'Indochine*, then *Bulletin de médecine vétérinaire indochinoise*. The last issue recorded in the National Library in Paris was published in 1925.

35.  For higher education in the French colonies, see Pierre Singaravélou, "'L'enseignement supérieur colonial': un état des lieux," *Histoire de l'éducation* 122 (2009): 71–92.

36.  H. Schein, "Recrutement et formation du personnel vétérinaire indigène en Indochine," *Revue de Médecine Vétérinaire Exotique* 1 (Oct.–Dec. 1928): 177–81.

37.  Archives Nationales d'Outre-Mer, Aix-en-Provence (ANOM), GGI 17680: "Epizooties: rapport sur le fonctionnement du service vétérinaire, zootechnique et des épizooties du Tonkin," 2ᵉ semestre 1908.

38.  See for example: G. Le Louët and Nguyên Van Dung (transl.), *Notions élémentaires de police sanitaire à l'usage des cultivateurs et éleveurs annamites* [Elementary elements of animal health policy for Annamese farmers and breeders], 1923 [Government of Cochinchina (NAV), Center no. 2, Goucoch, IA 4/146(1)]; A. Hubac, *Hygiène et maladies des animaux*

*expliquées au paysan annamite: Nói về vệ sinh và các bệnh loài vật nuôi* (Hanoi: Imprimerie Tonkinoise, 1925).

39. ANOM, GGI 17665, "Application de la loi du 21 juillet 1881 sur les épizooties en ce qui concerne la peste bovine," 1902/1907–08; Lepinte (1908), "Rapport sur le service vétérinaire, zootechnique et des épizooties de 'Indo-Chine'," 658–9.

40. The mode of injection and choice of correct timing were rather complicated. "Instructions pour l'emploi du sérum contre la peste bovine," *Bulletin Economique de l'Indochine* 4 (Feb. 1901): 125–9.

41. The method consisted of a simultaneous inoculation of a small amount of blood from a sick animal and serum. The first risk was an association of rinderpest with another disease in the sick animal that had not been diagnosed. Secondly, the susceptibility to infection varied, which involved properly estimating the serum dosage. A three-week rest period and monitoring of inoculated animals had to be observed. Last but not least, the breeders had to be well informed so that the method would not cause any animal losses. See: H. Schein and Jacotot, "La séro-infection: vaccination préventive contre la peste bovine," *Archives des Instituts Pasteur d'Indochine* 1 (1925): 48–56.

42. C. Kakisaki in Japan and W.H. Boynton in the Philippines were the first scientists who studied this method of vaccine preparation. See: P. Bergeon and J. Cèbe, "Au sujet de la vaccination antipestique: Expériences faites au laboratoire de l'Ecole Vétérinaire de l'Indochine à Hanoi en 1929," *Bulletin Economique de l'Indochine*, Sect. B, 33 (May 1930): 434B–445B; H. Jacotot, *Instituts Pasteur d'Indochine: La peste bovine en Indochine* (Saigon: Imprimerie Nouvelle Albert Portail, 1931), 52–64.

43. G. Roche, "Prophylaxie de la peste bovine en Cochinchine: campagnes antipestiques de 1930–1931 et 1932," *Bulletin Economique de l'Indochine*, Sect. B, 35 (Jan.–Feb. 1932): 793B–808B.

44. Bergeon, "Les maladies du bétail au Tonkin," *Revue de Médecine Vétérinaire Exotique* 5 (Jan.–Mar. 1932): 25.

45. See for example: "Etat du cheptel Indochinois," *Bulletin Economique de l'Indochine* 40, no. 4 (1937): 629–56.

46. G. Le Louët, "La production animale en Indochine," *Exposition coloniale internationale: congrès de la production animale et des maladies du bétail* (1931):107.

47. The first council was created in 1904. In 1906, a council for animal husbandry development in Indochina was also created (ANOM, GGI 15145).

48. NAV, Centre no. 2, Goucoch, 1A 4/152(1): "Procès Verbal de la Réunion de la sous-commission du 8/11/1904 du Conseil de perfectionnement de l'Elevage au Tonkin et en Annam."

49. ANOM, GGI 12 "Exportation des bovidés": rapport à Monsieur le Directeur de l'Agriculture, des Forêts et du Commerce de l'Indochine sur les moyens de prévenir la dégénérescence de la race bovine, Hanoi, March 23, 1907.

50.  Ch. Sarazin, "Le bétail indochinois sur les marchés de France et d'Extrême-Orient," *Bulletin Economique de l'Indochine* 19 (Sept.–Oct. 1916): 608.

51.  Auguste Dervaux, *L'élevage des animaux domestiques en Annam*, thèse de doctorat vétérinaire, Faculté de Médecine de Paris, 1929. Dervaux declared that this practice was conducted in Annam from 1917, and that more than 10,000 low-breeding quality males a year were eliminated.

52.  NAV, Center no. 2, Goucoch, IA4/152(2): Elevage, correspondances 1920–24; G. Le Louët, "L'élevage des bovidés en Cochinchine," *Bulletin Economique de l'Indochine* 31, no. 2 (1928): 111–19.

53.  Concerning the Indian community in Indochina during the French colonization, see Natasha Pairaudau, *French Indians in Indochina, 1858–1954* (Denmark: NIAS Press, 2016).

54.  Abel Lahille, "Le lait et les laiteries de Saigon," *Bulletin Economique de l'Indochine* 22 (Mar.–Apr. 1919): 199–213.

55.  Le Louët, 1928. Veterinarian-Inspector Schein who travelled to India was refused the purchase of Ongole-bred animals, which were replaced by Sind-bred ones.

56.  In this context, the percentage of mature cows in a herd giving birth to one calf once a year.

57.  G. Le Louët, "Essai sur les possibilités de l'élevage industriel du bétail en Indochine," *Bulletin Economique de l'Indochine*, Sect. B, 34 (July 1931): 561B; Roche, "Rapports des chefs des services vétérinaires des divers pays de l'Union pour l'année 1933," *Bulletin Economique de l'Indochine* 37 (Mar.–Apr. 1934): 312–33.

58.  NAV, Centre no. 2, Goucoch, III59/N21(19): Rapport d'ensemble sur l'élevage, 1937.

59.  Charles Evanno, "Les entreprises d'élevage au Tonkin," *Bulletin Economique de l'Indochine* 41, no. 2 (1938): 338.

60.  L.M. Feunteun, "Concours interprovincial d'élevage de My Tho (Cochinchine) 1937," *Bulletin Economique de l'Indochine* 41, no. 1 (1938): 115–20; Evanno, "Les entreprises d'élevage au Tonkin."

61.  Lebouc, "Rapports des chefs des services vétérinaires des divers pays de l'Union pour l'année 1933, II: Annam," *Bulletin Economique de l'Indochine* 37 (Mar.–Apr. 1934): 322.

62.  R. Baradat, "La foire de Prek Khpop," *Bulletin Economique de l'Indochine* 42, no. 2 (1939): 230–59, 244.

63.  Baradat, "Conditions d'élevage au Cambodge," 555–6.

64.  During the Vichy period, J. Brévié was one of the artisans behind the creation of the Office of Colonial Scientific Research (ORSC) in France (later on called ORSTOM, then IRD): Christophe Bonneuil and Patrick Petitjean, "Les chemins de la création de l'ORSTOM, du Front Populaire à la Libération en passant par Vichy," in *Les sciences coloniales: figures et institutions*, ed. P. Petitjean (Paris: ORSTOM Editions, 1996), 133. See

also: Pierre Singaravélou, "'L'enseignement supérieur colonial': un état des lieux," *Histoire de l'éducation* 122 (2009): 89.

65. ANOM, GGI Serv. Eco. 2524, Jules Brévié's letter to the Minister of Colonies, 1938.

66. These concessions would be granted gratuitously and title deed would finally be given on condition of the owner's purchasing one-third of the herd, fencing half of the grazing area with wire, crucial for grazing area rotation, and providing tubs for bathing the animals.

67. Havard-Duclos favored the second solution, which would definitively "cleanse" the territories and leave them "homogeneous."

68. B. Havard-Duclos, "Possibilités d'amélioration et de développement de l'élevage en Indochine," *Bulletin Economique de l'Indochine* 42, no. 6 (1939): 1125–70; 43 (1940): 12–45, 213–58.

69. ANOM, GGI Serv. Eco. 2525: "Envoi en Indochine de deux vétérinaires chargés d'étudier le développement de l'élevage colonial, 1939." The Ministry of Colonies sent two veterinarians to Indochina. The General-Governor of Indochina protested because this mission was at the colony's expenses and Havard-Duclos had just submitted his report. The Ministry answered that the new mission did not overlap with the Havard-Duclos' one as this was classified as a military secret. His report (kept in the ANOM, GGI Serv. Eco. 2524) was only published in the *Bulletin Economique de l'Indochine* after 1940.

70. Jacotot, "Note sur le développement de l'élevage et l'amélioration des espèces domestiques en Indochine," Nov. 11, 1940, ANOM, GGI Serv. Eco. 2529.

71. Annick Guénel, "The Conference on Rural Hygiene in Bandung of 1937: Towards a New Vision of Health Care?", in *Global Movements, Local Concerns: Medicine and Health in Southeast Asia*, ed. Laurence Monnais and Harold Cook (Singapore: NUS Press, 2012), 62–80.

72. G. Hardy and Ch. Richet, *L'alimentation indigène dans les colonies Françaises* (Paris: Vigot Frères, 1933).

73. G. Le Louët, "Consommation du bétail en Indochine," *Bulletin Economique de l'Indochine*, Sect. B, 34 (Dec. 1931): 1102B–13B.

74. Etienne Landais, "Sur les doctrines des vétérinaires coloniaux français en Afrique noire," *Cahiers de Sciences Humaines* 26 (1990): 37–9.

75. See, for example, the theses defended in France by: Savang Prom-Tep, *Facteurs sociaux et religieux dans l'élevage au Cambodge*, thèse pour le doctorat vétérinaire, Faculté mixte de médecine et de pharmacie de Toulouse, 1954; Dinh-Chinh-Vu, *L'élevage bovin au Viêt Nam*, thèse pour le doctorat vétérinaire, Faculté de médecine et de pharmacie de Lyon, 1955; Tran-Trong-Hieu, *Considérations sur l'élevage et l'amélioration du gros bétail au sud-Vietnam*, thèse pour le doctorat vétérinaire, Paris, 1962.

## CHAPTER 4

# Women's Health in Laos:
# From Colonial Times to the Present

*Kathryn Sweet*

In 2012 the poor state of women's health in Laos was in the spotlight due to the advancing deadline of the Millennium Development Goals (MDGs) and MDG 5 in particular, which aimed to improve maternal health by reducing maternal mortality rates and providing universal access to reproductive health services. The Lao People's Democratic Republic (Lao PDR) had for many decades one of the highest maternal mortality rates in the East Asia-Pacific region, few trained midwives, and comparatively low rates of access to contraception and other basic reproductive health services. It would be tempting to assume that these low indicators for women's health were the result of long-term neglect. This chapter questions that assumption by examining the numerous, often repeated, attempts from colonial times to the present to address women's health in Laos. It argues that the low indicators may be more usefully considered as evidence not of the absence of previous efforts but rather of their low sustainability, whether due to changes in health policy, administrative regime, or the composition and policy preferences of international donors that provide development assistance to Laos. This chapter focuses on three women's health interventions in particular: midwifery, more generalized maternal health care, and family planning services.

## Foreground

A key determinant of women's health and livelihood in developing nations is the number of children a woman bears, and the conditions in which she does so. High fertility is widely acknowledged to have a detrimental impact on a woman's health and well-being, especially in settings where she has a high workload, low income, and low nutrition. Unassisted delivery, without the services of a trained midwife, can heighten the risks of childbirth, most importantly that of maternal mortality. Unplanned pregnancies add to high fertility rates as well as expose women unnecessarily to the risk of maternal mortality. Family planning services have grown in popularity internationally, in part due to their potential to lower the maternal mortality rate and lifetime risk of maternal death by limiting the number of times a woman gives birth.[1] Such services can be especially effective in settings such as Laos, with limited health budgets to cover the cost of both basic and emergency care, a shortage of trained health personnel, and high fertility rates. Strategies to improve women's health therefore take account of the total fertility rate, the maternal mortality rate, the availability of trained midwives, and the contraceptive prevalence rate, defined as the proportion of married women currently using some form of contraception.

In 2005, the Lao PDR's total fertility rate was 4.07, one of the highest in the Asia-Pacific region.[2] The high total fertility rate was coupled with a low contraceptive prevalence rate of 35 per cent, which gave rise to other important aspects of women's health: one of the highest maternal mortality rates in the world, estimated at 405/100,000 in 2005, as well as very few trained midwife-specialists, and no training program for Lao midwives.[3] In a bid to meet its self-appointed MDG targets of significantly reducing the maternal mortality rate to 260/100,000 and increasing the contraceptive prevalence rate to 50–55 per cent by 2015, which were in fact unachieved targets of the National Population and Development Policy scheduled for 2010,[4] the Lao PDR's Ministry of Health launched a new "Strategy and Planning Framework for the Integrated Package of Maternal, Neonatal and Child Health Services" in 2009.[5] The framework included the prospect of free delivery in selected locations, and new specialist midwifery training through a "Skilled Birth Attendance Development Plan," which aimed to increase the number of trained midwives working in Laos tenfold from 140 in 2009–10 to 1,500 by 2015.[6] Significantly less fanfare surrounded the government's approach to providing universal access to reproductive health, which remained less clear.

Interestingly, many of the "new" policies put in place in the 2000s and 2010s and funded mainly by international development agencies were reminiscent of previous attempts to improve women's health in

Laos. However, it is difficult to discern in the recent policies the degree of acknowledgement or examination of previous attempts, or the factors that contributed to their failure or eventual unsustainability.

The international development sector globally has been frequently criticized for its ahistorical approach. Development scholar David Lewis argues that the sector has encouraged generalized, decontextualized initiatives which have been grounded in a seemingly "perpetual present."[7] Through the development sector's general decontextualization and neglect, or skewing of history, it has been possible for international donors to repeatedly implement strategies, plans, and projects in a 'one-size-fits-all' manner, in various locations around the developing world, whether or not previous approaches were successful or appropriate in individual settings. By the same token, it has been possible for developing nations to repeatedly request and/or accept international assistance to implement the same or similar policies and interventions over the course of decades, on the internationally-funded development merry-go-round. Historians of medicine and health development are well placed to contribute to informed debate about repeated health initiatives. However, while development theorists Michael Woolcock, Simon Szreter, and Vijayendra Rao note a readjustment within contemporary development circles, which now widely acknowledge that "history matters," they remark that very often historians continue to be absent from policy-making discussions.[8]

Women's health in Laos offers a textbook example of the "perpetual present" engendered by the development sector, where interventions have become a series of discontinuous episodes of similar, sometimes seemingly identical, policies implemented over the course of a century, first by the colonial regime, then by successive Lao governments, supported by financial and technical assistance from an ever-changing array of international donors. This practice has been enabled in part by the dearth of information that connects history and development activity in Laos: general histories of Laos devote limited space to developments in the health sector, and, conversely, contemporary health strategies, plans, and reports of the Lao government and international donor agencies devote limited attention to history.

This chapter revisits some of the key historical milestones in the repeated attempts to address women's health in Laos. The chapter charts the historical trajectory from colonial times to 2012 of initiatives in midwifery, more generalized maternal health care, and family planning training and service delivery. It begins by introducing recent statistics concerning women's health in Laos, and the policies introduced by the Lao Ministry of Health in the 2010s to improve the status of women's health and address MDG 5. It charts the initial steps to support women's health within the French colonial health service in Laos from 1904 to 1950, before turning to the Royal Lao Government's (RLG) resurrection of fading colonial initiatives in the years from 1950 to 1975, and the introduction of family planning services in the late 1960s with assistance from the World Health Organization (WHO), the United States Agency for International Development (USAID), and Filipino non-government organization (NGO) Operation Brotherhood. It then traces the changes and continuities in women's health training and service provision during the early period of the Lao PDR from 1976 to 1990, effected with assistance from United Nations agencies and a new suite of socialist nations, before examining the more recent period from 1991 to 2012, when assistance has been provided by an increasing number of international development agencies that currently include the World Bank, the Asian Development Bank, WHO, UNICEF, Luxembourg, South Korea, and NGOs Save the Children International and Médecins du Monde.[9] The chapter rounds up with a summary of key factors that have contributed to the seemingly weak sustainability of women's health initiatives. It advocates the acknowledgement and examination of previous initiatives and the reasons for their failure in the mid- to longer-term to inform and potentially improve present and future policies and actions in the health sector.

The chapter draws on archival research in the Archives Nationales d'Outre-Mer in Aix-en-Provence, France, the National Archives and Records Administration in Maryland, USA, the WHO Western Pacific Regional Office library in Manila, the Philippines, and the Lao National Archives Department in Vientiane, Lao PDR, as well as discussions with approximately 50 current and former health workers.[10]

## Women's Health in Colonial Laos, 1904–50

The French colonial administration began providing biomedical health services in Laos in the early years of colonization. In 1904, the Lao Medical Service (*Assistance Médicale au Laos*) gathered the four existing French *ambulances*, small clinic-cum-hospitals akin to present-day district hospitals and dispensaries, into a health system modeled on those of the larger and more established French Indochinese territories of Cochinchina, Annam, Tonkin, and Cambodia.[11] The full suite of staff and services was not provided in Laos, presumably due to its remote location, low population, and the limited funds available for colonial health efforts there.

Midwifery was virtually the only women's health service offered by the Lao Medical Service, apart from sporadic checks on the sexual health of female prostitutes. Maternity wards were attached to hospitals in the larger towns, but Lao women proved extremely reluctant to make use of them. They were perhaps dissuaded by the male environment of colonial hospitals in Laos, which were staffed predominantly by men from France and Vietnam. Lao women were under-represented as both health workers and patients in colonial Laos, similar to Khmer women in Cambodia.[12] The low representation of women in health staffing found its most extreme expression in Laos, where formal education rates were the lowest of all Indochinese territories. Even Lao men were poorly represented among health staff, as fewer Lao youth than Vietnamese immigrant youth accessed the colonial education system. Vietnamese staff, mainly employed as nurses but also as auxiliary doctors (*médecins auxiliaires*) and pharmacists (*pharmaciens auxiliaires*), outnumbered the few French doctors and the small but growing number of Lao auxiliary doctors who assisted them.[13] For example, in 1913, 25 of the 29 local (*indigène*) nurses employed by the Lao Medical Service were Vietnamese and only 4 Lao. All were male.[14] By 1929, 103 of the 146 nurses were Vietnamese, the others Lao, and 4 (whose nationalities were not stated) were female.[15] The ratio of Lao to Vietnamese staff began to even out during the 1930s, encouraged by affirmative action policies, although the proportion of female staff remained low until the 1950s.

The colonial health service was ill prepared to provide women's health services to Lao women. A maternity clinic was constructed at the main hospital in Vientiane in 1915, but there was no trained midwife.[16] A Chinese midwife from Cholon was posted to Vientiane from August 1916 to December 1917, but her contract was not renewed due to a budget shortfall.[17] The few women delivering in hospital facilities in the 1920s were Vietnamese. Of the 112 deliveries recorded at the Vientiane maternity clinic between February and December 1924, 110 were Vietnamese, 1 Chinese, and only 1 Lao[18]—whose Vietnamese husband reportedly forced her to attend the hospital.[19] In 1921 the Head of the Lao Medical Service observed:

> Only the Vietnamese women come to give birth in our *ambulances* [hospitals]. The Lao women never come. For a long time, the

women have been afraid and displayed excessive modesty in respect to our health facilities. To change that state of affairs, we need a doctor who knows the language and the customs, who can on certain occasions make house calls, and can convince them [Lao women] to accept care at the time of delivery. This service should not be allocated to the Head of the *ambulance*, who is already overworked.[20]

Again there were similarities with the Cambodian experience. In both Laos and Cambodia, Vietnamese immigrant town-dwellers formed the bulk of service users. They often had closer dealings with the colonial administration than members of the Lao or Cambodian communities, and were more likely to be familiar with its formalized system of bio-medicine. Moreover, in the hospital setting Vietnamese patients had the advantage of shared language, culture, and social relations with the pre-dominantly Vietnamese hospital staff.

The vast majority of Lao women chose to continue the practice of giving birth in the privacy and cultural familiarity of their own homes and village environments. They were attended by traditional birth atten-dants (*moh tam yae*) and/or female relatives, and observed local rituals designed to address the spiritual as well as physical elements of the birthing process, including the widespread Southeast Asian tradition of 'lying by the fire' (*you fay*) after the birth.

Despite the slow uptake of hospital-based midwifery by Lao women, the Lao Medical Service embarked on a series of measures to improve services. Affirmative action to recruit Lao nurses began in the mid-1920s.[21] A midwifery school was established in Vientiane in 1924,[22] and maternity clinics were constructed at each of the six main provincial hospitals as funds became available: Vientiane in 1915 as previously mentioned, Luang Prabang in 1924,[23] Pakse in 1931,[24] and Thakhek, Savannakhet, and Xieng Khouang in later years. Unlike other Indochinese territories, Laos had no maternity clinics located separately from hospitals (*maternités isolées*), possibly due to its smaller popula-tion and the lower demand for facility-based maternity services.

By 1930 five midwives were reported to be employed by the Lao Medical Service: three in Vientiane, one in Pakse, and one in Thakhek.[25] However, it proved difficult to find suitable Lao candidates for mid-wifery training, as students were required to have completed primary education and have basic literacy in French language. In 1924, the year the school opened, the Head of the Lao Medical Service remarked:

> It is extremely difficult to find in Laos young women who know
> how to read and write. Two of them [midwifery students], who
> came from Tranninh [the Vietnamese name for Xieng Khouang,
> frequently used by the French administration] at the beginning of
> June, are absolutely illiterate.[26]

Several of the early midwifery graduates were of mixed race: Lao-
French and Lao-Vietnamese, which is likely to have increased their
chances of entering the colonial education system.[27] But midwifery
training did not prove popular. By 1931, there was only one student in
first year, and two in second year.[28] The midwifery school faded out
after eight years of low-scale operations, closing its doors in 1932, at
the same time as the school in Phnom Penh. Both schools cited difficulties in recruiting students; however, the concurrent timing raises
the question of whether broader colonial policy played a part in the
closures.[29] Somewhat unusually, the Lao school re-opened in August
1940, under the supervision of a *médecin-capitaine* from the French
armed forces, who was unlikely to have had much experience in midwifery.[30] At this time, there were nine permanent midwives (*infirmières
sage-femmes titulaires*) and six non-permanent midwives (*infirmières
sage-femmes journalières*) working in the Lao Medical Service.[31]

On-the-job training opportunities for prospective Lao midwives
were also limited, as no French midwives were ever assigned to Laos.
A French doctor, Mme d'Ambert de Serilhac, was assigned responsibilities for maternal and child health and the monitoring of local prostitutes
at Luang Prabang hospital in 1924, but remained in Laos for only a
short time.[32] When a European female nurse was posted to Vientiane
in 1930, the Head of the Lao Medical Service complained that she
came at the price of two local *médecins auxiliaires*, suggesting they
would have been more appreciated.[33] It is unclear from archival records
whether the nurse was forced out due to sexism, unsuitability for the
job, or lack of on-going funding. Needless to say, there is no indication
of any sustainability in the practices she attempted to introduce.

In the immediate post-World War II period, the colonial administration established an Indochina-wide Social Welfare Service that promoted maternal and child health among local women. This initiative
included midwifery training in France for two young Lao women, who
were intended to serve as instructors on their return. Ultimately only
one travelled to France while the other remained in Laos to marry.[34]
A related initiative during the same period was the training of a cadre

of rural birth attendants (*accoucheuses rurales*) who, once trained, would return to assist births in their home villages. Disregarding the earlier difficulty of securing sufficient female midwifery students, and the continuing low education rates of women and girls, an ambitious plan set out to train a corps of approximately 120 women in 1949.[35] Interestingly, it did not appear to follow an earlier Vietnamese strategy of providing biomedical top-up training to already practicing traditional midwives, but rather training young women from scratch.[36] In 1950 the Lao government reported that its Practical Midwifery School in Vientiane offered two-year courses for midwives (*sages-femmes*) and six-month practical hospital placements for rural birth attendants.[37] There was no mention of the school's recent re-establishment, its patchy history, nor any discussion of how it intended to overcome the previous challenges of attracting and/or retaining midwives within the health system.

## Women's Health in the Royal Lao Government Period, 1950–75

Official structures to address women's health, notably maternal health care and midwifery services, were formalized in the years following national independence under the Royal Lao Government (RLG), and were supplemented by the adoption of family planning services in the late 1960s. Due to the absence of any baseline data, it is not possible to provide hard evidence that women's health improved during this period. However, it can be safely assumed that the health status of some Lao women did gradually improve as access to basic maternal health services expanded from the main provincial centers into districts and even some larger villages of rural Laos.

Responsibility for health services was handed over from the French colonial administration to the Royal Lao Government in early 1950, following the Franco-Lao Treaty of July 1949. The trained medical cadre inherited by the Lao Health Service (*Phanek Satharanasouk Lao*) was modest. A contemporary official publication lists a trained staff of 12 *médecins indochinois*, 10 newly graduated *médecins assistants*, 1 registered midwife (*sage-femme d'état*), 4 Indochinese-trained midwives (*sages-femmes indochinoises*), 11 midwives of unspecified level employed on contract, and 220 nurses.[38] The Indochinese midwives were reported to have completed two years of training at the colonial midwifery schools in either Hanoi or Saigon, presumably during the closure of the Vientiane school.[39]

The bureaucratic record is silent for much of the 1950s, with little information concerning developments within the Lao Health Service, which constituted one department within the larger Ministry of Cults [religion], Education, Health, Social Welfare and Information. From the mid-1950s accounts of international aid officials and technical advisers sketch a picture of women's health status. They suggest that women in Laos married young, bore many children, and risked high rates of maternal mortality. Alex Moore, a founding member of the United States Operations Mission in Laos, observed that there were "kids everywhere" when he arrived in Vientiane in 1954,[40] while anthropologist Joel Halpern observed in Luang Prabang in the late 1950s that women were pregnant every 18 months, and contraception did not appear to be known, even by "most of the educated officials."[41] He also noted that most women gave birth at home, despite a small maternity ward at Luang Prabang hospital staffed by a French doctor, a French nurse, and a Lao midwife.[42] A WHO report from 1956 conceded that the maternal mortality rate in Laos was unknown.[43] Tom Dooley, an American doctor who ran a series of small rural clinics in the late 1950s, hazarded a guess that approximately 20 per cent of Lao women died in childbirth.[44]

There was little local impetus for midwifery or maternal health care training throughout the 1950s, due to the limited nature of Lao government funding. Laos' budgetary situation was extremely strained as the nation became entangled in the First and then the Second Indochina War. As a result of the political situation and regular government budget deficits, international development assistance assumed an important role within the Lao Health Service (increasingly referred to as the Ministry of Health), as financial and technical assistance promoted and enabled medical education, training, and service delivery. The majority of international inputs were channeled through development assistance projects.

The Maternal and Child Health (MCH) Services project, a joint Lao Ministry of Health/WHO undertaking, was launched in 1959, at a time when WHO supported MCH projects in many developing countries in the region. At project termination in 1975 it was one of the longest-running health projects in Laos.[45] The project aimed initially to determine Laos' MCH needs, to improve and develop MCH services, and establish training programs for MCH personnel.[46] It was negotiated and agreed in the late 1950s, during Dr Oudom Souvannavong's tenure as Minister for Health. A graduate of the Medical Faculty at the University of Paris, he had the distinction of being Laos' first fully qualified doctor.

Moreover, his medical thesis of 1949 had mapped out a framework for improving maternal and child health care, with the goal of reversing the high mortality rates which he feared could lead to the depopulation of Laos.

For Oudom, maternal and child health care was the most important element of a social medicine policy. He advocated the provision of MCH services conforming to a "Western" system of obstetric care: antenatal, delivery, and postnatal care. However, he suggested that services should be simplified for the Lao cultural and financial environment, and acknowledged that while hospital births were preferable, they might not be realistic in the short term. Instead, he recommended that efforts be made to gradually persuade Lao women to give birth in health facilities.[47] Oudom also recommended that existing Lao *médecins indochinois* upgrade their skills by undergoing short-term overseas training in MCH and, more importantly, that efforts be made to bring traditional midwives into the health workforce.

It seems that few of Oudom's recommendations had been taken up before the commencement of the MCH project. In 1960 the Ministry of Health established an MCH technical service (*Service national de la protection maternelle et infantile*), no doubt prompted by the presence of the WHO-supported project, and by the early 1960s began to set aside financial allocations for MCH services.[48] A National MCH Centre established in 1960 offered antenatal and postnatal care, home visits, classes for mothers, vaccinations and a health education program. It also offered in-service training for provincial MCH staff who were progressively employed throughout Laos, and a training program for rural midwives.[49] It is unclear to what extent the WHO program for rural midwives replicated or continued the French-promoted program of 1949–50, because WHO documentation makes no reference to it. A WHO report from the time the project commenced stated that: "Mahosot Hospital in Vientiane had the only maternity ward" in Laos and, "there was no organized preventative and curative care for mothers and children in the country."[50] The WHO's statement thus acknowledged neither the colonial health structure that had by 1938 established six *maternité* clinics, nor the training of Indochinese midwives or rural birth attendants.

The RLG/WHO project set up MCH centers in the main provincial towns under RLG administration: Luang Prabang, Thakhek, Savannakhet, and Pakse, later expanding with US funding into smaller towns such as Houay Xay, Champassak, and Khong.[51] The only major provincial hospital not included in project activities was Xieng Khouang, as it was located within the area administered by the Patriotic Lao Front (*Neo Lao Hak Xat*) resistance movement from the early 1960s onwards.[52]

The MCH Services project was complemented by a WHO-supported Nursing Education project implemented from 1962 to 1976. This project was instrumental in enabling the education of Lao midwives and nurses to be conducted in-country in the French language, with students studying overseas only in rare cases. This development ensured greater standardization in the ranks of Lao midwives and nurses than was the case with Lao medical doctors, who studied overseas in a variety of countries, using differing medical systems and diverse languages.[53] The Nursing Education project focused on expanding the number of trained nurses and midwives in government service. It supported the development of rural midwifery schools in four provincial centers, and provided refresher training in MCH and midwifery for existing personnel.

Project documentation states that the technical advisors' brief was "to *start* [my emphasis] a nursing and midwifery school" at Mahosot Hospital.[54] As Mahosot was the site of the previous French colonial midwifery school established in the 1920s and revived in the 1940s, the WHO-supported school constituted an attempt to upgrade or rebrand the school but not the creation of an additional school. In the past, a steady supply of students and, presumably, funding had eluded the school and prevented its consolidation. In its reincarnation, the WHO took care of funding and the provision of instructors, but the challenge of attracting sufficiently educated and motivated Lao students remained.

Before admission, nursing students were required to have completed six years of primary schooling, the final three years in the French medium. In 1967, the project supported the introduction of two-year training courses for nurses (*infirmiers/infirmières auxiliaires*) in Vientiane and the provincial nursing schools, which was added to the existing two-year training for auxiliary midwives (*sages-femmes auxiliaires*). Two years later, in 1969, a three-year qualification for registered nurses (*infirmiers/ infirmières d'état*) and midwives (*sages-femmes d'état*) was introduced.[55] The first cohort graduated in 1972, adding to the small pool of Lao women who had studied midwifery in France on RLG and/or French government scholarships in the 1950s.[56] However, more flexible staffing options were required as the number of rural dispensaries increased in the mid-1970s. Training for nurse-midwives, a new category of health worker, was introduced into the provincial schools for this reason.

The RLG Ministry of Health's MCH and nursing services were supplemented by those of Operation Brotherhood, a Filipino NGO under contract to USAID's Public Health Division program in Laos from 1963–75. Operation Brotherhood ran a network of hospitals in rural Laos, in areas with zero or low levels of RLG health service coverage, but where there had often been modest medical presence in colonial times.[57] Its hospitals provided a range of clinical health services including midwifery, and mobile health teams conducted MCH outreach in rural areas.[58] Throughout the 1960s the NGO trained several cohorts of practical nurses who completed two-year courses in the English medium, through Lao interpreters. Operation Brotherhood did not train midwife specialists, but basic obstetrical and gynecological nursing skills were included in the curriculum studied by its more than 130 practical nursing graduates.[59] Training curricula and professional classifications were American-influenced, making it difficult to later reconcile Operation Brotherhood qualifications with those of the French-influenced Ministry of Health/WHO graduates.

USAID commenced its own Maternal and Child Health/Family Planning project in 1969, intended to support both the Ministry of Health and the Operation Brotherhood health network. Like the WHO beforehand, USAID project documentation did not acknowledge the MCH initiatives of other agencies and claimed that, despite the ongoing RLG/WHO project, "there were no RLG medical personnel trained in maternal and child health" when it began.[60] Also, despite its classification as a technical assistance project, it focused overwhelmingly on construction. The main project activities involved construction of a 200-bed MCH facility in Vientiane and 4 provincial MCH centers, and renovation of 11 rural facilities, as well as the seemingly unrelated expansion of the USAID medical warehouse.[61] USAID auditors displayed concern at the lack of consideration given to the Lao Ministry of Health's ability to provide the necessary human and financial resources to operate the expanded MCH facilities, once constructed.[62] A follow-up audit team found the initial concerns had been borne out:

> It had been assumed by USAID/Laos that the RLG would provide all necessary manpower to staff the hospital.... A staffing pattern for the Mahosot MCH Center was submitted to USAID/Laos by the RLG in August 1973, one month before the scheduled opening of the hospital which showed that...the hospital was lacking 112 nurses, or seventy three percent of the number required, and sixty

eight percent of the needed housekeeping staff.... To correct the staffing deficiencies at Mahosot, plans were made to transfer seventy nurses from the cities of Luang Prabang and Pakse to Vientiane.... Although the transfer...will solve the immediate staffing problem at the Mahosot MCH Center, new staffing problems are being created for the Pakse MCH Center which is nearing completion and should be operational in early 1974.[63]

The inputs of MCH training and infrastructure development resulted in slightly higher numbers of women delivering in health facilities, despite the contraction of the land area and population under RLG administration during the 1960s and 1970s as the Second Indochina War progressed. Between 1966 and 1973, deliveries in RLG health facilities increased from 2,835 nationwide to 3,270. Significantly more deliveries occurred in the home with the attendance of a medical worker or rural birth attendant.[64]

Family planning services were a new addition to development assistance programs during this period. Support for family planning had grown internationally throughout the 1960s, and joined the mix of MCH and nursing education initiatives in Laos by way of the USAID project in 1969. It was reinforced by the RLG/WHO's reformulated MCH and Family Health project in 1971. USAID, the largest international donor to Laos during this period, vigorously promoted family planning (and sometimes its more aggressive sibling, population control) in many developing nations, but was forced to adopt a gentler strategy in Laos.

USAID documents stated that the project would "introduce family planning concepts and practices to trainee midwives, nurses and doctors, and also to patients as a normal part of their medical consultation."[65] The agency claimed the initial impetus for family planning in Laos came from a group of elite Lao women, although it also conceded that their Lao mission had been "strongly urged [by USAID headquarters in Washington DC] to develop interest within the Lao government for a family planning program." Early efforts to introduce a program met with opposition from high-ranking members of the RLG. The Lao Prime Minister Prince Souvanna Phouma was on record as stating that Laos needed additional population, while another key figure in government reportedly claimed contraception was against "the religion" (presumably Buddhism) and RLG policy.[66] The political opposition movement, the Lao Patriotic Front, took a similarly strong position, claiming that family planning "destroyed the nation and the fine traditions of Lao society" (*tham-lay xat, tham-lay sangkhom anh-dee-ngame khong lao-hao*).[67]

Due to official resistance, family planning services were initially offered through non-government providers. From 1969–70 the Lao Family Welfare Association (LFWA) (*Samakhom Songkho Khobkhoua Lao*) was the sole provider of family planning services.[68] The LFWA was the local affiliate of the International Planned Parenthood Federation, and headed by Dr Maniso Abhay, the first Lao woman to qualify as a doctor and a former technical head (*médecin-chef*) of the National MCH Centre. By the early 1970s rural hospitals and dispensaries run by Operation Brotherhood and USAID also offered family planning services.

Strong lobbying of the RLG by the LFWA and foreign donors secured government endorsement of a national population policy in 1972, and the creation of a Commission for the Promotion of Family Well-being, headed by the Minister of Health. The Ministry of Health did not provide family planning services until 1974, during the short-lived administration of the Provisional Government of National Union, by which time family planning was available in 155 service outlets nationwide, including 75 Ministry of Health facilities and 80 non-government facilities.[69] The range of contraceptive methods on offer included contraceptive pills, injections, IUDs, condoms, diaphragms, spermicidal foams and lubricants, and explanation of the rhythm method. Tubal ligation (tubectomy) was available at larger hospitals.[70]

Much less is known about women's health efforts during this period in the "Liberated Zone," that is, in areas under the administration of the Patriotic Lao Front. We know that women's health services were included among the more modest services provided with support from the Democratic Republic of Vietnam and other socialist nations. One official report loosely classifies "Liberated Zone" health staff as medical workers, pharmacy workers, and midwifery workers.[71] A North Vietnamese health adviser confirms that MCH formed part of the practical training for grassroots Lao medics, some of whom were barely literate.[72] Such training was likely to have been conducted in the Vietnamese medium, through Lao interpreters. Some RLG-trained informants considered the technical skills and knowledge of medical staff from the "Liberated Zone" to be lower than their own.[73] These views should be understood in the context of the more recent introduction of, and lower opportunities for, basic education in the predominantly rural and ethnically diverse "Liberated Zone," as well as the difficulty of conducting technical education and training with minimal funding in areas that were often war zones.

Nationwide, female nursing students began to outnumber males in 1960s Laos, but there remained a relatively high proportion of male students in the Ministry of Health and Operation Brotherhood nursing schools compared to the experience of neighboring countries. Also, while basic education services expanded considerably in the postcolonial period, few ethnic minority students were in the school system, except in the "Liberated Zone." As such, the increased numbers of female staff in the nursing and midwifery professions were drawn almost exclusively from the Lao ethnic group.[74]

## Women's Health in the Early Lao PDR Period, 1976–90

Women's health policies and services underwent a significant reassessment following the change of government and the establishment of the Lao PDR in December 1975. The Ministry of Health planned to implement a Primary Health Care (PHC) policy, including MCH, throughout Laos to address the urban bias of the Lao health sector, and to improve access to basic health services for the comparatively poorer and ethnically diverse rural communities. It required a major increase in the numbers of rural health facilities and trained health staff, and a reliable budget to support the expansion. Due to the poverty of the Lao PDR, implementation of the policy was heavily dependent on the receipt of international donor assistance.

The PHC approach of providing basic health care as close to home as possible enjoyed widespread popularity internationally, particularly in socialist nations such as China, Vietnam, Cuba, and the Soviet Union. The WPRO's annual report for 1976 confidently announced changes underway in health policy and practice in newly socialist Laos: "The Lao PDR is organizing a system of primary health care, with supervision provided by local health committees and services at the periphery by village health workers. Nurses and midwives have received refresher training for their new functions in rural areas."[75]

The policy faced significant staffing shortages, a long-standing problem exacerbated by the numbers of educated Lao who departed the country as refugees post-1975. No figures are available on the exact number of trained health staff who fled Laos, although internal Ministry of Health reports from the late 1970s document the numbers of health workers fleeing Vientiane across the Mekong each month.[76] Martin Stuart-Fox, a well-known historian of Laos, reported that approximately

10 per cent of the population fled in the first decade of the Lao PDR, in what he termed "one of the most serious [losses of population] suffered in percentage terms by any modern state," and which was "remarkable for the fact that those who left constituted by far the majority of all educated Lao."[77]

Health staff who remained in Laos posed another problem. Professional classifications of staff trained in the various RLG, Operation Brotherhood, and Patriotic Lao Front health services were not equivalent. The diversity of medical standards and technical languages (French, English, Vietnamese, and Lao) used by the various training programs provided in Laos by the separate health services was further complicated by the high proportion of overseas-trained doctors, who had been exposed to an even wider range of approaches and languages.

Post-1975, Laos also had to contend with a reduction in international assistance to its health sector. All USAID-funded programs were terminated and the Operation Brotherhood hospital network was handed over to the Lao government in mid-1975. French assistance to the medical school ended in 1978 following a diplomatic wrangle between the Lao PDR and France. In the main, the terminated projects and departing technical advisers were replaced by new projects and advisers from the Soviet Union and Vietnam, and to a lesser extent, by those from Cuba, Czechoslovakia, East Germany, and Mongolia. The WHO continued to assist the Lao health sector, but its long-running projects in MCH Services and Nursing Education ended soon after the change in regime, reflecting changes in the new government's health policy priorities.

In its bid to expand PHC services, and presumably to save time and money, the Ministry of Health simplified professional categories and shortened training courses. New staff trained and deployed in the late 1970s and 1980s were later criticized for their low skills base, and many of the rural facilities were acknowledged to be non-operational due to lack of supplies, basic equipment and operating budgets, as well as staff. In 1992, a UNICEF publication reported that only 20 of the recorded 110 district hospitals in Laos were actually offering health services.[78]

Furthermore, women's health was not accorded the priority within the Lao PDR's PHC program that might be assumed on the basis of wider international practice. MCH work in the Lao PDR focused more often on children than on their mothers. Preventable childhood illnesses and immunization garnered attention, as did the construction of nurseries and childcare centers (*heuan fark dek*) in government workplaces.[79]

But family planning services ceased because the new government viewed them as a threat to national culture and population levels, and the topic was removed from the medical training curriculum.[80]

The Lao PDR replaced family planning with a pro-natalist policy that aimed to "improve the health of mothers and children, and promote *population growth* [my emphasis]."[81] An informant advised that in the mid-1980s nursing and midwifery students learned only "informally" about family planning because contraceptives were banned by the Ministry of Health and unavailable in government health facilities, but were smuggled across the border from Thailand, and in some cases mailed to family members in Laos by relatives residing overseas.[82]

After several years in the wilderness, a new MCH program was launched by the Ministry of Health in 1983, with financial and technical support from WHO and UNICEF.[83] The program followed in the footsteps of the ad hoc MCH efforts of the French colonial period and the RLG/WHO program running for 16 years from 1959–75. The concept of family planning, renamed and repackaged as "birth spacing," was tentatively accepted by the Lao government in 1988.[84] A MCH Institute was established in 1989 and a MCH hospital in 1993, presumably not dissimilar to the WHO-supported National MCH Centre of the early 1960s and the USAID-constructed MCH hospital of the early 1970s.[85] The new MCH program planned to expand services to provincial locations, just as the former RLG/WHO MCH project had done. In 1985, the Ministry of Health reported that it conducted MCH activities in six districts of Vientiane capital and three districts in Vientiane province and was planning expansion into a fourth, although no locations further afield than Vang Vieng were mentioned. Services included antenatal and postnatal checkups, delivery, and vaccinations for mothers and infants.[86]

Midwifery training was also re-introduced in the 1980s after almost a decade of neglect. According to UNICEF, training of auxiliary midwives started "around 1982" in some provinces, and a three-year specialist midwifery course was introduced (or rather, reintroduced) at the Medical Sciences Technicians' School (*Honghian Phet Sanh Kang*) in Vientiane in 1987.[87] Three cohorts of approximately 30 students each were accepted into the midwifery course from 1987 to 1989.[88] Before the third cohort completed its training, however, the course was merged with the generalist nursing course in order to produce a general purpose nurse-midwife, reminiscent of the nurse-midwife classification which emerged in the final years of the RLG period.

Once again, there was little mention of the past. And as before, the unreliability of external assistance budgets limited the extent to which the Ministry of Health could follow through on the implementation of its plans. This time, significant reduction in funding from the socialist countries squeezed Lao government budgets in all sectors, including health. The Ministry of Health coyly describes the decision to cease midwifery training in the late 1980s as being prompted by "a variety of reasons,"[89] but does not elaborate as to what they may have been.

## Women's Health in the Recent Lao PDR Period, 1991–2012

Women's health has featured consistently on the Lao government agenda since the 1990s, although policy support has been at times more rhetorical than practical in nature. A 1991 report from a WHO technical adviser cut through the rhetoric in its damning assessment of the state of maternal health care in the Lao PDR:

> Clearly, there is a lack of competent maternal services in most of the country, and people have no confidence in the public health services. The few obstetric wards in provincial hospitals are largely underutilized, particularly by rural women...the root of the problem is the insufficient attention given to pregnancy-related issues at all levels. Midwives in particular have been neglected both in their status and in their practical training: there should be more of them in the districts, with more support, more equipment, more appropriate training and more supervision.[90]

Despite the relaunch of the MCH program in the mid-1980s, health indicators made available after the first national census in 1985 suggested that the status of women's health in Laos was not improving. At the beginning of the 1990s, the Lao PDR had one of the highest fertility rates in the world. UNICEF calculated that in 1993 Lao women were giving birth, on average, to a phenomenal 7.1 children, and that the fertility rate was rising.[91] Increasing fertility was suspected to have been caused by a combination of at least three factors: changes in the social behavior of Lao women after the cessation of the war (they were marrying at a younger age and had an earlier onset of childbearing than their mothers), the government's pronatalist policy, and the resultant absence of contraceptive services.

The high maternal mortality rate was attributed to the shortage of midwives, their low status within the health sector, and their continued absence at most births. In 1995, only 7 per cent of births took place in a hospital or clinic with a skilled birth attendant (that is, a midwife or doctor) in attendance,[92] suggesting there had been little change in birthing choices since colonial times. In 1993 the maternal mortality rate was 660/100,000 live births.[93] While it was reported to have been reduced to 530/100,000 in 2000,[94] lifetime risk of maternal death in Laos remained one of the highest in the world at a 1/49 chance—a combination of the high maternal mortality rate and the high fertility rate. To put this figure in perspective, in the Asia-Pacific region, only women in Afghanistan and Timor Leste faced a higher risk.[95]

In response to the high incidence of maternal mortality, international agencies led by the United Nations Population Fund lobbied the Lao government to legalize (or rather, re-legalize) contraception. Few Lao health staff trained post-1975 were aware of the previous initiatives in family planning promoted by the LFWA, the RLG, USAID, and Operation Brotherhood in the late 1960s and early 1970s.[96] Two Vientiane hospitals began providing birth spacing services in 1991 in low-key pilot programs, offering pills, injections, IUDs, condoms, and tubectomy, but not diaphragms, gels, or spermicides, which had been available pre-1975.[97] International NGOs partnering with the Lao Ministry of Health, such as Save the Children Australia from 1992 and Family Planning Australia from 1998, supported expansion of services into selected provincial areas.[98] However, supply of contraceptives was irregular and services in no way comprehensive,[99] suggesting official ambivalence to family planning within either the leadership of the Lao PDR or its wider administrative structure, or perhaps both.

The cautious reintroduction of family planning resulted in the formulation of a National Birth Spacing Policy in 1995 and a 2005 revision titled the National Reproductive Health Policy, as well as a National Population and Development Policy in 1999 and Guidelines on MCH in 2004.[100] Actual service delivery was characterized by concentration in urban areas and limited outreach into rural areas, where the majority of the population resided. In 2000 the National Reproductive Health Survey found that the national contraceptive prevalence rate was only 29 per cent (or 32 per cent, when traditional methods of contraception are also included in the calculation), and that the unmet need for contraception was high at "about 40 per cent."[101] Fertility rates and maternal mortality rates remained high into the 2000s as more reliable national health statistics were formulated.

Under internal and external pressure to improve its efforts towards achieving MDG 5, the Lao Ministry of Health also decided to revive specialist midwifery training in 2009. This required rapid effort, as it was reported that in 2009 there were only 86 trained midwives working in the health sector nationwide.[102] These presumably included midwives from the three cohorts trained from 1987–91, and possibly some trained in the pre-1975 RLG period. The midwifery plan of 2009 aimed to train and deploy two levels of specialist midwives: community midwives, presumably more qualified than the rural birth attendants (*accoucheuses rurales*) of the French colonial period and similar to the rural auxiliary midwives of the RLG and early Lao PDR periods; and registered (high-level) midwives, slightly more qualified than the registered midwives (*sages-femmes d'état*) of the French and RLG periods and the midwife-specialists of the late 1980s.[103]

Some key improvements in women's health were discernable by 2012. The Lao Social Indicator Survey (LSIS) of 2012 found that along with rising incomes and education levels, the total fertility rate had declined to 3.2, contraceptive prevalence had risen to 50 per cent, and the unmet need for contraception hovered at 19.9 per cent, although it acknowledged inequalities by geographic area, age, and ethnicity. In addition, maternal mortality was estimated to have declined (from 660/100,000 in 1993) to 357/100,000 in 2012.[104] These achievements were countered by the Ministry's continued grappling with unreliable data, high variation in the quality of service provision, and weaknesses in the supply chain.[105]

As for the initiatives to improve midwifery services, a recent evaluation reported that the Ministry of Health target for the number of midwife-specialists to be trained in the past five years had been surpassed. It found, however, that the target had been achieved at the expense of quality. The evaluation report states:

> In the imperative to produce 1,500 midwives by 2015, the quality processes, crucial to ensure sustainable success of the plan had been neglected. Thus, the speed with which the numbers of midwives have been produced has not been matched by the progress in quality.[106]

Trained and suitably qualified midwifery teachers had been in limited supply, and as a result, both teachers and students were not confident of the skills they had learned during their studies. In other examples cited in the report, midwifery students recruited from non-clinical areas reportedly returned to these areas after completing the training, suggesting their participation may have been motivated more by the achievement of statistical targets than the delivery of improved midwifery services.[107] Such findings do not augur well for the future of midwifery services or women's health in Laos.

## Concluding Thoughts

Attention to women's health in Laos, and in particular, midwifery, maternal health care, and family planning, has gone through a series of waxing and waning cycles since the colonial period. Despite talk of "lessons learned," the international development sector has rarely acknowledged previous initiatives or overtly examined their attendant successes or failures in any depth before embarking on a renewed round of effort. Critics of development wryly comment that asking: "What happened last time?" is an awkward question for international development professionals, given the lack of institutional memory in terms of their engagement with the country setting and/or technical subject matter.[108]

Laos, as a developing nation heavily dependent on external financial assistance and technical human resources for much of its modern history, has been particularly vulnerable to changes in the international political climate, as these have determined the sources and longevity of the financial and technical assistance it receives. Rather than building on previous or existing women's health services, archival sources strongly suggest that the Lao governments of each period, and their respective international donors, created midwifery and maternal health care services anew. This practice raises serious questions about the sustainability of previous initiatives, and in particular, about their suitability in terms of cultural, geographic, and financial accessibility to the population of Laos. On the whole, women's health services in previous periods have reached only a small proportion of the Lao population. The reasons have ranged from the shortage of trained health staff, the concentration of health facilities in urban areas, inadequate government health budgets, and the discontinuities in the provision and policy focus of international development assistance, in addition to the challenge of identifying appropriate cultural entry points. Bursts of French colonial enthusiasm and funding were dampened by the few local nursing and midwifery trainees, and the similarly low levels of Lao women giving birth in colonial facilities. American zeal to construct MCH centers throughout Laos vastly outpaced the ability of the RLG/WHO projects to train health staff needed to staff the centers. And post-1975 increases in staff numbers have been accompanied by concerns about the quality of staff training and service delivery standards.

Prospects for women's health looked hopeful in 2012 when, for the first time since independence in the 1950s, Laos possessed a combination of political stability, an expanding human resource pool of secondary school graduates, and an increasing supply of government revenue after the World Bank upgraded the nation from being a Low Income Country to a Lower Middle Income Country.[109] Previously, the absence of one or more of these three necessary preconditions for the development of health services had repeatedly hampered attempts to improve women's health. The re-emergence of financial problems in the Lao public sector in 2013, and the resulting return to a reliance on international financial support, however, places the sustainability of achievements in women's health once again in jeopardy. Achievement of the women's health targets listed against MDG 5 may still prove possible within the extended timeframe afforded by the United Nations' Sustainable Development Goals (or SDGs), which replaced the MDGs on their expiry at the end of 2015.

A historical perspective that acknowledges and examines previous development initiatives shows that women's health in Laos has not been neglected, but rather has lacked the required follow-through to achieve sustainability. How long will the Lao PDR's current policies of promoting women's health, midwifery, and family planning remain in the spotlight this time? Will these policies succeed in gaining traction, or will they fade away after the MDG deadline has passed? At the time of going to press, a focus on nutrition appears likely to eclipse women's health as the initiative requiring a disproportionate amount of the Ministry of Health's finite human and financial resources. Will the increasing focus on nutrition be at the expense of the consolidation of improvements in midwifery, maternal health care, and/or family planning? Historical precedents suggest the likelihood cannot be discounted.

## Acknowledgements

I thank the National University of Singapore for partially funding this research. I would also like to thank Associate Professor Bruce Lockhart, Dr Pascale Hancourt-Petitet, the editorial committee, and two anonymous reviewers for their comments on earlier versions of this paper.

## Archives Consulted

Archives nationales d'outre mer (ANOM), Aix-en-Provence, France:
> Résidence Supérieur du Laos (RSL), Series S (Santé), Boxes 1–12, Records of the Lao Medical Service (*Assistance médicale au Laos*)

Lao National Archives Department (*Kom Samnao Ekasane Heng Xat*), Ministry of Home Affairs, Vientiane, Lao PDR:
> Documents from the RLG Ministry of Health, 1966–74
> Documents from the NLHX Central Health Committee, 1966–75
> Documents from the Lao PDR Ministry of Health, 1976–2000

World Health Organization's Western Pacific Regional Office Library, Manila, Philippines:
> Regional Committee reports, 1951–2000
> Budget Estimates, 1951–2000

## Interviews/Research Discussions

Ms A (anonymous), former OB and Lao PDR health worker, interviewed in Vientiane, Lao PDR on February 3, 2012.

Ms B (anonymous), former OB and Lao PDR health worker, interviewed in San Diego, USA on August 6, 2012.

Ms C (anonymous), Lao PDR and NGO health worker, interviewed in Vientiane, Lao PDR on December 17, 2012.

Ms D (anonymous), current Lao government health worker, interviewed in Vientiane, Lao PDR on June 2, 2012.

Perks, Carol, MCH/PCH Adviser from Save the Children International, interviewed in Sayabouly, Lao PDR on February 17, 2012.

Revilla, Jovit, former OB training supervisor, interviewed at Los Baños, the Philippines, on March 12, 2012.

## Notes

1. Carla Abou Zahr and Tessa Wardlaw, "Trends in Maternal Mortality in the 1990s," *Bulletin of the World Health Organization* 79, no. 6 (2001): 561–8.

2. National Statistics Centre, *Lao Reproductive Health Survey 2005* (Vientiane: National Statistics Centre and UNFPA, 2007), v.

3. WHO, *Human Resources for Health* (Vientiane: WHO, 2007), 10.

4. State Planning Committee, "National Population and Development Policy of the Lao PDR" (Vientiane: State Planning Committee, Nov. 1999), 5–6.

5. Ministry of Health, *Strategy and Planning Framework for the Integrated Package of Maternal Neonatal and Child Health Services 2009–2015* (Vientiane: Ministry of Health, 10 May 2009).

6. Ministry of Health, *Midwives in Lao PDR, Scaling up Skilled Birth Atten-dance: Putting Midwives at the Community Level towards Achieving MDGs for Mothers and Children*, Report 2012 (Vientiane: Ministry of Health and UNFPA, 2012), 4.

7. David Lewis, "International Development and the 'Perpetual Present': Anthropological Approaches to the Re-Historicization of Policy," *European Journal of Development Research* 21 (2009): 32–46.

8. Michael Woolcock, Simon Szreter, and Vijayendra Rao, "How and Why Does History Matter for Development Policy?" *Journal of Development Studies* 47, no. 1 (Jan. 2011): 71.

9. Ministry of Health, *Midwives in Lao PDR*, 6.

10. The anonymity of Lao health workers in Laos and overseas has been re-spected. It is also important to note that all demographic information used in the calculation of health indicators for Laos was based on estimations until 1985, when the first ever national census of Laos was conducted.

11. *Ambulances* were originally mobile field hospitals, but had become station-ary clinics by the time French colonial forces occupied Laos in the 1890s.

12. Sokhieng Au, *Mixed Medicines: Health and Culture in French Colonial Cambodia* (Chicago: Chicago University Press, 2011), 119.

13. *Médecins auxiliaires*, also referred to as *médecins indochinois*, were local medical staff who underwent four years of technical training at the Hanoi Medical School. They were trained to work as assistant doctors under the supervision of European (French) doctors, but due to ongoing staff shortages in Laos, they were often the only medically trained staff mem-ber in remote locations.

14. Archives nationales d'outre mer (ANOM), Résidence Supérieur du Laos (RSL), Series S, Box 3: Rapport annuel médical d'ensemble de 1913, Mar. 17, 1914, 7.

15. ANOM, RSL, Series S, Box 4: 1929 Rapport annuel, March 12, 1930. "*Indigène*" in this context refers to non-European "natives" or "locals," and thus includes immigrant Vietnamese with Lao, together with other Asian people.

16. ANOM, RSL, Series S, Box 3: Rapport annuel médical ensemble de 1915, Feb. 16, 1916, 3.

17. ANOM, RSL, Series S, Box 3: Rapport annuel 1917 de la Circonscription et de l'ambulance de Vientiane, Jan. 10, 1918, 4.

18. ANOM, RSL, Series S, Box 3: Rapport annuel de 1924 de l'Assistance médicale au Laos, [n.d.], 75.

19. Ibid., 78.

20. ANOM, RSL, Series S, Box 3: Rapport annuel de 1921 de l'Assistance médicale au Laos, [n.d.], 26.

21. ANOM, RSL, Series S, Box 3: Rapport annuel de 1924 de l'Assistance médicale au Laos, [n.d.], 116–17.

22. Ibid., 118.

23. Ibid., 23.

24. ANOM, RSL, Series S, Box 4: Rapport annuel de 1931 de l'Assistance médicale du Laos, April 20, 1932, 17.

25. ANOM, RSL, Series S, Box 4: Rapport annuel de 1930, August 12, 1931; and Kate Frieson, "Sentimental Education: *Les Sages-Femmes* and Colonial Cambodia," *Journal of Colonial History and Colonialism* 1, no. 1 (2000): 18–33.

26. ANOM, RSL, Series S, Box 3: Rapport annuel de 1924 [n.d].

27. ANOM, RSL, Series S, Box 4: AML Rapport annuel de 1930, Aug. 12, 1931, 10.

28. ANOM, RSL, Series S, Box 4: Rapport annuel de 1931, Apr. 20, 1932.

29. ANOM, RSL, Series S, Box 4: Rapport annuel 1935 [n.d.].

30. ANOM, RSL, Series S, Box 4: Laos. Assistance médicale: Rapport du 4e trimestre 1940, Mar. 25, 1941.

31. Ibid., May 25, 1940.

32. ANOM, RSL, Series S, Box 6: Assistance médicale 1925, [n.d.].

33. ANOM, RSL, Series S, Box 4: Rapport annuel de 1930, Aug. 12, 1931.

34. Grant Evans, *The Last Century of Lao Royalty: A Documentary History* (Chiang Mai: Silkworm Books, 2009), 264.

35. ANOM, RSL, Series S, Box 11: Letter of Lao Prime Minister Souvannarath to Lao Minister of Health, Kou Abhay, Jan. 18, 1949.

36. Laurence Monnais, "La médicalisation de la mère et de son enfant: l'exemple du Vietnam sous domination française, 1860–1939," in *Children's Health Issues in Historical Perspective*, ed. Cheryl Krasnick Warsh and Veronica Strong-Boag (Waterloo, Ont.: Wilfried Laurier University Press, 2005), 242–3; and Au, *Mixed Medicines*, 150.

37. *Laos: Mil neuf cent cinquante* (no publication details, undated), 100.

38. ANOM, RSL, Series S, Box 12: AML Rapport annuel de 1950, July 30, 1951, Table 5, 6, no page numbers.

39. *Laos: Mil neuf cent cinquante*, 98.

40. Alex Moore, *Un Américain au Laos aux débuts de l'aide américaine (1954–1957)* (Paris: L'Harmattan, 1995), 21.

41. Joel M. Halpern, *Aspects of Village Life and Culture Change in Laos* (New York: Council on Economic and Cultural Affairs, 1958), 98.

42. Halpern, *Aspects of Village Life*, 100.

43. WHO, *Budget Estimates, WP/RC7/5, Part I* (Manila: WHO, 1957), x.

44. Dooley observed that "many of those who survived [childbirth] were left horribly mutilated," presumably referring to the incidence of fistula. Tom Dooley, *Dr Tom Dooley's Three Great Books: Deliver Us from Evil, The Edge of Tomorrow [and] The Night They Burned the Mountain* (New York: Farrar, Straus & Cudahy, 1960), 151.

45. While initially funded by WHO, by 1969 the MCH Services project was funded by several international donors including UNICEF, the United States Agency for International Development (USAID), the Colombo Plan, the Asia Foundation, and the Dooley Foundation. It halted briefly in 1970 and restarted in 1971 as the Family Health/MCH Project. See WHO, *Regional Director's Annual Report to the Regional Committee, WPR/RC21/4* (Manila: WHO, 1970), 91 and WHO, *Regional Director's Annual Report to the Regional Committee, WPR/RC22/2* (Manila: WHO, 1971), 149.

46. WHO, *Regional Director's Annual Report WPR/RC21/4*, 90.

47. Oudom Souvannavong, "Une étude du problème medico sociale au Laos" (thesis for doctorat en médecine, Faculty of Medicine, University of Paris, 1949), 43–6.

48. WHO, *Budget Estimates, WP/RC10/4 Part I* (Manila: WHO, 1959), 24; WHO, *Regional Director's Annual Report to the Regional Committee, WPR/RC21/4*, 92–93; and WHO, *Budget Estimates, WP/RC12/4* (Manila: WHO, 1961), 57.

49. WHO, *Regional Director's Annual Report to the Regional Committee, WPR/RC21/4*, 93, and WHO, *Budget Estimates, WP/RC11/5* (Manila: WHO, 1960), 47.

50. WHO, *Regional Director's Annual Report to the Regional Committee, WPR/RC21/4*, 91.

51. Ibid., 92.

52. The Lao Patriotic Front (*Neo Lao Hak Xat*) is often referred to in English as the Pathet Lao or PL.

53. In 1966, some Lao nurses were studying in Saigon and Thailand. However, with the introduction of the Ministry of Health/WHO nursing and midwifery qualifications in 1967 and 1969, almost all Lao nurses and midwives studied in Laos. The exceptions were two registered nursing graduates from Canada and one from Australia in the late 1960s. In comparison, Lao medical students studied in countries as diverse as France, Cambodia, Thailand, Japan, the Soviet Union, Czechoslovakia, and Australia. See Lao National Archives Department (LNAD), Royal Lao Government (RLG)/ Ministry of Health (MOH), 211-004, Rapport statistique de lassistance médicale. Année 1966, Table P/6, no page numbers.

54. WHO, *Budget Estimates*, *WP/RC13/3* (Manila: WHO, 1962), 57.

55. WHO, *Regional Director's Annual Report to the Regional Committee, WPR/RC21/4*, 92–3.

56. Viliam Phraxayavong, *History of Aid to Laos: Motivations and Impacts* (Chiang Mai: Silkworm Books, 2009), 60. The duration of the midwifery course in France is unspecified, and Viliam lists 5 students every year from 1954 until 1959, totalling 25 students over the period. However, it seems more likely to have been 5 students who each studied a 5-year midwifery course.

57. For an account of Operation Brotherhood's activities in Laos in the years 1957–63, see Miguel Bernad S.J., *Filipinos in Laos*, with "Postscripts" by J. "Pete" Fuentecila (New York: Mekong Circle International, 2004). From 1969 OB hospitals were planned to be integrated into the RLG hospital network, but the move was hampered by Lao government staff shortages, inadequate government budgets to meet staffing and operating costs, and the ongoing fighting throughout much of the country.

58. Mrs Jovit Revilla, former OB training supervisor, interviewed at Los Baños, the Philippines, Mar. 12, 2012.

59. Summary of OB practical nursing curriculum, kindly provided by Mrs Cecile (Salarda) Datu, former OB training supervisor, interviewed in Manila, the Philippines, Mar. 23, 2012.

60. USAID, Audit report Maternal and Child Health Project (Washington DC: USAID, 1973), 2.

61. USAID, Audit report MCH Project 1971 (Washington DC: USAID), 22; and USAID, Audit report MCH Project 1973, 2.

62. USAID, Audit report MCH Project, 1971, 15.

63. USAID, Audit report MCH Project, 1973, 6.

64. LNAD, RLG/MOH, 211-004, Rapport statistique de l'assistance médicale. Année 1966, Table 4, no page numbers; and LNAD, RLG/MOH, 211-024, Rapport annuel des statistiques sanitaires, Année 1973, 84. Statistics from these two reports show that in 1966 there were an additional 6,741 home-based deliveries, and 5,766 in 1973, bringing the total number of recorded deliveries (there are likely to be many more unrecorded deliveries) to 9,576 and 9,484 respectively.

65. USAID, Termination Report for Laos (Washington DC: USAID, 1976), 104.

66. USAID, Termination Report, 103.

67. Lao PDR, Ministry of Health, Draft report on the health situation for the First Health Conference, Oct. 1–12, 1979 (*Hang lay-ngane saphap viak-ngane sathalanasouk you kong-pasoum-nyai khang thi 1, tae 1-12 toula 1979*), 3.

68. USAID, Termination Report, 107.

69. The Population Council, *Studies in Family Planning: Family Planning Programs: World Review 1974* 6, no. 8 (Aug. 1975): 229.

70. Lao Family Welfare Association, *Family Planning* [*Vang Phen Khob Khoua*] pamphlet (no publication details. Presumably Vientiane: LFWA, early 1970s), 5.

71. LNAD, Neo Lao Hak Xat (NLHX)/Central Health Committee (*Khana Sathalanasouk Sounkang*) (CHC), 23-05, Summary Report on the Health Situation, 1974 (*Saloup Saphap Sathalanasouk 1974*), 9.

72. Bui Van Y, "Public Health Support for Lao Friends during the Resistance Against the French," *History of Vietnam–Laos, Laos–Vietnam Special*

*Relationship 1930–2007*, Memoirs I (Hanoi: National Political Publishing House, 2012), 246.

73. Ms A (anonymous), former OB and Lao PDR health worker, interviewed in Vientiane, Lao PDR, Feb. 3, 2012, and Ms B (anonymous), former OB and Lao PDR health worker, interviewed in San Diego, USA, Aug. 6, 2012.

74. The Lao ethnic group is estimated to have represented a little over half of the population of Laos in the 1960s. It is not possible to cite official population statistics, because no population census of Lao was conducted before 1985, in large part due to the long-running, post-independence conflict.

75. WHO, *Regional Director's Report to the Regional Committee, WPR/RC27/3* (Manila: WHO, 1976), 5.

76. Reports of the Ministry of Health in 1979 and 1980 listed the number of health staff and students who fled each month. January 1980 was a particularly bad month for the ministry, as 35 low- and mid-level health workers were reported to have fled. See LNAD, Lao PDR/MOH, 23-04, Report on the situation and work of the Ministry of Health, January 1980 (*Lay-ngane saphapkane lae viak-ngane deuane 1/1980 khong kasouang sathalanasouk*), 2.

77. Martin Stuart-Fox, *Buddhist Kingdom, Marxist State: The Making of Modern Laos* (Bangkok: White Lotus, 1996), 168.

78. UNICEF, *Children and Women in the Lao People's Democratic Republic* (Vientiane: UNICEF, Apr. 1992), 135.

79. Ms C (anonymous), Lao PDR and NGO health worker, interviewed in Vientiane, Lao PDR, Dec. 17, 2012; and LNAD, Lao PDR/MOH, 23-17, Text of answers to foreign journalists: Summary of MCH work (*Bot neua-nay dob khamsamphat khong nak-khao tang pathet: Saloup viak mae lae dek)*, Mar. 11, 1985.

80. Khamphienne Philavong, Somboune Phomtavong and Saysavanh Ngon-vorarath, "Issues and Challenges of Public Health of 21st Century of Lao People's Democratic Republic," in *Issues and Challenges of Public Health in the 21st Century*, ed. Khairuddin Yusof, Wah-Yun Low, Siti Norazah Zulkifli, and Yut-Lin Wong (Kuala Lumpur: University of Malaya Press, 1996), 152.

81. WHO, *Budget Estimates 1982–1983 and 1984–1985, WPR/RC33* (Manila: WHO, 1982), 239.

82. Ms D (anonymous), current Lao government health worker, interviewed in Vientiane, Lao PDR, June 2, 2012.

83. UNICEF, *Children and Women*, 142.

84. National Statistics Centre/Lao Women's Training Centre/UNFPA, Report on the Fertility and Birth Spacing Survey in Lao PDR (LFPSS), UNFPA, Project No LAO/93/P02 (Vientiane: UNFPA, Nov. 1995), 7.

85. Stephen Holland, Chansy Phimphachanh, Catherine Conn, and Malcolm Segall, *Impact of Economic and Institutional Reforms on the Health Sector*

*in Laos: Implications for Health System Management* (Brighton, Sussex: Institute of Development Studies, 1995), 53.

86. LNAD, Lao PDR/MOH, 23-17, Text of answers to foreign journalists: Summary of MCH work (*Bot neua-nay dob khamsamphat khong nak-khao tang pathet: Saloup viak mae lae dek*), Mar. 11, 1985.

87. UNICEF, *Children and Women in the Lao PDR*, 143.

88. Ms D (anonymous), current Lao government health worker, interviewed in Vientiane, Lao PDR, June 2, 2012. Her statement is at odds with, but more credible than, the Ministry's statement that midwifery training ceased in 1986, given that she herself trained as a midwife specialist from 1987 to 1989. See Ministry of Health, *Midwives in Laos*, 4.

89. Ministry of Health, *Midwives in Lao PDR*, 4.

90. Catherine Spring, *Maternal Mortality in Lao PDR: Population Study, 1991* (Vientiane: WHO, 1991), 12.

91. UNICEF, *Children and their Families in the Lao PDR* (Vientiane: UNICEF, 1996), 103.

92. World Bank, *Lao PDR: Social Assessment and Strategy* (Washington DC: World Bank Human Resources Operations Division, Country Department 1, East Asia and Pacific Region, Aug. 15, 1995), 37.

93. Spring, *Maternal Mortality in Lao PDR*, 38.

94. Ministry of Health, *Strategy and Planning Framework*, 16.

95. Anna Scopaz, Liz Eckermann, and Matthew Clarke, "Maternal Health in Lao PDR: Repositioning the Goal Posts," *Journal of the Asia Pacific Economy* 16, no. 4 (2011): 600.

96. Admittedly, a UNICEF report from 1992 referred to a survey concerned with attitudes towards family planning conducted in 1974, "at a time when some contraceptive methods were available." See UNICEF, *Children and Women*, 99.

97. Nenita Balbuena, "Assessment and Evaluation of the Pre-project Activities, WHO Mission Report to Maternal & Child Health including Birth Spacing Project" (Manila: WHO, 1991), 2.

98. Carol Perks, MCH/PCH Adviser from Save the Children International, interviewed in Sayabouly, Lao PDR, Feb. 17, 2012. Also, from 2003 to 2005, I was employed as Family Planning Australia's project adviser to its Rural Women's Project, which ran from 1998 to 2005.

99. Khamphienne et al., "Issues and Challenges of Public Health," 152.

100. See Ministry of Health, "National Birth Spacing Policy," Vientiane, 1995; State Planning Committee, "National Population and Development Policy of the Lao PDR," Vientiane, Nov. 1999; Ministry of Health, "Regulations on Maternal and Child Healthcare," Vientiane, 2004; and Ministry of Health, "Reproductive Health Policy," Vientiane, Oct. 2005.

101. National Statistics Centre, *Lao Reproductive Health Survey 2000*, 36.

102. Scopaz et al., "Maternal Health in Lao PDR," 606.

103. Ministry of Health, *Midwives in Lao PDR*, 5.
104. Ministry of Health, *Lao PDR Lao Social Indicator Survey (LSIS) 2011–12* (Vientiane, 2012), iv, 66, 87.
105. UNFPA, "(Draft) Family Planning Situation Analysis," Vientiane, 2015, 2, 5.
106. Joan Skinner and Ketkaisone Phrasisombath, "Evaluation of the Midwifery Component of the SBA Development Plan, Lao PDR 2008–2012," Dec. 2014, 32.
107. Skinner and Phrasisombath, "Evaluation of the Midwifery Component," 35.
108. Raymond Apthorpe "Coda: With Alice in Aidland, a Seriously Satirical Allegory," in *Adventures in Aidland: The Anthropology of Professionals in International Development*, ed. David Mosse (New York/Oxford: Berghahn Books, 2011), 210.
109. http://www.worldbank.org/en/country/lao/overview.

## CHAPTER 5

# Learning to Heal the People: Socialist Medicine and Education in Vietnam, 1945–54

*Michitake Aso*

## Introduction

On October 15, 1950, the Hanoi Medical University's (HMU) opening ceremony was held in the Viet Bac, the northern stronghold of the communist-led anti-colonial forces called the Viet Minh. More than 40 students crowded into the reception hall, with portraits of Marx-Engels, Lenin, Stalin, and Ho Chi Minh adorning the walls. Đỗ Xuân Hợp, a leading Vietnamese surgeon, directed the ceremony. Hợp spoke of the escalating war situation and of the generosity and foresight of the Communist Party to open a school despite straitened circumstances. Students recalled this day as one of the most hopeful of that time.[1]

The Y50 medical students, those starting their education in 1950, composed one of several HMU classes that studied outside of Hanoi between 1947 and 1954. With nearly 40 students, the Y50 class was the second biggest class during these years (only Y52 with 80 students had more). These medical students were quite young, often 16 or 17 years old when Ho Chi Minh declared Vietnam's independence during the August Revolution that took place in the summer of 1945. Many of the medical students were caught up in the excitement of the revolution and recalled joining the Viet Minh out of youthful ardor and love of country—and not necessarily because they subscribed to communist ideology. While they may have never heard of Karl Marx, they did know Ho Chi Minh. Others were politically aware. Vũ Thị Phan, one of the rare female students, recalled growing up with the revolutionary stories of her great-grandfather and very much looked forward to becoming a party member.[2]

The Y50 class provides an exemplary location to study the politics and practice of socialist biomedicine in Vietnam. The potentially divided loyalties that existed were on display in a short pamphlet called "Thought, Function, and Direction of Vietnamese Revolutionary Medicine," published around 1954 by the Department of Military and Civilian Medicine in the Southern Region (*Sở Quân Dân Y Nam-Bộ*).[3] This pamphlet begins by describing the characteristics of "feudal imperialist" medicine. In essence, this medicine is "individualistic" (*riêng*).

> Feudal imperialists don't see that MEDICINE IS THANKS TO THE BLOOD AND GUTS EXPERIENCE OF THE PEOPLE struggling with nature [thiên nhiên], with sickness (mistakenly eating poison, poisonous mushrooms, being bitten by snakes), immeasurable pain, and countless deaths, only then can the experience of medicine be constructed. MEDICINE IS THANKS TO THE WORKING POWER OF THE MASSES OF THE PEOPLE TO STUDY, TO RESEARCH ACROSS THOUSANDS OF YEARS; THE HEALTH WORKER ONLY INHERITS THAT SCIENTIFIC PROFESSION [capitalization in original].

In opposition to "feudal imperialist" medicine, Vietnamese medicine had to be "scientific, ethnic, and of the masses" (*khoa học, dân tộc, đại chúng*). It had to be scientific, which meant attuned to advances coming out of the Soviet Union; it had to be ethnic, which meant paying attention to local experience and drawing from traditional medicine; and it had to be of the masses, which meant uncomplicated, non-hierarchical, not too technical, and most of all, not remote from the people (*tách rời quần chúng*).[4]

This pamphlet describes a commonly held image of socialist medicine in Vietnam and China during the twentieth century. In this image, socialist medicine is seen as holding a holistic vision of health, willing to share its authority over nature and the body with other traditions of medicine, is egalitarian and focused on the common good, and able to improvise with the technology at hand. In Vietnam during the First Indochinese War, political cadre promoted this ideal of medicine (and science) that was rarely achieved in practice. Rather, as the historian Xiaoping Fang has shown for barefoot doctors in the People's Republic of China, practitioners of socialist medicine were key conduits of a modernist vision of biomedicine in rural Asia.[5]

My chapter unravels the medical training received by Y50 at the Hanoi Medical University in order to explore the conflict between political and professional allegiances in socialist biomedicine during a formative moment. In addition to imparting skills and technical knowledge, as the introduction to this volume points out, education attempts to form professional identities and emotional dispositions. As the education of Y50 shows, the notion of what formed a "good" education differed between political cadres and medical doctors. For cadres, a "good" education focused on decolonizing the mind of trainees and bringing them closer to their patients and "the people." For physicians, a "good" education imparted technical skills and the professional values of biomedicine essential to prevent and treat wounds and diseases. Paralleling Jenna Grant's discussion of Cambodian medical doctors, socialist doctors in Vietnam held a modernist vision of their job, including an emphasis on surgery, pharmaceuticals, and technology, largely in line with contemporary norms of biomedicine.

These tensions played out in a number of ways. One issue over which medical educators came into conflict with the Party was its valorization of "Traditional Vietnamese Medicine" (TVM), which the Party found useful both for its low-cost therapeutic properties and for its role in promoting a national identity and legitimizing socialism in the eyes of the people. Only a few biomedical doctors at the HMU were familiar with TVM and they turned to it, letting the body heal itself, when biomedicine was too costly or unavailable. Even though the Y50 class included Hoàng Bảo Châu, probably the most famous practitioner of so-called Đông Y, or Eastern medicine, the Y50 generation's biggest contribution to Eastern medicine was to further infuse it with biomedical values, including an emphasis on knowing and controlling nature.[6]

Also at stake was the relationship between language and identity. After 1945, physicians who were responsible for medical education under the Viet Minh decided at first to teach in French, the colonial language. This decision made pedagogical sense as textbooks were in French and both students and teachers had extensive schooling in that language. As the Viet Minh began to receive outside aid, the political cadre emphasized the importance first of Chinese and then Russian as scientific languages, while the medical doctors who traveled to these countries looked to French- and English-language material for the latest in medical advances. For these doctors, the use of foreign languages in training students was necessary for professional competence. Employing French, for example, did not mark physicians as pro-French but instead signaled their participation in a cosmopolitan community of biomedical healers. Meanwhile, for many cadres, especially less well educated ones, speaking French was often equated with "Frenchness" and they viewed the minds of medical doctors as potentially still colonized.

Another issue that reveals political and professional tensions was who should become a medical doctor. For the Party, the ideal medical student had a proletarian background and was untainted by collaboration with the French, the Japanese, or anti-communist nationalists. For educators, the ideal student was well prepared linguistically for higher education in French, as well as able to handle the rough conditions of the battlefield. While in theory women, ethnic minorities, and poor males could enroll at the HMU, few had the prerequisites necessary to qualify for a medical education. Military service did offer a pathway for some poor boys to become doctors.

Given Vietnamese notions of authority, the model physician was male and belonged to the major ethnic group, the Kinh. Yet, as representatives of the state, medical doctors were also supposed to connect with patients who were only loosely controlled by its authority. In these cases, the colonial gaze of biomedicine could put a wedge between physicians and patients who put their stock in TVM, a phenomenon that had frustrated French medical doctors during the colonial era. Likewise, speaking French, or being Kinh and male, did not always serve to legitimize doctors' control over their patients' bodies. From the Party's perspective, a "well-educated" socialist medical doctor should be near to the masses. For their part, physicians often expressed a strong allegiance to the discipline of biomedicine and to its attendant social authority, a position that at times brought them into conflict with their ideal position as being close to the people.[7]

More broadly, medical education was an arena for working out goals and core values in government health care. In state-published medical manuals, cadres and physicians agreed that biomedicine was important to increase the health, productivity, and war-making capacity of the population. Furthermore, the circumstances of war often forced both sides to compromise as ideals were set aside for practices that "worked." As such, a study of professionalization opens a window onto the success and failures of the state-making project carried out by the Viet Minh during the First Indochina War. It is not surprising that the Viet Minh adopted a biopolitical approach to rule, as the historian Christopher

Goscha has recently argued, since biopolitics has been a normative state practice for quite some time. The more interesting question is how and to what degree the Viet Minh were able to implement their vision of health. With due respect to Goscha, my chapter shows limits to the Viet Minh's state-building efforts. Besides soldiers and cadres, male Kinh made up only a minority of the population and, I argue, most people either remained outside the orbit of biomedicine or only partially accepted the authoritative gaze of the biomedical doctor.[8]

My chapter draws from archival material held at National Archives III in Hanoi, Vietnam, and oral and published histories of medical doctors. The oral histories were collected by Vietnamese researchers between 2009 and 2013. These researchers also transcribed the interviews from digital recordings while the translations to English, and analysis, are my own. In order to study the place of medical doctors in Vietnamese society, my chapter draws from Science, Technology, and Society (STS) approaches. As Bruno Latour pointed out long ago, scientists and medical doctors are useful actors to follow because of their disciplinary allegiances and access to international and transnational networks, as well as their key position in the modern state.[9] The generational approach of sociologist Ming-Cheng Lo's *Doctors within Borders* offers another good analytical model. Lo's book shows that in Taiwan at least, a nuanced approach to different generations is necessary to understand how individual medical doctors responded to the twinned questions of nationalism and decolonization.[10]

After a brief introduction to the Hanoi Medical University and the Y50, my chapter is divided into five main topics that highlight different aspects of the Y50 experience. The first two sections tackle the question of medicine and politics directly. The first section shows that while cadres asserted the political aspects of medicine, doctors sought to define their job as purely technical. This strategy helped physicians retain independence in their field even as other intellectuals felt increasing state control over their activities. The second section looks at how students were taught to deal with their patients. The third section considers the more indirect politics surrounding the language of medical education. The fourth section considers the relationship between biomedicine and traditional medicine at the HMU. The final section examines the relationship between military and civilian medicine, or *Quân Y* and *Dân Y*, and how medical doctors established their social authority. During the First Indochinese War, treating soldiers was a priority and the Y50 learned how to treat war wounds. They spoke of the close relationship between military and civilian medicine, and the 1954 victory at Dien Bien Phu as one of the crowning achievements of their lives to that point.

## Y50 Goes to the HMU

The Hanoi Medical University, the first European-style medical school in Vietnam, was founded in 1902 as part of the Indochinese University in Hanoi. This school was designed only to train assistants to French medical doctors, rather than Vietnamese medical doctors who could work independently. Until the 1930s, France was the only place that Vietnamese could get a medical degree that would allow them to practice medicine in a capacity equivalent to their French colleagues.[11] These limitations meant that there was a large gap between the medical needs of French Indochina and what the French-controlled medical system could provide. By one historian's count, there was 1 biomedically trained doctor for every 67,000 people in Indochina in 1930 and according to another historian, the ratio was 1 to 157,000 people.[12]

The outbreak of the First Indochinese War, or the War of Resistance against the French, in 1946 pressed home the need for more medical doctors. After the end of World War II, the French government made clear its intentions to recapture political and military power in Indochina. The Indochinese Communist Party (ICP) led by Ho Chi Minh opted to resist French efforts to re-colonize Indochina. Among the coalition of anti-colonial forces that it largely controlled, called the Viet Minh, there were few medical doctors. Moreover, these doctors had a heavy double task: first, to keep soldiers fit enough to fight and second, to train the next generation of doctors.[13] Hồ Đắc Di, who had been a respected doctor in France, was chosen as the head of the HMU. Its curriculum focused on military medicine and the Viet Minh worked to integrate students into the framework of the military. Topics studied included field surgery, war wounds, internal military medicine, malaria, and various infections, with medical doctors and advanced students giving lectures.[14]

Among those educated at HMU between 1945 and 1954, Y50 was a transitional generation for at least two reasons. First, the Y50 took part in the process of decolonization, which played out during the war over three generations. The first generation, or the professors of the HMU after its move to the resistance zone in the Viet Bac, were fluent in both French and Vietnamese, but favored French in professional settings. Physicians in this generation formed part of the tiny minority to obtain medical degrees before 1945. The second generation, or the students in the Viet Bac including Y50, were fluent in both French and Vietnamese, but made the transition to Vietnamese in professional settings. This generation was greater in number and also had to overcome many hardships to obtain medical degrees. As well as intellectual and social challenges, this generation suffered from the material hardships of the resistance base. The third generation were the students trained in the post-1954 Democratic Republic of Vietnam. These students were less proficient in French, if they spoke it at all, and used Vietnamese as both personal and professional languages. Russian and Chinese were increasingly used as spoken second languages, while French and English were key reading languages. This generation was even more numerous and could advance quickly through the educational system.

The second reason that the Y50 generation was transitional is that they began their education during a time of increasing security for the Viet Minh, when the HMU had moved back from Trung Giáp to Chiêm Hoá in the Viet Bac and stayed there until the Viet Minh victory at Dien Bien Phu in 1954. Material conditions in the resistance zone were always spartan but 1950 represented an important turning point. By that time, the Viet Minh had established their base and they were able to resist intensified attacks of the French military. In addition, after the 1949 victory of the communists over the nationalists in China, medical supplies began to flow, or rather trickle, over the border. And with more settled conditions came better conditions for study and training.[15]

Many Y50 students came from what was termed the petty bourgeois (*tiểu tư sản, TTS*), which potentially put a barrier between these students and the workers and peasants according to Marxist theories. A female student from Y52, Nguyễn Thị Ngọc Toản, recalls that those students with "royal backgrounds" (*vương thành phần*) had to take political classes.[16] Some students faced difficulties in their careers because of their family and political backgrounds. For example, even though he was the leader of a medical unit, Nguyễn Duy Tuân was officially denied party membership in 1955, supposedly because he had not completely reported his resume (*lý lịch*). Tuân believes that the decision was due in part to a youthful indiscretion with the Nationalist Party (Đại Việt Quốc Dân Đảng) during the August Revolution of 1945; in addition, Tuân's great-grandfather had been a mandarin for the Nguyễn emperors, his grandfather and father had both served as officials in the French protectorate of Tonkin, and his mother had come from an important land-owning family.[17]

HMU students could hail from other types of elites. As the children of party cadres, medical doctors, and prominent revolutionary families, they often took leadership positions among the students. For example, Trần Mạnh Chu, a Y46 student, was the son of the medical doctor Trần Văn Lai, who was the first president of the administrative committee of Hanoi after the 1945 revolution. Chu headed the military medical unit where the Y50 performed their internships, namely Đội Điều Trị 5 (DDT5). The section heads included Hoàng Thủy Nguyên, Y49, son of Minister of Medicine Hoàng Tích Trí.[18] In keeping with the Communist Party's policy of a united front for independence, these students often kept their identity as cadre muted, if not completely secret.

The professors of these students included some of the most famous Vietnamese medical doctors. Nguyễn Mạnh Liên, a student of Y50, recalled studying surgery with Đỗ Xuân Hợp (*giải phẫu*) and Tôn Thất Tùng (*ngoại khoa*, focused on external injuries), internal medicine with Hồ Đắc Di, and bacteriology and parasitology with Đăng Vân Ngữ, among others.[19] The professors of Y50 often came from prominent intellectual families. Hồ Đắc Di, who was born in Hue in 1900, came from a prominent family and studied at Paul Bert School in Hanoi, after which he went to study in France in 1918 and graduated as a medical doctor. Not all professors were similarly privileged. Even though Tôn Thất Tùng, who was born in 1912, belonged to a branch of the royal family in Hue, he and his mother were fairly poor.[20] This did not stop Ho Chi Minh from teasing Tùng about his aristocratic background.[21]

## Politics or Technique?

Party cadres tried to enforce revolutionary politics on student doctors and they emphasized the need for doctors to have a class standpoint, especially after February 1951 and the official "communization" of the medical services.[22] For example, the pamphlet "Thought, Function, and Direction of Vietnamese Revolutionary Medicine" urged physicians to discriminate in their treatment of the exploiting class and the working class, an urgent question in the south.[23] Cadres asserted the importance of politics over medicine in other ways as well, and given incidents where criticism of party actions was repressed, one might expect a high level of interference in the ways in which doctors thought and worked.[24] Yet, the Party did not exert too much political pressure on HMU students initially, in part because of their essential role in military operations. Medical doctors, unlike humanists and social scientists, were rarely

thrown in jail for speaking out against the Party and the greatest conflicts arose concerning the distribution of resources. The Party, argued
doctors, allowed them a technical space somewhat shielded from politics
despite medicine's political character.

Many physicians trained in the resistance zone explain the restraint
of the cadre by pointing to the technical aspects of medicine. Nguyễn
Thúc Tùng, a professor at HMU who was called "Tùng Con" or Small
Tùng, to differentiate him from Tôn Thất Tùng, who was called "Tùng
Lớn" or Big Tùng, put it this way: "And the people like us, for example,
or like Tôn Thất Tùng, the Party only used us to do our profession."[25]
Tùng continued: "The Ministry of Defense or a Party Member, how
could they interfere in the work of a doctor?" Tùng further explained:
"Practically, they didn't have the time or the skill level, because they
didn't know anything about medicine…they were revolutionaries."[26] The
weakness of the Viet Minh's position meant that it depended on a united
front strategy that called for contributions from all patriots and during
the early years of the First Indochinese War, the Party simply could
not afford to alienate doctors, even if they held nationalist, rather than
communist, loyalties. Together, these factors can help explain why the
medical doctors felt relatively little political interference in their work.

This is not to say that politics did not appear at all in medical
education. In September 1951, at the opening ceremony for the second
year of Y50, portraits of communist world leaders were once again on
display.[27] Yet "politics" did not simply mean studying the collected
works of Marx or Ho Chi Minh. As Nguyễn Thúc Tùng put it, "Politics,
I studied it all day!" But by politics, Tùng wasn't referring to Marxism;
instead, he meant the "situation," that is, the First Indochina War.
"Studying politics didn't mean looking at Stalin with Lenin or Karl
Marx at all. At that time, politics was how to fight the French."[28] The
Party taught students "why the state did what it did, and to sympathize
with the state." In other words, "education was mostly about the issue
of patriotism," Tùng concluded, and "because of this [education], these
doctors were very conscientious and dedicated."[29] Even though medicine did not exist outside of politics, both teachers and students were
largely in agreement about the appropriate topics of study and the need
to apply medicine to military concerns.

At times the lack of resources did put strains on the relationship
between medical doctors and the state. For example, Tôn Thất Tùng
wrote to Phạm Văn Đồng, later the prime minister of the Democratic
Republic of Vietnam, imploring the Viet Minh leadership to deliver

more goods such as cotton gauze and anesthesia to the hospitals. Although Tùng was known as hot-headed, the tone of the letters is a bit surprising and his letters were quite direct. And in a 1953 letter to Anh Bẩy, Tùng argued that without new medical supplies, he would become a "croque-mort" or undertaker's assistant, rather than a doctor. In addition to the immediate need for treating cadre and fellow physicians, Tùng requested journals on medicine and surgery, and complained that "this year, [we] didn't have one issue!"[30] Some medical students were critical of the expedited nature of medical education, arguing that doctors were specializing too early and were weak in the basics. Finally, some doctors simply did not join the Viet Minh in the resistance zone, while others left because of difficult conditions.[31]

Conflicts over material resources somewhat decreased as the Party started to receive Chinese supplies and medical advisors after 1949. Although the Viet Minh began to receive supplies from the People's Republic of China, some medical doctors did not remember these supplies and their testimony speaks to the uneven impact of these goods at the time.[32] Chinese advisors were another question and students recall one lesson from the advisors about how and when to evacuate casualties. Another lesson involved changing the dressing and cleaning wounds, with the advisors using the slogan: "Left: clean"; "right: dirty." This meant that the left hand was kept clean, the right hand used for dirty things, and the two did not touch.[33]

Another potential source of conflict was the legacy of French colonial medical education. As with the French language, however, this legacy could be very useful for anti-colonial efforts. Nguyễn Thúc Tùng remembers a "good influence" from the colonial period because "French science was very good!"[34] Individual teachers were remembered fondly, including Pierre Huard, who taught at the HMU during World War II. Speaking about Huard, Tùng put it this way: "[We] must recognize that even though he…[and] those doctors, even though they were 'colonialist' [in French], in particular Huard…he was very good with the students."[35] Huard, a French naval doctor, taught students how to treat war wounds, and during the battle of Dien Bien Phu in 1954, Huard worked to evacuate wounded French soldiers while his former students did the same for the Viet Minh.[36]

Probably the most significant factor reducing conflict between biomedicine and politics was the disinclination of medical doctors compared with other intellectuals to question the decisions of the Party. In the education ranks, every group of students had a party member, often the child of trusted revolutionaries, who was the leader. In professional units, "there was one Party member, and that Party member was the leader. He was the leader about thought."[37] A few physicians who had "early enlightenment," such as Trần Văn Lai, could be political leaders. But often the cadre in the unit was a nurse, which put them in a lower position in the hierarchy than the doctors, thus mitigating their authority.

## How to be Close to the Patient

A key component of any medical education is how medical doctors imagine their patients. In the West, the medical anthropologist Claire Wendland argues that biomedical education is designed to desensitize medical doctors to the human in the patient and to emphasize the body as a mechanical and biological system. While this education does not produce the same result in all students, it transforms the worldview of the majority of them.[38] Students are not tabula rasa and they bring with them social markers such as gender, class, and ethnicity, which play an important part in the enculturation of the doctor-to-be and in forming the doctor and patient relationship.

In theory, education at the Hanoi Medical University was no different in this regard from its Western counterpart. Vietnamese medical doctors were supposed to view their patients, largely consisting of soldiers and cadres, as skin, blood, organs, and bones. Yet politically, physicians were urged to have a democratic attitude (*thái độ dân chủ*) and to view the patient as an equal participant in the healing process. It seems that party leaders had learned the lessons of colonial medicine well and they knew that medicine was an effective means to win the loyalty of the population. Most of the political education of medical doctors was aimed at convincing them of the importance of supporting their patients and "the people." In theory, Y50 students found themselves treating both Viet Minh soldiers and Vietnamese peasants, and expectations such as these meant that future medical doctors should be loyal revolutionaries.

The relationship between physician and patient was further strengthened by the war. Nguyễn Thúc Tùng remembered how "they [the students] went close to the soldiers in the forest. As a result of being close with the patients," Tùng continued, "the state…and the people…really had confidence in them."[39] Moreover, the continual interruptions to their education, the frequent time they spent feeling overwhelmed by the battlefield, and their powerlessness in front of many injuries meant that Vietnamese medical doctors were kept humble and affectively closer to their patients than otherwise would have been the case.

In addition to work on the battlefield, military and civilian medical doctors were charged with public health issues such as epidemics, maternal health, and general hygiene.[40] Malaria in particular received much attention. During the colonial era, Vietnamese doctors commonly viewed malaria as harmful for "our race" (*dân tộc mình*); similarly the Viet Minh viewed malaria as sapping the strength of the people to contribute to agricultural and military campaigns.[41] According to the Viet Minh pamphlet cited at the beginning of my chapter, the function of socialist medicine in fighting diseases such as malaria was "to pro-tect the health of the people against disease, to protect and increase the POWER TO STRUGGLE OF THE RACE [*dân tộc*], FORCE TO INCREASE PRODUCTION of the race, in order to allow the race to quickly reach independence, unity, democracy, and peace." In other words, medicine and the biopolitical project of the state were inextri-cably intertwined and followed the slogan "REVOLUTIONARY SCIENCE NOT FOR SCIENCE BUT ONLY FOR WELFARE OF THE PEOPLE."[42]

Such reasoning provided a powerful rationale for extending the reach of the socialist-state-in-the-making and one doctor observed that "wherever there is malaria, there is also the state."[43] Thinking about who was tasked with protecting the health of which people also helps clarify the relationship between physicians and patients. The rural sociologist Christian Lentz has shown how state-making in northwest Vietnam was often represented in dichotomous terms where the male and Kinh (the major ethnic group in Vietnam) elements were active, while the female and ethnic (Hmong, Thai) elements were passive.[44] Similarly in medical education, the ideal physician at the time was male and Kinh. Kinh dominated the ranks of the students and there was not much discussion of cross-ethnic treatments. Other than mass hygiene campaigns, non-Kinh ethnic groups were left to their own healing ways and even provided a source of "local" knowledge for male Kinh medical doctors.

Patriarchy was also a continuing problem and despite a Viet Minh ideology that called for gender equality, most HMU students were male. Y49, for example, had only 1 female (Nguyễn Thị Minh Vượng) out of 20 students, Y50 had 3 (Nguyễn Thị Bình, Trịnh Thị Mão, and Vũ Thị Phan) out of 39 students, and Y52 had 4 (Nguyễn Thị Ngọc

Toản, Mẫu Đơn, Quỳnh Giao, and Hà Thị Tư) out of 80 students.[45] Female medical students recount being teased and faced limitations that were reflective of broader trends in Vietnamese society.[46] Minh Vượng and Ngọc Toản both recount fondly how men went out of their way to protect them during difficult journeys to the Viet Bac; yet, their need for protection was seen as a potential liability. HMU directors had to find separate housing for the women and at times held them back from opportunities on the battlefield, a key place to gain experience, promotion, and the trust of superiors.[47]

In addition, class intersected with gender in determining who would become a medical student. The women who enrolled at HMU were either from the petty bourgeois or more elite backgrounds. Politically such backgrounds could be problematic, as shown by Ngọc Toản's account above. Yet, this background gave them access to good training at the high school level. In many ways, the low numbers of women overall were simply a continuation of Nguyen and colonial patterns of education, and reflected a lack of opportunities for the majority of women to achieve the prerequisites necessary to attend medical school, such as a high school education or battlefield experience.

For practical reasons, the Viet Minh could not afford to turn away qualified applicants and women played an important part in the medical corps.[48] In fact, the percentages of female enrollment during the late 1940s and early 1950s equaled the best rates for women at most medical schools in the United States during that time.[49] Women could also rise to prominent positions. Vũ Thị Phan, whose interest in malaria started when she witnessed the disease firsthand as a child, worked closely with Đặng Vân Ngữ and later became the head of the Institute of Malariology.[50] Many female students worked on the battlefield with the Quân Y, and by the 1960s female doctors, such as Đàng Thùy Trâm, were frequently sent to the south.[51]

As with medical supplies, doctors were in short supply for the many medical needs of the "liberated" zones. As Lentz points out, cadres and nurses (rather than doctors) were often called on to address the difficult medical conditions in the northwest.[52] Likewise, in the provinces of the Mekong Delta, maternal health and birthing were left to midwives. For example, a pamphlet for midwives on assisting birth suggests the limited contact between medical doctors and civilian patients, and the significant role of Southern medicine in giving birth and other important medical events. Likewise, Y50 doctors received little training in maternal health. With only a handful of women at the HMU, the question of access to, and social authority over, non-male, non-Kinh patients remained problematic for doctors, an issue further illustrated by the question of language.

## Authority over the Tongue

For any medical doctor trained before the 1950s, French was a necessary language. Hà Văn Mạo, who graduated from the HMU in 1952, stated bluntly, "At that time if you didn't know French then you couldn't study medicine."[53] Nguyễn Duy Tuân (Y47) and other medical students recall that French was still used in teaching in 1955 when the HMU moved back to Hanoi.[54] Yet, French was not simply a marker of French identity and French-speaking ability should not be read as a form of enacting "French-ness." Instead, French (and Chinese, English, and Russian) offered medical doctors access to international knowledge and a cosmopolitan identity that, while rooted in "Vietnamese-ness," allowed the doctors to travel in body and mind.

The reasons for the dominance of French in medical education were twofold: texts and teachers. First, professors continued to use colonial-era French manuals, including a textbook by Henri Rouvière on human anatomy and others from both France and Indochina.[55] These texts were essential as HMU instructors were familiar with them and had neither the time nor the resources to rewrite textbooks in Vietnamese. Even agreeing on a translation of technical words such as "spleen" or "tibia" from French into Vietnamese was a significant challenge. Đỗ Xuân Hợp, a major figure in the task of translation, translated tibia as "*xương chày*" (literally, "pestle" or "bell-stick" bone). This choice of words was judged to be "too creative" by critics who argued that Hợp should have drawn more heavily on Chinese roots to make this translation.[56] Second, teachers were key to the continued use of French. Even though Tùng, Di, and the other instructors could speak Vietnamese, their academic language was French. Y50 students recall Tùng using French terms throughout his presentation and Tùng's journals from that time were written largely in French.[57] As one historian colorfully put it: "For the majority of the professors at that time, lecturing in Vietnamese was as tiring as it would be to lecture in a foreign language today."[58]

According to the logic of an anti-colonial struggle, switching to oral and written Vietnamese in all facets of life was an important task.

Party cadres, many of whom also spoke fluent French, emphasized the need to speak Vietnamese and write in *quốc ngữ*, the Romanized alphabet, only. Among elite cadre, questions about a "colonized mind" seemed to be less prominent than practical concerns. Using French in official functions could drive a wedge between party members from lower class backgrounds and those from more elite families, and a central plank of the Viet Minh position was a selective rejection of colonial practices.[59]

Despite the links made between *quốc ngữ* and nationalism, teachers and students at the HMU seemed to have felt little need to work exclusively in Vietnamese.[60] Such a distinction shows the degree to which medicine was understood as a professional discipline with its own internal language. In order to rationalize the contradiction between political ideal and professional reality, medical students rendered foreign languages into technical instruments. In other words, medical students viewed foreign languages as intimately tied to their professionalization. Mạo, who worked as a teaching assistant for Y50, commented: "I initially studied foreign languages in order to consult professional material."[61] By treating language as a tool that could be used by anyone, the Viet Minh were able to retain their access to an extremely useful body of technical knowledge.

The switch to Vietnamese finally arrived for a practical reason: there were fewer and fewer students after 1945 who had enough French proficiency to study medicine in that language. Wartime conditions meant that school hours were cut and this led to a reduction in the number of foreign language hours. By 1952 or 1953, French had been eliminated completely from the curriculum. As a result, students entering the HMU in the 1950s could often read French but could not understand spoken French well enough to follow a lecture.[62] One doctor recalls: "the students from around [19]46, 47, even 45, they spoke French well already, they had passed their high school exam. But it is possible that the French level of the 1952 students was lower."[63]

There were also sound medical reasons for switching to Vietnamese in practice. Speaking Vietnamese, even during technical conversations, helped to bring medical doctors closer to those they were treating as well as to their assistants. While the 1948 plans for an assistant doctors' school called for an entrance exam testing the ability of candidates to translate Vietnamese into French, the nurses and assistants with whom doctors worked were unlikely to understand instructions in French.[64] Thus, it was vital to know how to describe procedures during the heat of battle in a way that could be understood by all. Yet, with the possible exception of Hợp, most professors would have continued to use French to teach if the students' ability to speak French had continued to be strong.[65]

Studying abroad after 1954 was a different matter and English, not French, Chinese, or Russian, was the language used to access international developments in medicine. Looking back, Small Tùng emphasized the diminishing importance of French in science, stating that "French was not the most important in science, primary was English."[66] Some medical students who spent a decade or more abroad became fluent in the language of their studies and some even served as translators for important political figures.[67] Reflecting the openness to learning foreign languages, many students and doctors who traveled to China or the USSR recalled the luxury of having access to journals from European countries and the United States.

## A Reorientation of Medicine

A key question that presented itself during the First Indochina War, which hinged on both political and medical considerations, was the appropriate relationship between *Đông Y* (Eastern medicine) or TVM, and *Tây Y* (Western medicine) or biomedicine. The historian C. Michele Thompson has convincingly shown that the roots of a "collaboration between western-trained Vietnamese physicians and members of the Vietnamese traditional medical community predate the founding of the *Quân Y* and the various organs of the national health care system of Vietnam."[68] The pamphlet called "Thought, Function, and Direction of Vietnamese Revolutionary Medicine" called for medical doctors to reject the tenets of biomedicine, while achieving good health for individuals and the population. Prevention, the pamphlet argued, was more important than curing and doctors were urged to increase the body's natural resistive capacity (that is, give up medical authority over the body and nature). This pamphlet clearly reflects the influence of Nguyễn Văn Hương, a biomedically trained doctor who came to appreciate the value of TVM.[69] Likewise, cadres tended to value Eastern medicine for both its ability to reach rural patients and its propaganda value. Yet, many biomedical doctors of the HMU preferred more technologically intense interventions. They were skeptical of Eastern medicine and were often discretely silent in their discussions of its efficacy.

Under French colonial rule, the categories of Eastern medicine and its definitional opposite, Western medicine, or biomedicine, developed simultaneously. Furthermore, Vietnamese society did not witness the wholesale rejection of healing traditions that occurred elsewhere in Asia.[70] Eastern medicine itself comprises two older, rather distinct entities—*thuốc bắc* (Northern medicine) and *thuốc nam* (Southern medicine). Northern medicine was based on the theory of yin and yang and the five elements. It had long been practiced by Vietnamese scholars well versed in the Confucian classics and represented a consolidated form of knowledge. By contrast, Southern medicine referred to a myriad of unsystematic practices involving local plants and herbs.[71]

The involvement of the Viet Minh in Eastern medicine and Western medicine had contradictory effects. On one hand, state approval gave Eastern medicine a significant new ally and was reciprocally used by the Viet Minh to gain legitimacy among rural populations. The colonial state had been at best tolerant of Eastern medicine, but the Viet Minh found in Eastern medicine a politically valuable form of knowledge that could be trumpeted as independent of colonial influence and a standpoint from which to criticize biomedicine. Even though Hoàng Bảo Châu argued that developing Eastern medicine institutions and practitioners was a long process and was still incomplete, Eastern medicine gained something close to parity with Western medicine in terms of official recognition.

Eastern medicine occupied an ambiguous position in socialist biomedicine and physicians and some cadres argued that the northern component of Eastern medicine still suffered from many feudal characteristics. Practitioners of Northern medicine also had the tendency to look down on practitioners of Southern medicine, with some Northern medicine doctors keeping their secrets to themselves and looking to make a private profit from their knowledge. Southern medicine came closer to the socialist ideal as it was a national (*dân tộc*) practice, one that helped localize (*địa phương hóa*) Northern medicine. It was also cheaper than either Western medicine or Northern medicine and its practitioners were almost all farmers as well.[72]

The involvement of the Viet Minh and the Hanoi Medical University doctors, however, worked to change Eastern medicine in many ways that contradicted the spirit of the practice. Viet Minh cadres criticized both Northern medicine and Southern medicine for a lack of scientific rigor and international awareness. These cadres argued that Northern medicine "did not go deeply into anatomy, bacteriology, physiology:

diagnosis is not based on methods of experimental science but only based on the two pulses and the theories of yin-yang and the five elements."[73] To address these weaknesses, cadres sought to *"khoa học hóa Đông Y,"* or scientize Eastern medicine and made a list of steps to incorporate Eastern medicine with Western medicine, which included matching a disease with a prescription, a rather reductionist approach.[74] Viet Minh pamphlets also emphasized that Eastern medicine knowledge was produced through struggling with nature *(thiên nhiên)* and over-coming disease and death, a historical interpretation which had more to do with dialectical materialism than any tradition of Northern medicine or Southern medicine.

Eastern medicine also played an ambiguous role in Y50 medical education and in histories of the HMU.[75] While most doctors recognized the need for Eastern medicine and agreed with its political aims, even Hoàng Bảo Châu, who studied with Y50 and eventually became a leading authority on traditional medicine in Vietnam, started his study of the field rather by accident. He initially volunteered to go to China to study traditional medicine not out of a concern for traditional medi-cine but mostly because he wanted to travel. In addition, many doctors saw only a limited role for Eastern medicine and the petty bourgeois background of many Y50 students meant that they were more comfort-able with biomedicine than with Vietnamese traditional medicine. While Small Tùng admitted some use for diarrhea and headaches, he recalls being taught to think that for malaria, "the many plants didn't have any value at all." The same doctor said that the soldiers also did not believe in those plants and that everybody hoped to have quinine.[76] And when Tôn Thất Tùng wanted to take care of an ailing Hồ Đắc Di, he requested modern vitamins to deal with the effects of malnutrition.[77]

In the south, Eastern medicine may have been more widely used as Nguyễn Văn Hưởng, the director of the Southern Medical Service, was favorably disposed to medications inspired by this tradition.[78] Two handwritten pamphlets produced by the Office of Military Medicine of the Western Interregional Division (approximately the Mekong Delta) and dated 1954 show a desperate lack of materials and ingenious ways devised to deal with this lack. The first pamphlet, entitled "Methods to Keep in Place and Not Have to Change Dressing for a Long Time," recommends using the stalks of banana trees *(bẹ chuối)* to preserve the dressings of wounds.[79] The second pamphlet, on "Diagnosing War Wounds," offers a quick, simple diagnostic guide on determining the character and extent of the wound and the best way to deal with it.[80]

While there was neither time nor the expertise needed to teach Eastern medicine at the HMU, this form of medicine was useful to the Viet Minh. It offered a critique of biomedical practices and was cheap, easy to understand, and available to bring to the battlefield.

## Away from the Individual, Towards the Collective

"The First Vietnamese School of Medicine was militarized from its beginning," states Christopher Goscha.[81] Y50 doctors recall much overlap between *Quân Y* (military medicine) and *Dân Y* (civilian medicine). Several factors contributed to this overlap, including the education provided in the Viet Bac. Nguyễn Thúc Tùng pointed out how "all of the military and civilian doctors studied together under the responsibility of Tôn Thất Tùng…in the forest."[82] The First Indochina War dictated much of the educational agenda and the same Y50 professor cited earlier recalled the Ministry of Health's slogan: "before anything else, study what you need most directly."[83] This meant that techniques relevant to soldiers—treating head injuries and performing rapid field surgery—were emphasized over concerns more relevant to civilians or to education in the basic sciences. All physicians were supposed to be partisan, and in the case of enemy soldiers, only if the soldier surrendered could doctors take care of them.[84]

Yet, there were differences between civilian and military medicine. HMU students may have been called to serve on the battlefield during their first year, but the process of militarization took time. For example, as late as May 1950, both civilian and military medicine existed as a separate school for military medicine had been created after 1945.[85] Medical doctors in military and civilian medicine followed slightly different career tracks and military doctors were more integrated into the Party structure. Furthermore, although doctors were supposed to treat both military and civilian Vietnamese, and the two branches shared equipment, soldiers received priority among all doctors.

After 1950, the war with the French dramatically intensified, which meant that the Y50 students were constantly traveling to the war front to conduct surgery on the battlefield. For the most part, they studied for a few months, traveled to the front, then returned for more study, as there was a desperate need for anyone who could properly treat a wound. Many students argued that the combination of self-study and practical experience gave them a good education and an understanding of the military. Material shortages both created a strong rationale to share resources and powerful incentives not to do so. In May 1950, the Ministry of Health acted to further integrate its efforts with those of the military, ordering provincial health branches to provide set amounts of pharmaceuticals, bandages, and other supplies to the local military units.[86]

A report summarizing the findings of a 1954 conference held by the Department of Military and Civilian Medicine in the Southern Region tells a different story. This report reviewed the successes and failures of 1953 and set an agenda for 1954. It was critical of the effort to integrate civilian and military medicine in the south in particular, and of efforts to establish a medical presence in general. In 1953, the Viet Minh had four objectives in the southern region: (1) increase activity behind enemy lines; (2) launch guerilla warfare; (3) improve material conditions and the morale of the people; (4) politically re-educate cadres and military leaders. In terms of medicine, military doctors were criticized as arrogant and looking down on civilian medicine, which in the south was largely composed of Eastern medicine doctors, "sorcerers" (*thầy pháp*), and other types of local healers. The medical service was also failing to deliver health care as doctors did not do enough to ensure hygiene, cure diseases, or produce pharmaceuticals. The intertwined goals for the following year were to push the war and to provide for the people's health. The report emphasized that "building a professional awareness would serve politics."[87]

A second report emerging from the same 1954 conference (or a similar one) set out a more detailed agenda for the reform of military-civilian medicine. According to this second report, the medical corps was neither following the revolutionary line nor creating an organization capable of fighting a guerilla war. More concretely, medical personnel suffered from a number of drawbacks in their approach to medicine. These drawbacks included: individualism, a parochial viewpoint, an authoritative and functionary attitude towards the people, overspecialization, and an unwillingness to be reassigned to distant, dangerous battlefields. These drawbacks, along with organizational problems, had led to underdeveloped medical services in many places and an almost complete separation between civilian and military medicine in practice.[88]

Was there really a difference between the cooperation of military and civilian medicine in the north and the south? This question is a difficult one to answer without the necessary archival documents, but it is possible to speculate. In the south, the Viet Minh had a weaker presence overall and were less effective at mobilizing coalitions and holding territory. In terms of medicine, neither medical doctors nor students in the south had an institution such as the HMU to rally around if they chose to follow the Viet Minh. The level of medicine in the southern resistance zone also appears to have been at a rather low level. And significantly, perhaps, the director of the Southern Medical Service, Nguyễn Văn Hương, leaned more towards nationalism than communism.[89]

One event that widened the gap between the medical services in the north and south happened in the spring of 1954 at the battle of Dien Bien Phu. This battle resulted in many wounded soldiers and gave an opportunity for Y50 to get experience working directly with patients. As with earlier fighting, broken bones and gangrene from wounds presented important problems for the medical doctors. Tôn Thất Tùng took charge of the medical aspects of the battle that is seen by many of the participating physicians as a crowning moment for the Viet Minh medical services.

## Conclusion

My chapter has traced the education of a generation of Vietnamese medical doctors. It has focused on Y50, or the medical class of 1950, trained in zones of resistance in the war against the French that lasted from 1946 to 1954. An examination of the training and perspectives of these students shows that they were professionalized in a Western way. That is to say, they viewed medicine through the lens of a biomedical moral order: reductionist rationality, authority over nature and the body, individualism, and technological orientation.[90] There were exceptions, and some biomedical doctors did in practice pay more attention to Eastern medicine and were less technologically oriented. But these practices were due to the exigencies of war, and doctors emphasized over and over that these were less than ideal adaptations to difficult conditions. Such adherence to a biomedical order as held by the Y50 should not be surprising. These doctors by and large retained the skills, professional identities, and moral values imparted to them by their French-educated, cosmopolitan Vietnamese teachers. This does not make the Y50 doctors less interesting for students of Vietnamese history. As Claire Wendland has recently argued, African doctors trained in biomedicine are no less "African" than their herbal doctor counterparts.[91] With over 100 years of biomedicine in Vietnam, surely the same can be said of Vietnamese doctors. One of the most interesting aspects of the Y50 is that they held biomedical moral values yet in practice, they showed a more flexible attitude.

Through Y50, my chapter also explores the relationship between politics and science in Vietnam at the beginning of the Cold War. It looks at this relationship by analyzing how medical doctors interacted with political cadres and state structures. The Y50 generation is a particularly fruitful one for studying questions of politics and science for the following four reasons. First, there was the question of language and whether French or Vietnamese would be used in medical instruction. Second, there were the issues of class, gender, and ethnic divides in healing practices and physician-and-patient relationships. Third, tensions arose between Party cadres and scientists regarding the distribution of state resources. Fourth, the medical doctors' contribution to military medicine meant that they escaped the worst repression.

Four conclusions emerge from my study regarding science and politics in medicine. First, the Y50 generation shows that the Party did not initially play a significant role in medical education. Second, medical doctors were almost exclusively preoccupied by wartime needs. Nearly all medical education, and indeed intellectual production, was directed towards military ends. Even though Vietnamese medical doctors were quite innovative with regards to military techniques, they could not follow lines of "pure" research. Third, insofar as medicine helped the Viet Minh gain legitimacy among the people, training medical doctors contributed in important ways to the state-making project. Fourth, the state was able to co-opt medical doctors and they presented little challenge to political authority except in technical matters. As a result there seems to have been little direct censorship or repression of scientists. In this way, the Viet Minh during the First Indochinese War differed from the Chinese Communist Party during the Cultural Revolution. Regarding scientific matters, medical doctors were largely left to their own devices.

## Acknowledgements

This chapter was developed during two conferences of the History of Medicine in Southeast Asia (HOMSEA) hosted in 2012 in Surakarta, Indonesia, and 2014 in Manila, the Philippines. The gracious hosts of both conferences made them exceptional experiences. I thank National Archives No. 3 (TTLT 3) in Hanoi and the CPD (Trung Tâm Di Sản

Khoa Học) for their help in locating material for my chapter. I also want to thank C. Michele Thompson and two anonymous reviewers for their helpful comments on earlier drafts.

## Notes

1.  Văn Ngạc, Cảnh Cầu Nguyễn, Mạnh Liên Nguyễn, Đỗ Trinh Trần, Long Tạ, Quý Tảo Nguyễn, and Bá Thả Đoàn, *Lớp Sinh Viên Đại Học Y Khoa Niên Khóa 1950 Trong Khánh Chiến Chống Thực Dân Pháp* (Hanoi: Trường Đại Học Y Khoa Hà Nội, 2007), 26.
2.  Vũ Thị Phan, interview, Oct. 23, 2009. For early political awareness, see also Nguyễn Thị Ngọc Toản, interview, June 19, 2013.
3.  TTLT 3, Ủy Ban Kháng Chiến Hành Chính Nam Bộ, 1945–55, HS 988, Tu-Tuong Nhiem-Vu Duong-Huong Cua Y-Hoc Cach-Mang Viet-Nam.
4.  Ibid.
5.  Xiaoping Fang, *Barefoot Doctors and Western Medicine in China* (Rochester, NY: University of Rochester Press, 2012). Of course, the barefoot doctor movement started in 1965 was quite different from medical doctors fighting with the Viet Minh during the First Indochina War. The barefoot doctors were much more numerous, less well trained, and worked in a time of social upheaval but not in a war involving foreign powers. See also Shaun Kingsley Malarney, "Germ Theory, Hygiene, and the Transcendence of 'Backwardness' in Revolutionary Vietnam (1954–60)," in *Southern Medicine for Southern People: Vietnamese Medicine in the Making*, ed. Laurence Monnais, C. Michele Thompson, and Ayo Wahlberg (Newcastle upon Tyne: Cambridge Scholars Publishing, 2012), 107–32.
6.  See C. Michele Thompson, "Medicine, Nationalism, and Revolution in Vietnam: The Roots of a Medical Collaboration to 1945," *East Asian Science, Technology, and Medicine* 21 (2003): 114–48. Thompson demonstrates the cooperation between the Viet Minh and practitioners of TVM. Yet, the attitude of the majority of Y50 students and teachers seems to have been one of skepticism. This issue is discussed further below.
7.  For colonial-era issues of social authority, see Sokhieng Au, *Mixed Medicines: Health and Culture in French Colonial Cambodia* (Chicago: University of Chicago Press, 2011).
8.  Christopher E. Goscha, *Vietnam: un état né de la guerre, 1945–1954*, translated by Agathe Larcher (Paris: A. Colin, 2011).
9.  Bruno Latour, *Science in Action: How to Follow Scientists and Engineers through Society* (Cambridge, MA: Harvard University Press, 1987).
10. Ming-Cheng Lo, *Doctors within Borders: Profession, Ethnicity, and Modernity in Colonial Taiwan* (Berkeley, CA: University of California Press, 2002).

11. Laurence Monnais, *Médecine et colonisation: l'aventure Indochinoise 1860–1939* (Paris: CNRS Editions, 1999). Medical education was a bit more advanced in the Dutch East Indies. Hans Pols, "Tending to the Nation: Medicine, Nationalism, and Decolonisation in the Dutch East Indies 1900–1950," unpublished manuscript.

12. The historians are David Marr and Ngo Vinh Long respectively. Cited in Thompson, "Medicine, Nationalism, and Revolution," 122. These rates are comparable to those for Malawi from 2000 to 2007. Claire L. Wendland, *A Heart for the Work: Journeys through an African Medical School* (Chicago: University of Chicago Press, 2010), 54.

13. See Goscha, *Vietnam*, 2011, especially Chapter 5, "La médecine sur la brèche." As Goscha points out, only a minority of medical doctors chose to follow the Viet Minh to the resistance zone.

14. Ngạc, et al., *Lớp Sinh Viên*, 37.

15. There are many good accounts of the political and military events of the First Indochina War, including Mark Atwood Lawrence, *Assuming the Burden: Europe and the American Commitment to War in Vietnam* (Berkeley: University of California Press, 2005).

16. Tôn Thất Bách, Khang Lê Văn, and Lanh Nguyễn Ngọc, *100 Năm Đại Học Y Hà Nội: Năm Tháng và Sự Kiện* (Hà Noi: Trường Đại học Y Hà Nội, 2002), 152. Ngọc Toản was the sister-in-law of Đăng Vân Ngữ according to Goscha.

17. Nguyễn Duy Tuân, *Trưởng Thành Trong Thử Thách* (Hà Nội: Self-published, 1998), 3–5, 25, 73–4. Tuân also mentioned that his family's house was confiscated and had not been returned.

18. Ngạc, et al., *Lớp Sinh Viên*, 41.

19. Nguyễn Văn Huy, Phi Nga Mai, Kim Ngân Phạm, and Thị Trâm Nguyễn, *Di Sản Ký Ức Của Nhà Khoa Học*, Vol. 1 (Hà Nội: Nhà Xuất Bản Tri Thức, 2011), 18. For a list of professors, see Ngạc, et al., *Lớp Sinh Viên*, 21.

20. Ngạc, et al., *Lớp Sinh Viên*, 59–65.

21. Michitake Aso and Annick Guénel, "The Itinerary of a North Vietnamese Surgeon: Medical Science and Politics during the Cold War," *Science Technology & Society* 18, no. 3 (Nov. 2013): 294.

22. Goscha, *Vietnam*, 216–17.

23. TTLT 3, Ủy Ban Kháng Chiến Hành Chính Nam Bộ, 1945–55, HS 988, Tu-Tuong Nhiem-Vu Duong-Huong Cua Y-Hoc Cach-Mang Viet-Nam.

24. See Kim Ngoc Bao Ninh, *A World Transformed: The Politics of Culture in Revolutionary Vietnam, 1945–1965* (Ann Arbor, MI: University of Michigan Press, 2002), especially Chapter 4, "Intellectual Dissent," 121–63.

25. Nguyễn Thúc Tùng, interview, June 2, 2013.

26. Ibid.

27. Ngạc, et al., *Lớp Sinh Viên*, 56.

28. Nguyễn Thúc Tùng, interview, June 2, 2013.

29. Ibid.

30. TTLT 3, Phủ thủ tướng (PTT), 2849, "Tập Thư Trao Đổi Giữa Bác Sỹ Tôn Thất Tùng Với Đ/C Phạm Văn Đồng, Trần Quý Kiên, Anh Bảy Về Tình Hình Tổ Chức Và Phương Tiện Chữa Bệnh Năm 1953." The letter to Phạm Văn Đồng was addressed to Anh Tô on May 19, most likely 1953, and that to Anh Bảy on Nov. 28, 1953. It seems that the latter was the alias for Phạm Hùng, the assistant of Lê Duẩn.

31. Nguyễn Thúc Tùng, interview, June 2, 2013. See also Trần Ngọc Ninh, *Một Chút Lịch Sử: Y Khoa Đại Học Đường Sài Gòn: 1954–1975* (Montreal: Hội Y sĩ Việt Nam tại Canada, 2002).

32. Ngạc, et al., *Lớp Sinh Viên*, 65–7.

33. Ibid., 39, 42.

34. Nguyễn Thúc Tùng, interview, June 2, 2013.

35. Ibid.

36. Ibid.

37. Ibid.

38. Wendland, *A Heart*, 15–21. See also Pols, "Tending to the Nation," especially Chapter 5.

39. Nguyễn Thúc Tùng, interview, June 2, 2013.

40. TTLT 3, Ủy Ban Kháng Chiến Hành Chính Nam Bộ, 1945–55, HS 988, To Chuc Va Le Loi Lam Viec, 6–7.

41. TTLT 4, 3723, "Elaboration d'une notice de prophylaxie contre paludisme, Etudes des docteurs Moreau, Antoine, Đăng Văn Dư sur drainage et anti malarien, 1937–38." See also Michitake Aso, "Patriotic Hygiene: Tracing New Places of Knowledge Production about Malaria in Vietnam, 1919–75," *Journal of Southeast Asian Studies* 44, no. 3 (Oct. 2013): 423–43.

42. TTLT 3, Ủy Ban Kháng Chiến Hành Chính Nam Bộ, 1945–55, HS 988, Tu-Tuong Nhiem-Vu Duong-Huong Cua Y-Hoc Cach-Mang Viet-Nam.

43. Nguyễn Thúc Tùng, interview June 2, 2013.

44. Christian Cunningham Lentz, "Mobilizing a Frontier: Dien Bien Phu and the Making of Vietnam, 1945–1955" (PhD diss., Cornell University, 2011), 338.

45. These numbers vary slightly according to counting methods. For example, Khoa Niên Khóa 1950 lists only 39 students in the class but other sources list 40. See Ngạc, et al., *Lớp Sinh Viên*, 227–30. Bách, et al., *100 Năm*, 2002, 145–50. For slightly different numbers, see Goscha, *Vietnam*, 2011, 202.

46. Vũ Thị Phan, interview, Oct. 23, 2009.

47. Minh Vượng in Bách, et al., *100 Năm*, 2002, 146–7. Nguyễn Thị Ngọc Toản, interview, June 19, 2013.

48. Karen Gottschang Turner and Hao Thanh Phan, *Even the Women Must Fight: Memories of War from North Vietnam* (New York: John Wiley & Sons, Inc., 1998).

49. Judith Walzer Leavitt and Ronald L. Numbers, eds, *Sickness and Health in America: Readings in the History of Medicine and Public Health* (Madison: University of Wisconsin Press, 1978), 103.

50. Bộ Y Tế, *Bệnh Sốt Rét: Phòng Chống và Tiêu Diệt Sốt Rét Ở Việt Nam, 1958–1975* (Hà Nội: Viện sốt rét ký sinh trùng và côn trùng, 1976).

51. Đàng Thùy Trâm, *Last Night I Dreamed of Peace: The Diary of Dang Thuy Tram* (New York: Harmony Books, 2007).

52. Lentz, "Mobilizing a Frontier," 125; 127n121.

53. Huy, et al., *Di Sản Ký Ức*, 197.

54. Tuân, *Trưởng Thành*, 43. See also Bách, et al., *100 Năm*, 178–81.

55. Authors include Testut, Saroste Carillon, Sergent, Patel, Forgue, and Quenu. Ngạc, et al., *Lớp Sinh Viên*, 27.

56. Bách, et al., *100 Năm*, 180.

57. Ngạc, et al., *Lớp Sinh Viên*. Aso and Guénel, "The Itinerary," 291–306.

58. Bách, et al., *100 Năm*.

59. Ninh, *A World Transformed*, 18–20.

60. Ibid., 102.

61. Huy, et al., *Di Sản Ký Ức*, 198.

62. Bách, et al., *100 Năm*, 179.

63. Nguyễn Thúc Tùng, interview, June 2, 2013.

64. TTLT3 PTT 639, "Buôi Họp Của Bộ Y Tế, Bộ Quốc-Gia Giáo-Dục Va Quân-Y-Cục Để Thảo Luận Vê Việc Tổ-Chức Trường Y-Sĩ Việt Nam," 4.

65. Bách, et al., *100 Năm*, 181.

66. Nguyễn Thúc Tùng, interview, June 2, 2013.

67. Ibid.

68. Thompson, "Medicine, Nationalism, and Revolution," 121.

69. TTLT 3, Ủy Ban Kháng Chiến Hành Chính Nam Bộ, 1945–55, HS 988, Tu-Tuong Nhiem-Vu Duong-Huong Cua Y-Hoc Cach-Mang Viet-Nam.

70. Thompson, "Medicine, Nationalism, and Revolution."

71. C. Michele Thompson, *Vietnamese Traditional Medicine: A Social History* (Singapore: NUS Press, 2015). See also Hoang Bao Chau, "The Revival and Development of Vietnamese Traditional Medicine: Towards Keeping the Nation in Good Health," in *Southern Medicine*, ed. Monnais, Thompson, and Wahlberg, 133–51.

72. TTLT 3, Ủy Ban Kháng Chiến Hành Chính Nam Bộ, 1945–55, HS 988, Buc Tho Than Kinh Goi Cac Ban Dong-Nghiep Eastern Medicine.

73. Ibid.

74. Ibid.

75. Discussed in Bách, et al., *100 Năm*.

76. Nguyễn Thúc Tùng, interview, June 2, 2013.

77. TTLT 3, PTT, 2849, "Tập Thư Trao Đổi Giữa Bác Sỹ Tôn Thất Tùng Với Đ/C Phạm Văn Đồng, Trần Quý Kiên, Anh Bảy Về Tình Hình Tổ Chức Và Phương Tiện Chữa Bệnh Năm 1953." Letter to Anh Tô on May 22, 1953.

78. Thompson, "Medicine, Nationalism, and Revolution," 131. See also Goscha, *Vietnam*, 212–4.

79. TTLT 3, Ủy Ban Kháng Chiến Hành Chính Nam Bộ, 1945–55, HS 988, Phuong Phap Giu Yen Va De Lau Ngay Khong Thay Bang, 14–15.

80. TTLT 3, Ủy Ban Kháng Chiến Hành Chính Nam Bộ, 1945–55, HS 988, Chan Doan Thuong Tich Chien Tranh.

81. Goscha, *Vietnam*, 203.

82. Nguyễn Thúc Tùng, interview, June 2, 2013.

83. Ibid.

84. TTLT 3, Ủy Ban Kháng Chiến Hành Chính Nam Bộ, 1945–55, HS 988, Tu-Tuong Nhiem-Vu Duong-Huong Cua Y-Hoc Cach-Mang Viet-Nam.

85. Bách, et al., *100 Năm*, 2002, 147.

86. TTLT 3 PTT 2768, "Thông-Tư Về Viềc Câp Thuốc Cho Bô-Đôi Đia-Phương," June 12, 1950.

87. TTLT 3, Ủy Ban Kháng Chiến Hành Chính Nam Bộ, 1945–55, HS 988, Nghi Quyet An Hoi Nghi Quan Day Y Nam Bo, 9.

88. TTLT 3, Ủy Ban Kháng Chiến Hành Chính Nam Bộ, 1945–55, HS 988, To Chuc vaf Le Loi Lam Viec, 2.

89. Goscha, *Vietnam*, 212–14.

90. Wendland, *A Heart*, 2010.

91. Ibid.

## CHAPTER 6

# The Expansion and Transformation of Medical Education in Indonesia During the 1950s in Jakarta and Surabaya

*Vivek Neelakantan*

Between 1945 and 1957, as Southeast Asian nations declared de facto independence from colonial rule, their primary concern was to create a strong and healthy population, a necessary prerequisite for economic development. Thus, public health became a significant component of nation-building not only in terms of resurrecting a strong and healthy nation free of disease, but also in ensuring increased respectability of individual nations on the world stage. Due to an acute shortage of doctors, countries of the region were unable to address pressing public health concerns such as the control of endemic diseases, particularly malaria, tuberculosis, yaws, and leprosy, which vitiated the overall productivity of the population.[1]

Like any other newly independent Southeast Asian nation, Indonesia also had its share of public health problems when it declared independence in 1945. It suffered from an acute shortage of physicians. Most Dutch physicians had left, and to compound the shortage, the Indonesian medical schools only graduated a modest number of fewer than 30 physicians annually. Indonesia attempted to remedy this shortage of physicians by changing the curricula at the existing medical schools and by founding new schools on the outer islands. The Indonesians had inherited the Dutch model of medical education, a model that followed the German model which emphasized research and individual study, allowing students to sit their examinations whenever they felt adequately prepared. Starting in 1952, proposals were made to refashion the medical curricula based on the American system, which fostered problem-solving and critical thinking, and introduced cohort-based rather than individual examinations. Universitas Indonesia (UI) in Jakarta and Universitas Airlangga (UNAIR) in Surabaya affiliated themselves with the University of California medical school in order to implement the American model. In reality, the choice between the Dutch and American models of medical education was constrained by local health care priorities within Indonesia, budgetary limitations, and Cold War politics. This chapter explores how Indonesia managed to respond to its public health problems such as a high prevalence of maternal and infant mortality, malnutrition, and endemic diseases, by increasing the rate of graduation of physicians from its medical schools.

The 1950s coincided with the Cold War in Southeast Asia. At the time, the British, French, Dutch, American, Soviet, and Chinese models of medical education, which often competed against each other, were emulated, transformed, or rejected in specific local contexts. Indonesia refashioned the medical curricula in Jakarta and Surabaya based on the curricula prevalent in North American medical schools. This was part of the larger strategy of the US and international aid agencies, particularly the Rockefeller Foundation and the China Medical Board, to win the loyalty of Indonesian leaders in the fight against communism. The Indonesian leaders were initially suspicious of international aid initiatives in medical education as infringements on the country's hard-won political sovereignty. In this chapter, I argue that the transformation of medical education in Indonesia based on the American model was a result of the balance between nation-building priorities and Cold War politics.

Language was a major inhibiting factor in Indonesian medical schools' transition from Dutch to American curricula. Due to its association with the anti-colonial struggle, Bahasa Indonesia replaced Dutch as the medium of instruction in Indonesian medical schools; however, textbooks were published either in English or German—languages foreign to most local students. Several obstacles impeded the implementation of the American model, in particular a lack of infrastructure and a shortage of qualified teachers. Further, the transition from the Dutch to the American model was unevenly implemented, in particular at UNAIR, due to inadequate administrative support from the Ministry of Education. Since there was hardly any process of selection to enter the medical school, annual attrition rates remained high, especially during the premedical year. Cohort-based teaching could not be successfully implemented due to a shortage of Indonesian academic staff. By 1969, the American model proved unsustainable at UNAIR and the medical school reverted to the Dutch curriculum, whereas its counterpart at UI continued to follow the American model.

## Medical Education in Jakarta: Transition from the Dutch to the American Model

From 1927 to 1942, the medical faculty at Batavia (Geneeskundige Hoogeschool, GHS) and subsequently at the UI in Jakarta (1950–54) followed the Dutch model of medical education, which itself followed the German model. According to the Dutch model, while students were required to finish a prescribed set of courses, examinations were individually administered and could be taken whenever the student felt prepared. The curriculum was rigorous: it emphasized extensive theoretical grounding in the natural sciences followed by a written examination. After completing the course of study, there was an oral examination.[2] As a result, approximately 80 per cent of the students failed the examinations.

The Dokter Djawa School, which was the outcome of initiatives to organize medical education in Batavia, started in 1851.[3] That year, Willem Bosch, head of the Netherlands Indies medical service, organized the training of local medical professionals to be employed as vaccinators. The training course lasted two years. The medical graduates were awarded the title of *Dokter Djawa* (Javanese doctor), which distinguished them from the university-trained Dutch physicians. In the beginning, Malay was the language of instruction, but it was replaced by Dutch in the mid-1870s, because the teachers at the school were convinced that Malay did not suffice as a language of scientific instruction. In 1875, the duration of the training program was raised from two to seven years, of which two years were devoted to a basic foundation in science and five to medical training.[4] In addition, starting in 1890, students were given outpatient training for surgery and eye diseases.

In 1902, the school was renamed STOVIA (School ter Opleiding van Inlandsche Artsen; School for the Education of Native Physicians) and the curriculum was revised once again. STOVIA students who successfully passed all of their examinations were awarded the title of *Inlandsch Arts* (Native Physician). In 1913, the NIAS (Nederlandsch-Indische Artsen School; Netherlands-Indies Physicians School) was established in Surabaya; it followed the STOVIA curriculum. Students who successfully completed their medical training at the NIAS would be conferred the title of *Indisch Arts* (Indies Physician; from that date, the STOVIA also awarded this degree).[5] In 1927, the GHS opened in Batavia, awarding the same medical degrees as universities in the Netherlands. At that time, the STOVIA no longer accepted new students, but students who had already enrolled could finish their studies or transfer to the GHS. The NIAS did not change; consequently, there were two courses of study open to students in Indonesia.

At the beginning of the Japanese occupation in 1942, the medical schools at Jakarta and Surabaya were closed for one year. In 1943, the Japanese established the Ika Daigaku (Medical School) in Jakarta. The duration of medical education in Ika Daigaku was five years.[6] Thirteen STOVIA and GHS graduates, including Bahder Djohan, Boentaran Martoatmodjo, and Soetomo Tjokronegoro, were appointed as lecturers at the Ika Daigaku. They also became members of the Izi Hoko Kai, which was a precursor to the Indonesian Medical Association (Ikatan Dokter Indonesia) that was established soon after independence in 1950. The duration of medical study at the Ika Daigaku included one year of practical training.

Soon after the defeat of the Japanese in the Pacific War in August 1945 and the proclamation of Indonesian independence on August 17, 1945, the Balai Perguruan Tinggi Republik Indonesia (Institute of Higher Education of the Indonesian Republic), with faculties of medicine and law, was inaugurated by Soetomo Tjokronegoro.[7] In early October 1945, the Dutch returned to the Indonesian archipelago and the Netherlands Indies Civil Administration (NICA) established control over Jakarta. Due to the political uncertainty in the period that followed, the Indonesian Faculty of Medicine was transferred to Yogyakarta and Klaten in central Java, then under the control of the revolutionaries.[8]

In 1946, the Dutch established the Nooduniversiteit (Emergency University) in Jakarta, with faculties of medicine, law, humanities, agriculture, and technology. In 1947, its name was changed to Universiteit van Indonesië. Gradually, as the Dutch reasserted their control over the Indonesian archipelago, they established faculties of mathematics and physics in Bandung (within the former Technical College buildings), faculties of veterinary medicine and agriculture in Bogor, a second medical faculty in Surabaya, and a faculty of economics at Makassar—all of which were affiliated to the newly established Universiteit van Indonesië.[9] The Universiteit, which was then under Dutch control, was able to continue its educational programs uninterrupted until December 1949.

During the first and the second Dutch military actions (1948–49), the activities of the Indonesian Faculty of Medicine, which were under the control of the revolutionaries at Klaten, were disrupted as no buildings could be provided for lecture rooms or laboratories.[10] The Sultan of Yogyakarta offered the residence of the Crown Prince for housing the medical school. With support from the Sultan of Yogyakarta and the Jajasan Balai Perguruan Tinggi Gadjah Mada (Institute of Higher Education, Gadjah Mada, a private foundation), a private university was founded in November 1949. It comprised a faculty of medical science, dentistry, pharmacy, agriculture, and veterinary science, with Sardjito, a STOVIA alumnus (1915) and bacteriologist as the first president (1950–61).[11] Like the medical faculty at Jakarta (1950–54) and its counterpart at Surabaya, which maintained the Dutch model of medical education between 1954 and 1960, the UGM medical school also continued the Dutch model until 1965.[12] In 1950, the Universiteit van Indonesië was renamed Universitet Indonesia (UI), then Universitas Indonesia in 1954.[13] By now, the Republic of Indonesia had three medical schools, that is, the Faculty of Medicine at Yogyakarta (UGM), the Faculty of Medicine at Jakarta, and the Faculty of Medicine at Surabaya, under UI administration from 1950 to 1954, which was amalgamated with UNAIR in 1954.

From 1950 to 1954, the UI medical schools at Jakarta and Surabaya followed the Dutch medical model. Technically, any student who passed the high school examination was accepted into the premedical year. Consequently, the number of students who were admitted into the premedical year, plus a number of students who had to repeat classes, exceeded by far the physical capacity of the available classrooms.[14] The premedical curriculum was a burden for the medical schools at Jakarta and Surabaya as the instruction in botany, zoology, chemistry, and physics did not strictly constitute a part of the medical curriculum. Teachers were recruited on a part-time basis from other institutions such as the School of Natural Sciences or the School of Technology, and could not therefore devote their full attention to developing a strong academic foundation among aspiring medical students.

Unfortunately, during the early 1950s, there was a steady exodus of Dutch lecturers and other scientists to the Netherlands as the monthly remuneration of Dutch academics in post-independent Indonesia could not keep pace with the rising inflation. This was exacerbated by the Indonesian Decree (1946) stipulating that all academic lectures had to be delivered in Indonesian.[15] Many of them had experienced considerable hostility and were eager to leave the country. Running medical schools became very difficult as vacancies could not be filled by Indonesian academics. The number of physicians who graduated from the medical schools at Jakarta and Surabaya was small (estimated at less than 30 for the early 1950s). Most of the new medical graduates preferred to work as private practitioners in urban areas where salaries were higher. In the early 1950s, the Indonesian government recognized that its most acute needs were to raise the levels of health care and medical education.

As a way out of this situation, in 1952, Professor of Pathology Soetomo Tjokronegoro (Universitas Indonesia) approached Francis Scott Smyth, the chairperson of the Foreign Graduate Student Committee on the Committee of Education, University of California, San Francisco (UCSF), with a proposal to affiliate the UI Faculties of Medicine at Jakarta and Surabaya with UCSF, with a view to remodel the medical curriculum based on the American model. Together, Tjokronegoro and Smyth attacked the question of how Indonesia could increase the supply of Indonesian medical professionals.

During the 1950s, Indonesia was the focus of several international aid-based organizations including the Technical Cooperation Administration (TCA) of the American government, Australian Aid (administered through the Colombo Plan), the World Health Organization (WHO), and private philanthropies such as the Ford Foundation, China Medical Board, and the Rockefeller Foundation. At the time, the Soviet Union loaned US$110 million to Indonesia for general economic and social development, and to establish a faculty of technical education in Amboina.[16] The interest of Western agencies in Indonesia was due to its geopolitical significance in the Cold War, particularly after the communist victory in mainland China. Moreover, the US was apprehensive of the spread of communism to Southeast Asia. As a preventative strategy, it used technical assistance, particularly Harry Truman's Point Four Program, to advance the economic and social development of newly decolonized Southeast Asian nations, especially Indonesia. In 1951, Indonesian foreign minister Achmad Subardjo committed Indonesia to Section 511a (Economic and Technical Assistance of the US Military Security Act), that is, to US technical assistance without sanction from the parliament, giving rise to a general fear that Indonesian foreign policy would become entangled with the politics of the Western Bloc.[17]

Indonesians were initially skeptical of accepting any kind of American aid, including education personnel, for fear that technical aid had political or military strings attached to it.

A major problem that international aid agencies operating in Indonesia, in particular the Rockefeller Foundation and the China Medical Board, had to grapple with was the development of basic medical education or the building of research capacity.[18] The China Medical Board elected to emphasize basic medical education that would orient future doctors to public health problems in Indonesia, whereas the Rockefeller Foundation concentrated on developing Indonesia's capabilities in biomedical research. The China Medical Board directed its efforts towards developing medical education on the island of Java, the political nucleus of Indonesia. Soedjono Djoened Poesponegoro, Dean of the Medical School and Professor of Pediatrics, had tried to secure the assistance of the Rockefeller Foundation for the UI medical school for much of the 1950s, but his requests had always been declined.[19] The Rockefeller Foundation was unwilling to offer fellowships to Indonesian physicians studying abroad during the 1950s due to the unsettled political conditions in the country.

The affiliation of the medical school at UI with UCSF was implemented in a volatile political context charged with Cold War politics. E. Ross Jenney (Chief of the US Technical Mission to Indonesia and Head of the Public Health Division from 1950–53) proposed "adoption" of Indonesian universities by their American counterparts as part of the technical assistance program. The Indonesian Ministry of Education and Culture expressed reservations regarding the use of the word "adoption," stating that this signified the subservience of Indonesian universities to their American counterparts.[20] For this reason, the word "adoption" was dropped from the American proposal when the question of affiliating the UI medical school with the UCSF was proposed in 1952.[21] But problems arose on the American side. The regents of the University of California argued that the local medical faculties were too burdened with returned World War II veterans and with upgrading the existing medical faculties to meet the requirements of the local population. They also questioned the feasibility of transplanting the American medical education model to the Indonesian medical schools given that Indonesia's public health conditions differed drastically from those in America.[22] As a result of mutual misgivings, no agreement could be brokered for affiliating the two universities at the official level, although there was some progress.[23] Smyth was initially unprepared to advocate affiliation between the two faculties as the regents of the University of California lacked sufficient information related to the health conditions of Indonesia. In anticipation of the proposal to affiliate, in 1953, Dr Thomas Nathaniel Burbridge of the UCSF, Department of Pharmacology, was sent to Jakarta to reorganize the department of pharmacology at UI. His visit was sponsored by the China Medical Board.

The memorandum of understanding between the University of California Medical School and Faculty of Medicine at UI was officially signed on June 29, 1954 and effective from July 1, 1954 to June 30, 1957. Completely financed by the ICA (International Cooperation Administration), it involved affiliating the faculties of medicine at both institutions. As per the provisions of the contract, 31 American medical educators with expertise in basic medical and clinical fields were deputed to Indonesia for periods ranging from six months to seven years.[24] The University of California team of visiting lecturers offered assistance to the medical faculty of UI in the selection of prospective medical students and the reorganization of the medical curriculum. The latter could not be implemented until 1955 as American lecturers could not be recruited on such short notice.

On December 17, 1954, the UI medical faculty appointed a committee consisting of Sarwono Prawirohardjo, Professor of Obstetrics and Gynecology; Soedjono Djoened Poesponegoro; Edwin Schultz, Chairman of the University of California-Field Staff and Visiting Professor of Pathology; Sutarman, Professor of Physiology; Satrio, Associate Professor of Anatomy (Minister of Health in Indonesia between 1959 and 1966); Raden Mochtar, Associate Professor of Public Health; and Sujito Danusuproto, Associate Professor of Physics.[25] The function of this committee was to propose changes to the medical curriculum and increase the supply of doctors. The committee proposed that the duration of medical training be reduced to six years and specifically recommended the introduction of the American model, in particular, the periodic assessment of the students' performances in tests administered by the course instructor. The medical school's adoption of the American curriculum in 1955 was intended to foster problem-based experiential learning and initiate cohort-based—rather than individual—examinations, so that an entire batch of doctors could graduate from the medical school each year.

Prior to the affiliation of the UI medical school with its counterpart at UCSF, the UI raised the following two questions with the Curriculum Development Committee of the medical school:[26]

(a) Will the American model of medical education be oriented towards teaching or research?

(b) Will the development of the new curriculum be focused on training students to diagnose and treat individual diseases, or will it emphasize the social aspects of health care?

The vision of the Curriculum Development Committee was to increase the number of students graduating from the medical school each year without compromising the quality of medical education. The Committee observed that Indonesia had to mobilize physicians who would address the exigencies of national reconstruction and development, and meet the aim of resuscitating a strong and healthy population free of disease. The new curriculum would educate physicians who were capable of carrying out rural and community health programs. But the main goal of affiliating the UI medical school with its counterpart at UCSF was to train teachers of the former to a high level of competence so that they would be able to educate large numbers of medical practitioners. This would in turn generate a multiplier effect, according to John S. Wellington, Associate Dean of the UCSF Medical School.[27]

The American medical model originated in the mid-nineteenth century. Medical educators in the US de-emphasized didactic teaching by lecturers, advocating instead that medical education produce problem-solvers and critical thinkers who could evaluate information independently.[28] Clinical research required making meticulous bedside observations of patients. In every department of the medical school, there was congruence between teaching required courses and the specific research interests of the teaching faculty.[29] Instructors were passionate about teaching the students research problems they themselves had encountered when pursuing their own research. The medical curriculum in the US was arranged logically—preclinical subjects, namely anatomy, biochemistry, physiology, bacteriology, and pharmacology, oriented the medical student for clinical study.[30] The courses undertaken during the preclinical and clinical years were intended to familiarize the medical student with the basic processes governing the functioning of structure, function, and behavior of the human organism in health and disease. Instruction emphasized active learning through small group discussions in which students mastered problem solving skills. A great deficiency of the American model was the scant attention devoted to issues such as preventative medicine, occupational medicine, and the doctor-patient relationship. In Indonesia, however, public health was incorporated

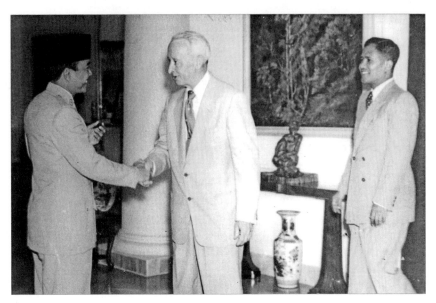

**Figure 1.** Breaking the ice: President Soekarno (left) receives Professor Francis Scott Smyth from the University of California, San Francisco on August 25, 1952 (Album Idayu 811, *Perpustakaan Nasional Image Collections*, used with permission).

into the revised medical curriculum following the initiative of Raden Mochtar to sensitize future medical students to public health problems relevant to Indonesia.

The most noticeable change associated with the switch from the Dutch to the American curriculum at the UI medical school was the structuring of the lectures. Under the old approach prior to 1955, lectures were delivered in a didactic style with very little input from the students. The number of hours devoted to premedical, preclinical, and clinical subjects was flexible; and students could choose not to attend classes. Teaching at the premedical level largely emphasized anatomy and histology; there was no integration of the lectures with laboratory work. With the introduction of the American model in 1955, lectures were structured around the semester. At the preclinical level, the teaching hours dedicated to physiology and biochemistry equaled those of anatomy and histology, with the objective of deepening the student's conceptual understanding of metabolic processes.[31] Beginning in 1955, training of medical students in public health commenced during the preclinical (second) year and included instruction in public health theory, medical ecology, demography, home economics, social anthropology, and statistics. During the third year, students were trained in the prevention of infectious diseases, health education, interpretation of epidemiological data, and smallpox vaccination. Theoretical training in public health thus synchronized well with practical training such as administering vaccinations. At the commencement of clinical study (the fourth year), students received instruction in social medicine. During the clerkship period (fifth year), students would be posted in maternal and child health centers in pilot demonstration projects and would subsequently discuss their field experiences in class. Students also conducted surveys related to the impact of socio-economic factors affecting the general health at the household level. In the sixth year, they undertook internships in public health lasting two months, worked as general practitioners and held discussions with regency health officers on public health questions.

Firman Lubis, formerly Professor of Public Health and Preventive Medicine at UI, recounts in his memoir *Jakarta 1960-an* that during his student days at the Faculty of Medicine, UI, subsequent to the introduction of the American model, practicals supplemented lectures in biology, chemistry, and physics even during the premedical year.[32] Medical training was intensive as students had to prepare themselves for periodic tests by consulting recommended readings in the library. They had difficulty in following textbooks as these were published either in English or German, both foreign languages to most of them. With the commencement of preclinical study, students were oriented to the theory of public health and had practicals in anatomy. In the third year, they were introduced to biochemistry with a special focus on enzymes, vitamins, and metabolism. Although medical students were introduced to various aspects of public health in the preclinical year, the teaching of epidemiology and public health statistics was unsatisfactory as the majority of students lacked a strong mathematical foundation to comprehend the lectures.[33] Attrition rates were consequently as high as 80 per cent per cohort.

Clinical instruction at UI—aimed at facilitating comprehension of the lectures—was fragmented into watertight compartments, often led by faculty members who jealously safeguarded their disciplinary boundaries.[34] Clinical training in pediatrics, midwifery, and surgery afforded an opportunity for medical students to apply theoretical knowledge gained during the first three years of premedical and preclinical study through careful bedside observation of patients.[35] During internship training in midwifery, students studied cases of septic abortion at Rumah Sakit Tjipto Mangoenkoesoemo, the UI medical school's teaching hospital. Soon after attending such cases, the lecturers would organize students into small groups and initiate discussions centering upon the socioeconomic factors affecting the prevalence of septic abortion and associated risks and the necessity of introducing birth control as a prophylactic measure.[36] The Department of Obstetrics and Gynecology at UI initiated a pilot project using midwives to train *dukun bayis* (traditional birth attendants) in scientific birthing practices. Medical students assisted midwives during obstetrical emergencies. The clinical training of medical students at the UI thus afforded an opportunity for problem-based experiential learning that sought to situate public health problems within their broader socioeconomic contexts and develop pragmatic solutions.

Under the affiliation, a number of Indonesian students received advanced instruction at UCSF. Wellington interviewed 36 Indonesians who had undergone one-year postgraduate training in pathology and clinical medicine in late 1967, in order to gauge the relevance of the American model of medical education to Indonesia. His interviews revealed that trainees were disappointed on return to Indonesia as they acutely perceived a difference between conditions in American medical schools and medical practices in Indonesia.[37] They were unable to apply the basic principles learnt during their training, especially critical thinking, on return to Indonesia as students were not habituated to independent learning and using the library. In the words of one interviewee: "A national inferiority complex still constitutes a problem and causes too much paralysis of thinking when confronted by authority."[38] The quote illustrates that Indonesian students were accustomed to uncritically following what was taught in the lecture. *Adat* (tradition) also decreed that students never ask questions of their teachers. Trainees also faced colleague resistance in introducing new ideas extant in American medical schools.[39]

The introduction of the American curriculum at UI since 1954–55 was criticized by Slamet Iman Santoso, president of UI from 1958–65, in his biography *Warna Warni Pengalaman Hidup* (*Colorful Life Experiences*). According to him, the execution of the American model at UI was such that if students failed even a single course, they had to repeat the whole year. The high standards of the American curriculum could not be sustained as most lectures were delivered by graduate assistants. With the introduction of the American curriculum in 1954–55, the number of physicians graduating from the medical school more than doubled. Yet, a decade later, Indonesia continued to suffer from one of the lowest ratios of physicians to total population in the world, estimated at 1 doctor per 25,000 people. This roughly translated into 4,000 doctors for a population of approximately 100 million.[40] For these reasons, Indonesian physicians had a much greater social role compared to countries where the ratio of physicians to the total population was much higher.

Between 1955 and 1967, the combination of a pervasive mobilization mentality and a conceptualization of health as an important component of nation-building created a niche for Indonesian physicians as agents of social change. In his memoir, Satrio recollects that during the 1959 smallpox outbreak in Jakarta, he mobilized medical students from UI to undertake mass vaccination campaigns.[41] At the time, Chinese Indonesian physician Tan S. Hien (a 1958 alumnus from the UI medical school) was posted in a Community Rural Health Demonstration Project in Lemah Abang, funded by aid from the US.[42] Hien observed that doctors enlisted for compulsory public service were forced to supplement their meager incomes through private practice. During his routine visits to health centers in and around Lemah Abang, he noted that paramedical personnel had used scare tactics to prevent villagers from being examined by doctors and charged informal fees. They feared that competition from doctors would affect their lucrative private practice. But, in some cases, paramedical personnel would be trained by physicians as the latter were in short supply during the late 1950s.

Whereas 157 students graduated under the new curriculum at the UI medical school in 1959, in contrast to 59 a year earlier, it would be wrong to conclude that the increase in the number of graduates had a positive impact on the quality of health services that the population of Indonesia could access for three reasons. First, newly graduated physicians did not immediately enter the public health services for assignment to rural areas as many of them chose to pursue postgraduate training in medicine. Those who completed their postgraduate training became teachers in the medical faculties not only at UI, but also in new medical schools, especially those in Medan, Bukittinggi, and Makassar. Second, the need for medical manpower in Indonesia was tremendous. By the mid-1960s, although Indonesia's population had grown to over 100 million, the total number of physicians, including those in teaching and public service, was no more than 3,000. Given Indonesia's unfavorable doctor-to-patient ratio, even a doubling of the number of physicians would have only a minuscule impact on the quality of health services that the country's population could access. Third, in order for effective delivery of health services, Indonesia needed not only large numbers of physicians but also the training of paramedical personnel.

## Medical Education in Surabaya

The history of medical education in Surabaya began in 1913 with the establishment of the NIAS, the curriculum of which was similar to the STOVIA and continued until the outbreak of the Pacific War in 1941. From 1942 until the first Dutch military action (1948), medical education in Surabaya was suspended. In 1948, the Dutch established the Faculteit der Geneeskunde (Faculty of Medicine), which was then affiliated to the Universiteit van Indonesië under the leadership of A.B. Droogleever Fortuyn, who was Professor of Genetics and Veterinary Science.[43] Soon after the transfer of sovereignty to the Indonesian Republic in December 1949, the medical faculty at Surabaya was transferred to the newly established UNAIR and continued to employ the Dutch model of medical education until 1960. As incoming medical students were admitted as soon as they graduated from high school without being competitively selected through an entrance examination, nearly 60–70 per cent of students failed the premedical and preclinical courses annually.[44]

Beginning in 1955, academics from the medical faculty at the newly constituted UNAIR, particularly M. Soetojo (Professor of Surgery and Visiting Scholar in 1955) and Oey Hway Kiem (Lecturer of Physiology), proposed introducing the American medical curriculum. Their aim was to advance the development of problem-based learning so that students could apply principles learnt in the classroom to solve concrete problems such as reducing maternal mortality and malnutrition among infants.

The contract to affiliate the UNAIR medical school with the University of California medical school remained suspended until 1959 due to the strained US-Indonesian relationship following Soekarno's move towards "guided democracy" and the abrogation of Indonesian parliamentary institutions.[45] As a result, the existing contract of the University of California with the UI medical school came under scrutiny in the US. Due to the volatile political situation, Soedjono Djoened Poesponegoro recommended that Dr Smyth cancel his visit to Jakarta in 1958, work out a phase-out program with the UI medical school, and sign a contract affiliating the UNAIR and the University of California medical schools.[46] Despite the strained political relationship and UNAIR medical school Dean J.C. Kapitan's unexpected demise in October 1959, the UNAIR medical faculty signed a six-year contract (1960–66) with the University of California to restructure the curriculum.

The introduction of the American curriculum at UNAIR was constrained by several financial and administrative bottlenecks which were largely attributable to the high inflation rate, the depreciation of the rupiah in 1960, and the procedural difficulties encountered in securing counterpart funding from the University of California, which was disbursed in rupiahs. By 1960, the University of California had disbursed 7.5 million rupiahs (equivalent to a little less than US$70,000) via the Indonesian Ministry of Education, a sum that was inadequate considering the prevailing inflation rate of approximately 100 per cent and the eightfold depreciation in the international exchange value of the rupiah between 1952 and 1959.[47]

The academic heads within the medical school had little say in the annual budget that was proposed by the Dean of the UNAIR Medical Faculty and sent to the Ministry of Education, Jakarta, for approval. The centralization of the administrative apparatus at Jakarta proved a hindrance to the timely disbursement of funds requested by various departments of the medical faculty. As the UNAIR lacked a microbiology department, personnel from the East Java Provincial Laboratory undertook training of medical students in this subject. As such, a microbiology department at UNAIR had to be built from scratch. For these reasons, the American model was introduced piecemeal into the UNAIR medical school between 1959 and 1964.

The new curriculum was first implemented in 1959 for the sixth year.[48] The introduction of the American model in the sixth year, prior to the reconstruction of the premedical and preclinical levels of study, was somewhat premature—sixth-year students, who had been schooled according to the Dutch curriculum, were not adequately prepared for the clerkships. By 1964, the American curriculum was fully implemented at UNAIR. It involved the shortening of the duration of the preclinical courses from 18 months to 12 months, the addition of public health and psychiatry, as well as instruction in anatomy, physiology, and biochemistry.[49]

The implementation of the American model at UNAIR was impeded by the passive resistance of medical students who opposed the introduction of English-language medical textbooks. The Student Senate of the UNAIR medical school had a stronger nationalist orientation compared to its counterpart at UI, and viewed the introduction of English-language textbooks with suspicion, especially with the deteriorating US-Indonesian relationship in 1959.[50] In January 1965, the Student Senate of the Medical Faculty at UNAIR urged the Indonesian government to abrogate the affiliation of the UNAIR medical school with the University of California. It also supported President Soekarno's proposal to withdraw Indonesia from the UN.[51] The activities of the UNAIR Student Senate strained the affiliation project, so much so that towards mid-1965, the USAID (United States Agency for International Development) office in Jakarta instructed the University of California to withdraw its academic staff from Indonesia.[52] In 1966, the affiliation of UNAIR medical school with the University of California officially ended, although the American curriculum persisted until 1969.

Twelve physicians graduated every year from the UNAIR medical school prior to 1959. Between 1964 and 1967, with the complete restructuring of the curriculum based on the American model, the medical school managed to graduate 188 physicians each year.[53] The American model was unsuited to Indonesian conditions, especially at UNAIR, whereas this was not true at UI. While students at UI had to pass an entrance test followed by a psychometric test prior to gaining admission to the medical school, the same was not true for UNAIR.[54] Incoming medical students at UNAIR were admitted soon after they graduated from high school. As a result, they lacked the verbal skills critical to success in the medical school. The American curriculum intended to foster problem-based learning through intensive student participation in coursework and written examinations. UNAIR students, however, were not only unaccustomed to initiating discussions in the classroom but also lacked an adequate command of English. Even with the introduction of periodic tests, structured readings, and academic discussions in the classroom, medical students continued to view study only as a means of passing examinations. As the American curriculum was unsuited to the prevailing academic climate at the UNAIR medical school, in 1969 it was abrogated in favor of the older Dutch model. In contrast, the UI medical school has been continuing the American model since 1955.

## Conclusion

After independence, the Indonesian government enlisted the support of the China Medical Board, the Rockefeller Foundation, and the UCSF to strengthen the foundations of medical education and research, increase the number of medical school graduates, and improve the availability of physicians for the rural areas of the country. The transformation of the existing medical curricula at the UI and UNAIR faculties of medicine in Indonesia into one based upon the American model, as well as the establishment of new medical schools, especially in the outer islands of Sumatra and Sulawesi, were two strategies employed to increase the number of graduating physicians. But a combination of nationalist anxieties about ensuring Indonesia's technological autonomy amidst divergent pulls of the Cold War, the foreign exchange crisis during the late 1950s, and bureaucratic bottlenecks led to measures that regulated international aid. Such measures circumvented institutional autonomy, particularly with reference to the UNAIR medical school.

With the introduction of the American model of medical education, Indonesia succeeded in doubling the number of physicians graduating from its medical schools annually. But the country continued to suffer from serious problems in making health services available and physicians faced high expectations from the local population. Whereas Indonesia focused on redressing the shortage of doctors by founding new medical schools and increasing the supply of doctors, for the CMB and the Rockefeller Foundation, the emphasis was not so much on the number of physicians graduating annually from the medical school as much as the quality of teaching. Deans of Indonesian medical schools often faced political pressure to increase the output of physicians, even at the cost of producing few teachers.

Meanwhile, Indonesian physicians who had undergone postgraduate training in the US during the 1950s and 1960s drew a clear line of demarcation between the curriculum at UI based on the American model and medical education in the US. The trainees were disappointed that they could not actually apply their expertise gained in the classroom due to a shortage of medical supplies, infrequency of autopsies, and colleague resistance. After the introduction of the American model, students learned to responsibly state their opinions and assert their rights, yet both the faculty's and students' adjustments to the American model was not without conflict.

Unfortunately, for a variety of reasons, the transformation of the medical curriculum based on the American model at Jakarta and Surabaya failed to maximize the output of physicians. Several problems were encountered: the new curriculum was implemented unevenly across the medical faculty at UNAIR. As there was hardly any screening of applicants, students with a weak medical background were often enrolled at premedical and preclinical levels. Attrition rates were consequently high. Cohort-based learning could not be fully implemented at UI and UNAIR due to a shortage of lecturers who elected for private medical practice in urban areas where remuneration for physicians was considerably higher. For these reasons, the transformation of medical education in Indonesia based on the American model remained constrained.

Even today, the ratio of Indonesian doctors to the total population is among the lowest in the world, as it was during the 1950s. Since 1995, there has been a 25 per cent decennial growth in the number of Indonesian physicians graduating from the country's medical schools. Yet, newly graduated doctors are unable to get jobs in public health centers or *Puskesmas* as they are forced to make under-the-table payments to local functionaries. In medical schools, the huge number of applicants has created wonderful money-making opportunities.[55] As such, the key to improving Indonesians' access to health care lies in curing the country's political ills such as corruption, collusion, and nepotism, rather than expanding the training programs for physicians and midwives.

## Archives

Parnassus Archives, University of California at San Francisco. *Projects in Medical Education: Indonesia Papers 1951–1966.*
Rockefeller Archive Center. File 02.1961. *General Correspondence*, Series 652 A.

## Notes

1.    Vivek Neelakantan, "The Campaign against the Big Four Endemic Diseases and Indonesia's Engagement with the WHO during the Cold War, 1950s," in *Public Health and National Reconstruction in Southeast Asia: International Influences, Local Transformations*, ed. Liping Bu and Ka-che Yip (Abingdon: Routledge, 2014), 154–74.
2.    Thomas Neville Bonner, *Becoming a Physician: Medical Education in Britain, France, Germany, and the United States, 1750–1945* (Baltimore: Johns Hopkins Press, 2000), 254–5.
3.    Liesbeth Hesselink, *Healers on the Colonial Market: Native Doctors and Midwives in the Dutch East Indies* (Leiden: KITLV, 2011), 83.
4.    Ibid., 265.
5.    Mus Harianto, *90 Tahun Pendidikan Dokter di Surabaya* (Surabaya: Fakultas Kedokteran Universitas Airlangga, 2003), 9.
6.    S. Somadikarta, Tri Wahyuning, M. Irsyam, and Boen Sri Oemarjati, *Tahun Emas Universitas Indonesia: Dari Balai ke Universitas*, vol. 1 (Jakarta:

Universitas Indonesia Press, 2000), 32. Soetomo Tjokronegoro, who graduated from the GHS in 1936, was a professor of pathology at Balai Perguruan Tinggi from 1945–47. Sarwono Prawirohardjo graduated from GHS in Gynecology in 1937.

7. Somadikarta et al., *Tahun Emas Universitas Indonesia*, 12–13.

8. Sardjito and Asikin Widjajakusumah were the leading academics of the medical faculty of Balai Perguruan Tinggi. Sardjito conducted preclinical lectures at Klaten whereas Asikin Widjajakusumah was in charge of clinical training at Solo.

9. Somadikarta et al., *Tahun Emas Universitas Indonesia*, 15.

10. Sardjito, *The Development of the Universitas Gadjah Mada (UGM)* (Jogjakarta: Universitas Gadjah Mada, 1958), 6–7.

11. Ibid., 8.

12. Ibid., 11. The Dutch model of medical education was implemented at UGM from 1949 onwards, after the faculty of medicine was inaugurated, and the system continued into the mid-1960s. The American model of medical education was introduced only as late as 1965.

13. I prefer to use the name Universitas Indonesia (UI) to avoid confusion.

14. Universitas Indonesia, Fakultas Kedokteran, *Laporan Perkembangan Pendidikan Dokter Pada Fakultas Kedokteran Universitas Indonesia* (Jakarta: Fakultas Kedokteran Universitas Indonesia, 1960), 19–26. Of the 626 students attending premedical classes in 1954, 301 failed the premedical examination and were forced to repeat an academic year. For the academic period from 1951–52, only approximately one-sixth of the premedical students managed to qualify for the preclinical stage of medical education, including those who had attempted the premedical examinations more than once. At the preclinical level, approximately one-seventh of the candidates (38 out of approximately 280 candidates from 1951–54) managed to qualify for entry into the clinical courses. At the end of the seventh-year examination, of the over 600 students who attended premedical classes at UI, only 20 to 30 physicians managed to graduate from the medical faculties at Jakarta and Surabaya, a number that was grossly insufficient to meet the needs of Indonesia's growing population estimated at approximately 80 million in the early 1950s.

15. Adam Messer, "Effects of the Indonesian National Revolution and the Transfer of Power on the Scientific Establishment," *Indonesia* 58 (1994): 41–68, 56.

16. Lannes Bruce Smith, *Indonesian-American Cooperation in Higher Education* (East Lansing, MI: Institute of Research on Overseas Programs, Michigan State University, 1960).

17. Anne M. Schmidt, "History of the University of California School of Medicine Affiliation with Medical Faculty of Universities at Djakarta and

Surabaya," in *Projects in Medical Education: Indonesia Papers 1951–1966*, Parnassus Archives, 12.

18.  "Indonesia Diary," File 02.1961 *General Correspondence*, Series 652 A, RAC (Rockefeller Archive Center).

19.  "Excerpt from Richmond K. Anderson (RKA): Dr R Soedjono Djoened Poesponegoro, Jakarta," File 02.1961 *General Correspondence*, Series 652 A, RAC.

20.  Firman Lubis, *Jakarta 1960–an: Kenangan Semasa Mahasiswa* (Jakarta: Masup, 2008), 160.

21.  Ibid.

22.  Francis Scott Smyth, "University of California Medical Science Teaching in Indonesia," *Journal of Medical Education* 32, no. 5 (1957): 344–5.

23.  Schmidt, "History of the University of California School of Medicine," 28. Until 1954, the politics of the Cold War influenced the decision whether or not to affiliate the faculties of medicine at Jakarta and Surabaya with the University of California. Even by February 1954, the regents of the University of California were undecided regarding the proposal to "affiliate" the University of California with the medical faculties at Jakarta and Surabaya, forcing UI to "negotiate with other institutions" (according to the wired correspondence between the Indonesian ambassador at Washington and Dr Smyth on February 26, 1954). At the same time, Indonesian diplomats were trying to establish their presence in Moscow, forcing the regents of the University of California to expedite the affiliation contract.

24.  E. Harold Hinman and Clifford A. Pease, "International Assistance to Medical Education," *Journal of Medical Education* 36 (1961): 1047.

25.  Schmidt, *History of the University of California School of Medicine*, 34–5.

26.  John S. Wellington and Ruth Boak, "Medical Science and Technology," in *Indonesia: Resources and their Technological Development*, ed. Howard W. Beers (Lexington: The University of Kentucky Press, 1970), 165–79.

27.  Smith, *Indonesian American Cooperation*, 80.

28.  Kenneth Ludmerer, *Time to Heal: American Medical Education from the Turn of the Century to the Era of Managed Care* (New York: Oxford University Press, 1999), 6.

29.  Ludmerer, *Time to Heal*, 37.

30.  Ibid., 66.

31.  *Report on the Development of Medical Education at the School of Medicine University of Indonesia Djakarta* (Djakarta: Fakultas Kedokteran Universitas Indonesia, 1960), 31.

32.  Lubis, *Jakarta 1960–an*, 169.

33.  Ibid., 178.

34.  Ibid., 272.

35.  Ibid., 280.
36.  Ibid., 296.
37.  John S. Wellington, "Indonesian Physicians Studying Abroad," *Journal of Medical Education* 43 (1968): 1185.
38.  Ibid., 1186.
39.  Ibid., 1188.
40.  Ibid., 1191.
41.  Satrio and Mona Lohanda, *Perjuangan dan Pengabdian: Mosaik Kenangan Professor Dokter Satrio, 1916–86* (Jakarta: Arsip Nasional Republik Indonesia, 1986), 190–4.
42.  Tan S. Hien, "Memoirs of Tan S. Hien," in *Memoirs of Indonesian Doctors and Professionals: More Stories that Shaped the Lives of Indonesian Doctors*, ed. Tjien Oei (Bloomington: Xlibris Corporation, 2010), 134–56.
43.  Agus Harianto, Urip Murtedjo, et al., eds, *90 Tahun Pendidikan Dokter di Surabaya* (Surabaya: Universitas Airlangga, 2003), 10–11.
44.  David Opdyke, "The Indonesian Medical Student and his Relation to Modern Medical Education," *Journal of Medical Education* 39 (1964): 755–61. For the period between 1952 and 1957, the medical school at Surabaya graduated only 63 physicians.
45.  US-Indonesian relations became strained following the Tjikini attempt on Soekarno's life in February 1957. In 1958, Sjafruddin Prawiranegara of the Masjumi party proclaimed a rival government in Padang, Central Sumatra, which denounced Soekarno's "guided democracy" and demanded regional autonomy based on faith in God. In February 1958, the Indonesian government accused Allen Pope of flying rebel planes into Central Sumatra and northern Sulawesi.
46.  Schmidt, *History of the University of California School of Medicine*, 74.
47.  Ibid., 93. The international exchange value of the rupiah had fallen eight-fold from 11.4 rupiahs to a dollar in 1952 to nearly 90 rupiahs in 1959–60.
48.  Mohammed Zaman, "Tugas Workshop Dalam Rangka Perkembangan Fakultas Kedokteran," *Madjalah Kedokteran Surabaya* 5, no. 4 (1968): n.p.
49.  Zaman, "Tugas Workshop."
50.  See Vivek Neelakantan, "Health and Medicine in Soekarno Era: Social Medicine, Public Health and Medical Education, 1949–1967" (PhD diss., University of Sydney, 2014), 205.
51.  Schmidt, "History of the University of California School of Medicine," 135.
52.  Ibid., 141–2.
53.  Ibid., 133.
54.  Lubis, *Jakarta 1960–an*, 103.
55.  Elizabeth Pisani, "Medicine for a Sick System," *Inside Indonesia* 111 (Jan.–Mar. 2013), accessed at http://www.insideindonesia.org/write-for-us/medicine-for-a-sick-system.

CHAPTER 7

# "Cambodian Pathology": Imagining Modern Biomedicine in the Cambodian-Soviet Medical Journal, *Revue Médico-Chirurgicale de l'Hôpital de l'Amitié Khméro-Soviétique* (1961–71)

*Jenna Grant*

> A scientific article is not of course a description or a distraction. It is a means of pressure on readers, convincing them to change what they believe, what they want to do, or what they want to be.[1]

In 1961, the Khmer-Soviet Friendship Hospital in Phnom Penh published the inaugural issue of its medical journal, the *Revue Médico-Chirurgicale de l'Hôpital de l'Amitié Khméro-Soviétique* (*The Medical-Surgical Review of the Khmer-Soviet Friendship Hospital*).[2] The hospital had opened only the year before, but there was much to show and to tell; it was the largest hospital in Southeast Asia at the time, a *vaste cité médicale* built by the USSR with state-of-the-art equipment and training from Soviet physicians. The journal (hereafter the *Revue*) contains case studies, epidemiological reports, comparative studies of treatments, and other discussions of clinical and experimental activities underway at the new hospital. The *Revue* also aims beyond the hospital—an indication of its intended prominence—to characterize health and medicine in Cambodia. Articles co-authored by Cambodian and Soviet physicians describe the particularities and universalities of a wide range of conditions—not only "tropical diseases"—and demonstrate the use of new medical technologies and techniques.

194

However, the articles do not just describe. Following Latour's sentiment that opens this chapter, the articles configure what Cambodian biomedicine should "want to do" and what it should "want to be." The *Revue* was published annually until 1969, with a final issue in 1970/71; yet despite its short life, it indicates much about the state of biomedicine in Cambodia at the time and imaginings of what future Cambodian biomedicine might be. The *Revue* enacts a biomedicine that is simultaneously Cambodian and cosmopolitan, a collaborative endeavor addressing the practical problems of the population, central to nation-building in a precarious though optimistic time. The *Revue*'s end in 1971 indicates just how precarious the arrangements that supported its publication were, and just how fleeting was the vision that biomedical knowledge production is important to new nations. Nonetheless, through practices of research, writing, and reading, the *Revue* taught how to be a doctor in post-independence Cambodia.

As a Cambodian-Soviet collaboration written in French, the *Revue* is a particular iteration of how biomedical training in Cambodia has always involved people, technologies, and politics that are both immediate and faraway. The *Revue* came into being during a time in Cambodian history when biomedicine was a key part of decolonization, and medicine practices—building hospitals and health centers, training professionals, publishing texts—are modes of nation-building and diplomacy. The Soviet model prioritized high-tech urban hospitals for training, care, and research, but it was only one model among others available at the time. Choosing a Soviet model over others—a Chinese system of barefoot doctors, for example—was a choice about Cambodia's postcolonial medical *and* national identity. Through analysis of this overlooked journal and the conditions in which it emerged, I seek to contribute a more nuanced understanding of Cambodian biomedicine in the 1960s than currently exists. If this is a Cambodian case study, it is also a study of a postcolonial relationship between Cambodia and the USSR. Thus, I also seek to show histories of medicine in which the Other of Southeast Asia is not easily categorized as "the West."

The *Revue* is unique in that it is a set of documents in which biomedicine was made experimental and knowable. Other medical practices, such as clinical care in public and private sectors, official policies, health statistics, or "black market" medicine may contradict the vision projected in the *Revue* of a scientific and high-tech biomedicine. Though I care very much what the Cambodian and Soviet authors write in the

*Revue*, my goal is not to assess the scientific validity of conclusions, appropriateness of treatment techniques, or effects on health policy. I write that the *Revue* "enacts" Cambodian biomedicine to foreground my perspective that the *Revue* brings a form of Cambodian biomedicine into being through particular discursive techniques, and in entanglement with social relations. This chapter, then, is an articulation of some of these techniques and relations. I see the *Revue* enacting, through its articles, images, prefaces, and authorship patterns, one form of medical practice among a multiplicity that existed in Cambodia at the time.

In the first section of this chapter, I sketch Cambodia's health system, including relevant domestic politics, and describe the construction of the Khmer-Soviet Friendship Hospital (hereafter KSFH). The discussion is based on analysis of primary sources—health-related materials from the National Archives of Cambodia (NAC) and Bophana Audio-visual Resource Center (Bophana Center); interviews and informal conversations—as well as secondary sources, particularly the work of anthropologists Anne Guillou, Ing-Britt Trankell, and Jan Ovesen. In the next section I describe the journal, highlighting discursive practices that define and imagine Cambodian medicine. I consider how authors characterize the diseases which burden Cambodians and the techniques for diagnosing and treating them as both similar to diseases and techniques of other nations or regions, and also particular to Cambodia; how advertising demonstrates development of a domestic pharmaceutical industry and engagement with the international therapeutic marketplace; and how, in prefaces and speech extracts, government officials highlight geopolitical relations as well as Cambodian medicine in relation to international medical science. This section is based on analysis of ten volumes of the *Revue*, which are located at the NAC. Despite my attempts otherwise, I was unable to interview contributors.[3]

I conclude with a critical reflection on the present moment: given that "medical diplomacy" has renewed currency today within the field of global health, might the *Revue* have something to tell us about possibilities for collaborative knowledge production? Here I follow a convention in postcolonial studies of looking to decolonial experience as a form of modernity in its own right, not in comparison to or deviation from a Euro-American ideal. Rather than the typical frame, which finds the situation in the postcolony lacking,[4] the *Revue* points to an alternative to contemporary forms of medical diplomacy marked by biosecurity and military humanitarianism.

## Biomedicine and Nation-Building in Sangkum Cambodia

Today, KSFH is commonly referred to as "Russian Hospital" in Khmer. It is still one of the largest government hospitals in Cambodia, and after decades of faded glory, parts of it are now being renovated. In the 1960s it was a spectacular demonstration of the government's commitment to improve public health and the medical system. This was apparent to Cambodians outside the fields of medicine or politics. A diplomatic official who was an education student at the time told me he remembers the hospital as a source of national pride.[5]

## Sangkum Modernity

The hospital was opened five years into the Sangkum era. The *Sangkum Reastr Niyum* (the People's Socialist Community) is both the political party and the ideology of Prince Norodom Sihanouk.[6] The Sangkum dates from 1955, Sihanouk's abdication of the throne to run for election two years after independence from France, to 1970, when his overthrow by General Lon Nol initiated civil war.[7] Sihanouk and official publications often refer to Sangkum ideology as "Buddhist socialism" or "Khmer socialism." Margaret Slocomb's analysis of state publications of the 1960s illuminates how Sangkum policymakers rejected Marxism because of its universality; instead, they argued that Cambodia's socialism must be particular to Cambodian morality, tradition, and history.[8] Cambodia's Buddhist socialism was officially described as following the "middle way," emphasizing social equilibrium, mutual assistance, and individual merit. Practically speaking, this meant a state-controlled economy but without land collectivization, and mixed ownership in some domains that would allegedly stimulate private savings and investment and protect the vulnerable from exploitation by foreign and national capitalist elites. Thus, Slocomb suggests, the Buddhist value of "the middle way" performed as an ideological foundation for both capitalist-socialist "duality" in Sangkum domestic policy and non-alignment in foreign policy.[9]

In addition to maintaining power, Sihanouk's most pressing concerns were to protect Cambodia from Thai and Vietnamese territorial incursions and stay out of the US/Vietnam war.[10] In terms of foreign policy, Sihanouk enacted a vigorous internationalism and neutrality. Cambodia joined the UN, Sihanouk attended the non-aligned movement and its conference in Bandung, and various Sangkum mouthpieces, such as *Cambodge d'Aujourd'hui* and reels of *Actualités*, documented the pomp of his many official visits to countries new and old, on both sides of the Cold War. These publications also documented the intense cultural production during the Sangkum in the domains of architecture, literature, education, public works, music, film, art, and medicine.[11] However, the later years of the Sangkum were marked by rapid depletion of public finances, increasing corruption, and persecution of those who advocated alternatives to the Sangkum.[12]

The KSFH was an exemplary gift, but it came at a time when gifts were available to newly independent nations. Sihanouk utilized the public face of neutrality to accept technical assistance and development aid from diverse sources, including the United States, China, France, the USSR, Japan, Czechoslovakia, Poland, and Yugoslavia.[13] He managed to obtain much of this aid in the form of grants and projects rather than loans. The United States was by far the largest donor, funding primarily the military but also infrastructure, education, and health projects. However, Sihanouk tired of the conditions of US aid, whose support of Thailand and South Vietnam imperiled domestic and regional security. In 1963 Sihanouk rejected US aid and in 1965 he severed diplomatic relations. Diplomatic relations with the USSR were severed during the subsequent regime, the Khmer Republic, in 1973.[14]

## Biomedicine During the Sangkum

Improving public health and the health system through constructing buildings and training health professionals was central to Sihanouk's national development agenda.[15] In 1955 there were 119 hospitals, district health centers, commune infirmaries, and dispensaries in Cambodia. Fourteen years later, in 1969, there were 656 of these health facilities, including an over fourfold increase in hospitals. Between 1955 and 1967 the number of pharmacies increased from 24 to 300 and the number of rural birthing centers from 60 to 644.[16] However, these numbers may be misleading: scholars suggest new buildings and their technologies were emptied of medicine, staff, and equipment soon after their opening in order to furnish the next inauguration.[17] While Phnom Penh received hospitals equipped with modern technologies, the "theatrical symbol par excellence of Sihanouk's modernism,"[18] facilities and care for the rural population were still lacking. Nonetheless, the spectacular increase in the number of medical institutions shows how, at a symbolic level, the health of the population was intimately linked to the vitality of the nation-state; the state was investing much of its energy and resources in a modernist bio-developmentalism.

*Actualités* and promotional films from the Sangkum include medicine in the national development project. A 24-minute Khmer language film about women's roles during the Sangkum depicts women manufacturing pharmaceuticals in a factory, operating an x-ray machine, assisting in surgery, and performing experiments in a medical laboratory (in addition to sowing rice, dancing, teaching, playing basketball, sailing, painting, and performing military exercises).[19] An undated *Actualité*, most likely from the early 1960s, devotes two of its five chapters to health-related activities: women being trained in "modern midwifery" (*wetyia chmop tumnup*) at a Phnom Penh training center, and "[a] day at the Takmao Health Center" informing us that the US/WHO/Cambodia are working together for prevention and treatment. In addition to breast-feeding mothers, a maternity ward, and children receiving vaccinations, we are also shown that the center has a lab and microscopes so that "health will rise up and blossom" (*sathiaronaq sokhaphibal luhk loah*).[20] Newsreels from the beginning of the Khmer Republic also depict health activities but not in the idiom of "national development." Rather, we see reel after reel of blood donations, military hospitals, and physical rehabilitation for soldiers, reflecting the government's focus on the civil war.[21]

The KSFH project made the USSR the first nation to rival the French in their influence over the Cambodian medical field.[22] KSFH was a state-of-the-art hospital, providing surgical procedures never before done in Cambodia, such as on the heart and goiter. Of the four main biomedical projects established during the 90-year period of French colonization—the military health service, the civilian health service or Assistance Médicale, the medical school, and the Institut Pasteur—the medical school and Institut Pasteur continued operation after independence. Decolonization of the medical system, and medical education in particular, was a slow process.[23] The language of medical training and administration remained French and physicians continued to train in France. The French built the large, modern Calmette hospital in Phnom Penh in 1959, but there was dispute between the Cambodians and the French as to who was in charge.[24] In contrast, KSFH was under Cambodian management.[25]

## Doctors During the Sangkum

As in other domains during the Sangkum, the health sector contained a combination of socialist and capitalist features. There was government control but doctors engaged in private clinical activities in addition to their government jobs, such that the medical profession existed in "ambivalent symbiosis" with the state, a term used by John Iliffe to describe the relation between the medical profession and the state in post-independence Kenya, Uganda, and Tanzania.[26]

Guillou's work on the medical profession from colonial times to the 1990s offers the most detailed study of medicine during the Sangkum era.[27] In complement to Iliffe's study, Guillou argues that, during the Sangkum, doctors developed a unique and "ambiguous" socio-professional role in Cambodian society, what she calls "*les médecins fonctionnaires-entrepreneurs*," combining government bureaucrat (*fonctionnaire*) and entrepreneur in private practice.[28] With this new category comes a more highly valued social status for physicians and other health workers. Guillou argues that under the Protectorate, few were attracted to join the medical profession because of the long duration of study, control by the French (often relayed through Vietnamese superiors), association of the medical profession with an unpopular civil service, and low pay. Before 1946, the year the École des Officiers de Santé was established in Phnom Penh, students had to go abroad to study medicine. During the Sangkum, the length of study came to be viewed as an investment, the association with the state guaranteed a form of protection, and the ability to open private practice made it lucrative. Guillou argues that this new socio-professional category emerges without conscious or collective action on the part of doctors. She identifies only three efforts on behalf of the profession—the Royal Society of Medicine of Cambodia, the Superior Health Council, and the Medical Association—and judges them quite poorly as short-lived, inconsistent, or ineffective in advocating for doctors' collective interests.[29] My analysis of the *Revue* attenuates this assessment; even if there is little evidence that writing for or reading the *Revue* brought forward a long-lasting professional identity, the journal takes the voice of, and addresses itself to, a Cambodian medical profession.

## Sangkum Medical Publications

The NAC hold a limited number of medical texts produced during the Sangkum, suggesting at least some effort at medical communication on the part of health workers or, at least, the government. The Ministry of Information published a French-language periodical, *La Santé Publique au Cambodge*,[30] of which two issues remain. These issues, from 1962 and 1964, contain short non-specialist articles and many photographs of buildings, babies, medical technologies, and of course, Sihanouk. They open with a famous quote from the *Hospital Edicts* of Jayavaraman VII, the Angkorian ruler who built medical stations and much of Angkor, and whose image Sihanouk often invoked.[31] The Royal Society of Medicine published a bulletin[32] containing research articles about different illnesses, and a few photographs, microphotographs, and drug advertisements. This bulletin bears the closest resemblance to the *Revue* in terms of content. In 1962, Kim Vien, director of the *Revue* from 1966–69, and V.A. Daniline, a Soviet physician at KSFH, published a small pamphlet on electrocardiography.[33] An unnamed entity published the *Bulletin of the Association of Health Workers*, a document that contains short, practical articles in Khmer on health and professional topics.[34] This is not an exhaustive survey of 1960s health-related publications; the archival record is incomplete. But from what is available at NAC, the *Revue* is the most sustained and significant health-related publication of the 1960s.

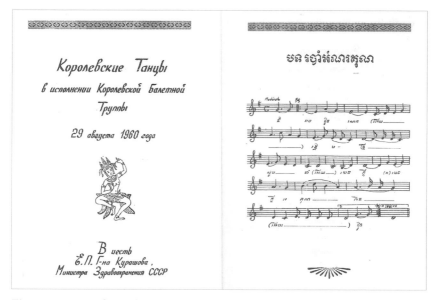

**Figure 1.** Page from the dance program for the inauguration of the Khmer-Soviet Friendship Hospital, August 29, 1960. (National Archives of Cambodia, Box 312).

## Building the "Vaste Cité Médicale"[35]

The idea for the Khmer-Soviet Friendship Hospital was initiated during Sihanouk's 1956 state visit to Moscow, the year diplomatic relations between the two nations were established.[36] In 1957 Sihanouk signed an agreement with then USSR Ambassador to Cambodia, Alexander S. Anikin, stating that the USSR would build a 500-bed hospital in Phnom Penh as a donation to the people of Cambodia. The buildings, which the Minister of Health praised as "like a huge bird with two wings,"[37] were designed, constructed, and equipped by the USSR. Construction began in 1958 and the hospital was completed and inaugurated in a large public ceremony on August 29, 1960, an impressive turnaround time for a project of that size and complexity.[38] According to the inauguration program, written in Khmer, Russian, and French (see Figure 1), the opening ceremonies included a performance of Khmer dance by the Royal Ballet Corps and a song composed specifically for the occasion, giving thanks to the Soviet Minister of Public Health, S.V. Kourachov, and the people of the USSR.[39] The first two verses of the song are:

> Welcome to his Excellency, the Minister,
> please convey our sincerest thanks
> to the people of Russia, our friends,
> who have the generosity to help the Cambodian nation.
>
> Friends, you have given the gift of a hospital,
> a great building of 500 beds,
> all the equipment needed for care,
> and treatment of all types of diseases…

The hospital had 7 units: general medicine (150 beds), surgery (60 beds), maternity (40 beds), women's health (20 beds), tuberculosis (120 beds), infectious disease (60 beds), and pediatrics (50 beds), in addition to a radiotherapy ward (10 beds).[40] Of the 500 beds, 200 were for patients able to pay a fee and 300 were for free medical care of the poor, monks, and civil servants who earned less than 25,000 riel. Outpatient consultation would be free for all patients.[41] The USSR pledged to donate medicine for 2 years, 24 staff (doctors, nurses, technicians, and translators), and 20 scholarships for Cambodians to study medicine in the USSR.[42] The financing and support of this institution was a significant act of "medical diplomacy" in the words of physician and historian Rethy Chhem,[43] who completed some of his medical training at the Soviet

Hospital in the late 60s. Nonetheless, Guillou writes that "the gift is a little poisoned,"[44] because, despite free medicines and Soviet technical experts, Cambodia was responsible for operational costs, and as the decade progressed, those costs were difficult to support.

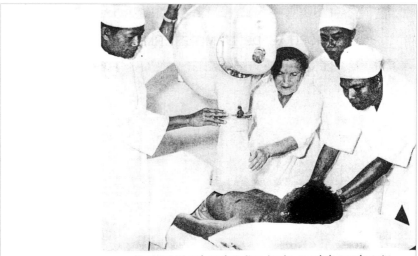

Le nouvel Hôpital est doté d'une bombe au cobalt pour le traitement des tumeurs malignes (ci-dessus).'

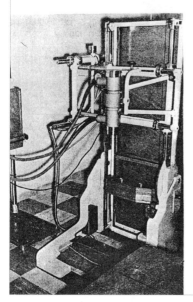

### RADIOLOGIE

L'Hôpital est doté de 7 appareils de radiodiagnostic modernes. Outre l'examen radioscopique cet appareillage permet de prendre à 0m,50 des photos de pointage par séries et par panorama qui donnent une idée exacte de la dimension du foyer lésionnel. De plus il permet de prendre des clichés par couches, indépendamment de la profondeur du foyer lésionnel, ce qui est particulièrement important dans les diagnostics des affections des viscères thoraciques. Enfin les médecins ont à leur disposition un appareil à rayons X portatif permettant d'effectuer toutes les opérations au chevet du malade.

Le service de radiologie est également équipé d'appareils de radio-thérapie. La bombe au cobalt pour le traitement des tumeurs malignes qui exige une installation complexe pour assurer la sécurité du personnel est installée dans ces bâtiments. Au cours du traitement le malade est constamment surveillé par une installation de télévision et demeure en contact avec le médecin traitant.

Une salle de radiographie de l'Hôpital

**Figure 2.** Radiologic devices, from *Cambodge d'Aujourd'hui* (July–August 1960): 37.

The opening of the hospital was covered in detail in the July–August 1960 issue of *Cambodge d'Aujourd'hui*. Figure 2 is a page from this feature dedicated to radiology. It tells how the new hospital is equipped with seven modern radiologic devices for diagnosis and for therapy, including a portable x-ray machine and a cobalt machine used to treat tumors. This state-of-the-art past contrasts with hospital conditions 50 years later: when I showed Figure 2 to staff in the imaging ward of KSFH in 2010, an older doctor gestured down the hall and joked, "They are the same x-ray machines."[45]

## The *Revue*

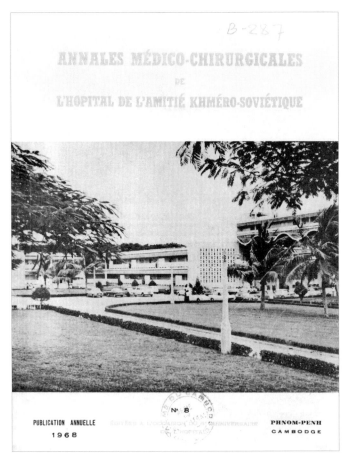

**Figure 3.** *Annales Médico-Chirurgicales de l'Hôpital de l'Amitié Khméro-Soviétique* (1968).

The 10 volumes of the *Revue* ranged between 138 and 290 pages of articles (with an average of 214 pages), and between 170 and 299 pages in total length, including tables of contents, prefatory material (preface, foreword, speech extracts), and advertising. Issues contain between 21 and 63 articles, on average 48 per issue. Articles range in length from 1 page to 22 pages with the majority of articles between 4 and 5 pages. Approximately 227 people contributed to the journal in its lifetime.[46] It seems that mostly men worked on the *Revue*.[47] In addition to authors of articles, contributors included the editorial board (directors, secretaries, treasurers, advisors), translators (all Russian), authors of the preface (six Ministers of Health over ten years), and even Prince Sihanouk, whose hospital inauguration speech extracts were included in the 1962 and 1963 issues, and letters to KSFH Director Kim Vien in the 1967 and 1968 issues. In addition to articles, sections of the journal included Director Kim Vien's four foreword between 1966 and 1969, and brief reviews of literature and recent theses in *Lu pour vu* and *Extrait du thèse*. These latter two categories can be seen as explicit efforts to form an audience of scientific readers, or consumers of medical texts.

The different types of articles included observations, case studies,[48] experiments (e.g., testing outcomes of local anesthesia, ether oxygen, and combined), investigations (e.g., testing hospital employees to determine blood pressure norms for Cambodians), epidemiological research, and studies that characterize a condition in Cambodia and compare it to other places (e.g., polio in South Vietnam, the US, France, and Cambodia). The images in the journal include photographs, x-rays, drawings, and microphotographs (photographs taken through a microscope to create an enlarged image). The composition of sections shifted from volume to volume. For example, sometimes surgery was combined with anesthesia, sometimes it was on its own. Tuberculosis was a consistent area of concern, reflecting the fact that over one-fifth of hospital beds were reserved for TB patients. Figure 4 represents the five most prominent subject areas of the journal (in terms of page numbers) over the decade.

Patterns of authorship[49] and the way contributors are credited show the rise of Cambodian control of the journal over the decade, reflecting the planned phase-out of Soviet mentorship and, more abruptly, the advent of civil war. During the 1960s and 1970s, countries with limited resources often looked to international collaboration as a way to build their research programs, and compared to resource-rich countries, a higher proportion of their publications are co-authored.[50] However,

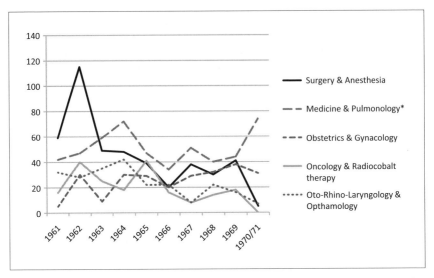

**Figure 4.** Topics in the *Revue* according to number of pages, 1961–70/71
(*Pulmonology includes tuberculosis).

despite a high volume of scientific publications, Soviet co-authorship
to the extent seen in the *Revue* seems to have been rare. According
to a study of scientific citations in 1973, the USSR produced the third
highest number of scientific publications (after the US and UK), but
the percentage of Soviet co-authorship with scientists from other countries was substantially below average in all fields, including clinical
medicine.[51] Early issues of the *Revue* were co-authored by Cambodians
and Soviets and credit Soviet translators. Soviets appear in the masthead
as a director and as editors. By 1966, names of Soviet contributors
(referred to only as "Soviet medical experts," not by name) have been
moved to the bottom of the masthead. In 1967, only translators appear
in the masthead, though Soviets continue to author articles. By the
1970/71 issue, there is only one contributing Soviet author.

The final issue is reduced in content and there is a significant turn-
over in Cambodian contributors, presumably due to the 1970 coup and
subsequent changes in government staff. For example, Thiounn Thoeun,
Director and senior surgeon at the hospital, Advisor to the *Revue*,
author or co-author of 63 articles between 1961 and 1969, and Dean
of the Faculty of Medicine at the University of Health Sciences, does
not contribute to the 1970/71 issue, presumably because he joined the
Khmer Rouge in 1970. Thiounn taught at a hospital in Kampong Cham

during the civil war, returned to KSFH, called "17 April Hospital," during Democratic Kampuchea (DK), and became DK Minister of Health.[52] Thiounn was unique in his refusal to act as *fonctionnaire-entrepreneur*; though some doctors joined the Khmer Rouge, the majority did not. If we follow Guillou's assertion that for most doctors, the entrepreneurial spirit was as compelling, if not more, than the spirit of public service (imperfectly realized within the state bureaucracy), we can see why doctors may not have been enamored of a leftist politics, nor leftist politicians of doctors.

## Advertising Biomedical Commodities

With the 1966 issue the *Revue* became the *Annales*, and the first advertisements for pharmaceuticals appear.[53] In 1966 these ten advertisements were exclusively from French laboratories, and each ad was stamped with an authorization from the *Office de Diffusion Médicale*. In later issues, ads appeared with or without this authorization, or with the name *Centre Khmer de Documentation Pharmaceutique et Médicale* in 1967, and *Centre de Documentation et Diffusion des Produits Pharmaceutiques* in 1968. In 1967, Soviet, West German, and Swiss companies placed ads in the *Revue*, in addition to French companies and multinationals such as Roche and Bayer. In 1968, an East German company placed an ad, and in 1969 Cambodian[54] and Japanese companies began to advertise in the journal. The majority of advertising in the *Revue* was for pharmaceuticals, though ads for vitamins, Japanese sutures, Cambodian cosmetics, and a Dutch/US nutritional supplement also appeared in later issues. The ratio of content pages (articles and reviews) to total pages (table of contents, prefatory material, advertising) changed; from 1961 to 1966 content was between 93 per cent and 97 per cent of total journal pages and between 1967 and 1970/71 this ratio declined to between 81 per cent and 87 per cent, reflecting primarily the increase in number of ad pages.

The ads can be read as instructions for how a modern doctor should stock one's cabinet. Ads for locally manufactured serums and painkillers appeared next to ads for newly developed and internationally popular benzodiazepines.[55] The co-presence of domestic and foreign products in the *Revue* circulates an image of a cosmopolitan Cambodian medicine: the global therapeutic market is integrated into Cambodian biomedicine and, through domestic production of its own products, Cambodian biomedicine integrates into the global market.

## Enacting Cambodian Biomedicine

> Readers will appreciate the value of this issue because each one, whether clinician or specialist, is certain to find the articles interesting or useful, because of the particularity of Cambodian Pathology, or because of their value from a diagnostic or therapeutic point of view.[56]

In the Preface to the 1968 issue, Minister of Health and Dean of the Faculty of Medicine Tip Mâm writes that the articles are "interesting or useful" because of the particularity of "Cambodian Pathology," as well as the articles' diagnostic and therapeutic value. She praises the "dedication, selflessness and valuable scientific spirit" of Cambodian doctors and their Soviet colleagues. How did authors enact the diseases and conditions particular to Cambodia, or "Cambodian Pathology?" Writings about place, nation, climate, and ethnicity show how authors characterized their research and how they situated their work in relation to international medicine. I searched the journals for uses of terms that referred to a specific identity, such as *Cambodge* and *Khmer*, and terms that indicated being part of a larger collective or process, such as *pays*, *tropique*, *développement*, *progrès*, *monde*, *international*.[57] The most productive words in terms of the frequency of their use and elaboration of medical issues are *Cambodge* and *pays*. First I describe techniques of defining conditions in Cambodia, including a focus on hygiene, and second, I describe techniques of relating conditions in Cambodia to other places through citation and comparison.

Articles mentioning "Cambodia" do so in cursory fashion or as the framework of the article. An example of the former is a brief mention of how public opinion in Cambodia tends to confuse tuberculosis with pulmonary hemorrhage (*l'hémoptysie*),[58] or how, thanks to modern methods of anesthesiology at the hospital, operations on the thorax were possible for the first time in Cambodia.[59] Another common example is an introductory or concluding sentence which situates the topic within Cambodia, such as Guilevitch et al. beginning their case study of ablation of a goiter with the statement: "in Cambodia, pathologies of the thyroid gland occupy an important place compared to other illnesses."[60] In an article co-authored with the Director of Institut Pasteur du Cambodge, authors describe how they diagnosed two young girls with oc-Thalassemia by first ruling out certain conditions such as leishmaniasis: "*Au Cambodge la leischmaniose n'existe pas.*"[61] The authors note that latent oc-Thalassemia has been described in literature on Southeast Asia, but their cases differ in that they were not latent but active, serious illnesses.

When the term "Cambodia" is used to frame an article, it does so in various ways. The *Revue* contains many articles that seek to characterize a certain condition by describing various aspects of a disease (epidemiology, treatment, outcomes) in Cambodia. The 1963 extract of Chhéa Thang's thesis examines polio.[62] Thang claims that the importance of polio is underestimated in both the public and medical domain due to a lack of statistics, which are based on a lack of diagnosis. Thang discusses characteristics of the virus, its epidemiology, hygiene practices, and cases at KSFH and at Kantha Bopha.[63] In the section on hygiene (*bref rappel de l'hygiène de l'habitat au Cambodge*), Thang describes Cambodia as a small country of six million people in the Mekong Delta with a tropical climate. As with the majority of developing countries, according to Thang, Cambodia suffers from inadequate rules of hygiene and problems of water and waste.[64]

In an article on xerophthalmia, Dr. Ung Péang analyzes 34 cases of eye problems seen at KSFH over a nine-month period, finding that xerophthalmia is the most common condition, which is similar to the situation in other parts of Asia.[65] Xerophthalmia is caused by lack of vitamin A, but all patients were from rural areas where leafy green vegetables rich in carotene are actively cultivated. Ung identifies two causes: (1) customs and beliefs—the majority of rural Cambodians, not just the poor, feed infants rice meal without meat, fat, or vegetables because it is thought that these foods are not good for infants and will cause a swollen belly;[66] and (2) high rates of gastrointestinal trouble. Ung notes that despite the frequency of xerophthalmia in Cambodia, his findings are more optimistic than those of the WHO, with a lower proportion of blindness and death. He attributes this to the fact that Cambodians are aware of the condition, that people are concerned about eyes and thus bring children to the hospital early in their illness, and that Cambodian women breastfeed for a long time.

Ung and Thang are not unique for their attention to hygiene; other articles defining a disease or condition in Cambodia also contain at minimum a sentence or two about hygiene and health education, perhaps reflecting the preoccupations of French colonial medicine, Soviet public health, or the field of "tropical medicine" more broadly. In an article on intestinal parasites, Dr Krioutchkov and Mr Tauch Kramam analyze cases from the biology lab at KSFH along with research from the Epidemiology Service of the Ministry of Health conducted among inhabitants of Kraing Kor village, in Kandal province.[67] The authors classify types of parasites in a large table and discuss treatment and prevention, including "health education." In the section "Prophylaxis and the battle against illnesses of intestinal parasites," the authors actually *provide* health education, contrary to the typical practice of making a vague statement that it is "necessary." Krioutchkov and Tauch describe in detail a method of layering fecal matter together with soil to make compost, including measurements of ideal volume and temperature: "*Cette méthode est facilement applicable au Cambodge. Elle est simple et efficace.*"[68] Their elegant combination of laboratory science, epidemiology, and hygiene resembles late nineteenth-century Pasteurian styles of writing described by Latour.[69]

Though the meanings and implications of "hygiene" are not uniform in the *Revue*,[70] in some articles the concept de-racializes sickness by attributing causes to modifiable behaviors rather than something inherent to a race or to the poor.[71] "Hygiene" in nineteenth- and early twentieth-century Europe and its colonies was a mode of disciplining, and in some cases dehumanizing, the poor and non-white.[72] Some work has been done on hygiene in the colonial period,[73] but a genealogy of "hygiene" is required; it is a keyword in 1960s Cambodian medicine and offers a means to situate Cambodia-focused studies in relation to other projects in anthropology and the history of postcolonial medicine.

In order to characterize Cambodian Pathology, some authors compare techniques, practices, and prevalence to those in other countries or regions. Tracing citations is one way to see how authors situate their research within a larger body of scholarship. Authors in the *Revue* cite works published in Russia, Italy, France, the United Kingdom, Germany, and the United States, and connect their own findings to studies of other places, for example, hypertension in Ethiopia and Japan.[74] In an article on uterine rupture during labor, Leao Thean Im compares cases of rupture per 1,000 births in Argentina, Germany, the USSR, Finland, Italy, France, Morocco, Pondicherry, "*Afrique Noire*," Cambodia, and the US (from lowest to highest).[75] The number of citations increases over the decade, with a few names embedded in article texts in 1961 and lists of works cited at the end of articles in 1968.

Despite significant scientific output, Soviet scientists were rarely cited internationally during the Cold War,[76] and in this regard, the *Revue* represents a less-lopsided engagement with relevant literatures. Drs. Kostenko, Nop, and Khim write that in the 18 months since the opening of the urology service, cases at KSFH correspond to "*la bibliographie médicale classique*" in that two conditions predominate—cancer and condyloma.[77] The authors cite scientific research from the Institute of Epidemiology and Microbiology in Kiev on the viability of trichomonas in various environments. Pridvijkine and Heng Kong Kimseng's 1961 article classifies skin conditions in Cambodia based on chart reviews of 1,500 patients at KSFH.[78] After a brief mention of similarities to the USSR (high frequency of bacterial skin infections or *pyodermites*) and "tropical countries" (frequency of the parasitic condition, achromia, and *tokelau*, a fungal infection), the authors describe the particular situation in Cambodia. In Cambodia, "tropical achromia" is the most common parasitic condition, while in *les pays de climat tempéré*, ringworm (*l'epidermophytie*) is more common. The authors also distinguish between Cambodia's inhabitants' susceptibility to certain conditions, such as photosensitivity disorders (*photodermatoses*): Khmers, Vietnamese and Chinese are adapted to heatstroke (*l'insolation tropicale*) while Europeans living in Cambodia often present with first- and second-degree sunburns. Further on, the authors note that what distinguishes syphilis cases in Cambodia compared to Europe and North America is the predominance of advanced stage disease. They conclude with a statement about international and domestic significance: their findings are of general scientific importance, and also have the ability to aid the Health Service in its goal of preventive health care.

In this section, I have presented different techniques of enacting Cambodian biomedicine in the *Revue*. Defining prevalence rates, treatments, behaviors, and norms for Cambodia is one set of techniques. Here, hygiene comes forward as a key concept. Citing and comparing findings to research in other places is another set of techniques, demonstrating for *Revue* authors and readers, Cambodian and Soviet, how to situate their work in relation to, and thus participate in, international medico-scientific discourse.

## Picturing Cambodian Medicine

The images in the *Revue* work with the text and as arguments in their own right to define the contours of modern Cambodian medicine.[79] The photographs, drawings, x-rays, and microphotographs usually come at the end of an article, but in some issues, particularly later ones, they are integrated within the body. The images are never credited and it is hard to know what went into their production. Authors refer to images as illustrations of what the text describes, such as anatomical drawings, and as evidence of treatment success, often photographs and x-rays.

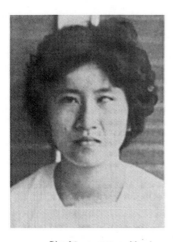 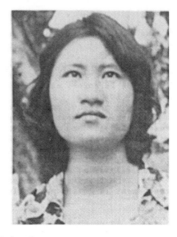

Strabisme concomitant convergent de l'oeil gauche de 50º.
La malade C.N. avant et après l'opération.

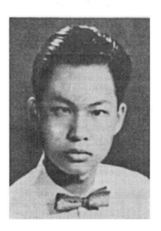 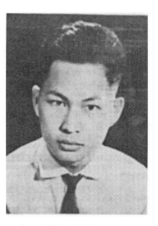

Strabisme concomitant convergent de l'oeil gauche de 40º.
Le malade U.L. avant et après l'opération

**Figure 5.** Before/After: photographs of patients with strabismus, from Karach and Tep Than, "Traitement Opératoire du Strabisme Concomitant," *Revue Médico-Chirurgicale de l'Hôpital de l'Amitié Khméro-Soviétique* (1962): 260–5.

Images in the *Revue* depict bodies and body parts, organ systems, treatment procedures, equipment and devices, and are frequently arranged in sets of before/after, normal/pathological, and inside/outside. Figure 5 is an example of the before/after type of image: the photographs on the left depict a man and a woman with strabismus, a condition where the eyes are not properly aligned. On the right, the images show the same

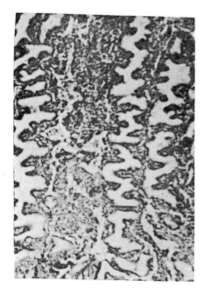 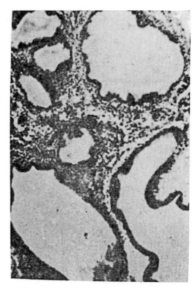

Fig. 1-a
Phase de prolifération normale.

Fig. 1-b
Phase d'hyperplasie glandulo-kystique.

**Figure 6.** Normal/Pathological: Microphotographs of uterine cells, from Inn Sunlay and Alexandrova, "Les hémorragies Utérines Dysfonctionnelles," *Annales Médico-Chirurgicales de l'Hôpital de l'Amitié Khméro-Soviétique* (1966): 42–9.

individuals after corrective surgery. Normal/pathological is demonstrated by the microphotographs in Figure 6. These images appear at the end of an article on dysfunctional uterine bleeding. According to the captions, the microphotographs depict normal uterine cells (on the left) and cells with hyperplasia (on the right). The biopsy came from a 46-year-old woman from Kampot. Many photographs in the *Revue* (and in other health-related publications of the Sangkum) depict equipment and devices. Figure 7 is one example from 1961: a photograph of equipment for delivering oxygen treatment for intestinal parasites, and on the right, a patient receiving treatment. Pairs of images showing the inside and the outside of the body are particularly compelling displays of biomedical knowledge. Karach and Kozlova include the two images in Figure 8 in their 1962 article, "Foreign bodies in the eye." First, an x-ray of the head, showing a large object in the eye, and second, a photograph of the foreign body removed, next to a ruler in order to show its precise size.

In addition to educating readers about available techniques and devices, images in the *Revue* perform three overlapping types of work:

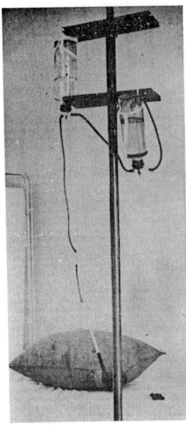

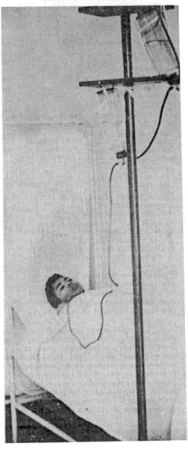

Le traitement des parasites
intestinaux par l'oxygène

Introduction de l'oxygène
dans le duodénum

Remplissage des bouteilles
d'oxygène.

**Figure 7.** Equipment and devices: Treatment of Intestinal Parasites with Oxygen, from Ngo Béng Tuot and Daniline, "Utilisation d'oxygène dans le Traitement de la Parasitose Intestinale," *Revue Médico-Chirurgicale de l'Hôpital de l'Amitié Khméro-Soviétique* (1961): 53–5.

they reveal ordinarily unseen bodily processes, they provide evidence of treatment success, and they indicate technological expertise. In multiple ways, they buttress the diagnostic, therapeutic, and explanatory power of biomedicine, and by extension, its practice by the authors and at the hospital.

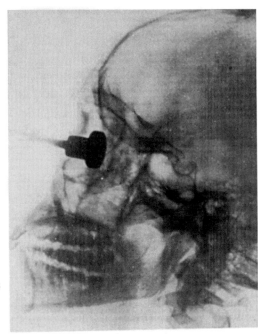

**Figure 8.** Inside/Outside:
Images from Karach and
Kozlova, "Les Corps Étrangers
dans l'orbite," *Revue Médico-
Chirurgicale de l'Hôpital de
l'Amitié Khméro-Soviétique*
(1962): 270–2.

Photo N° 1 : la radiographie
avant l'opération

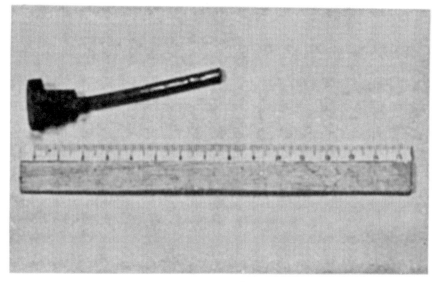

Photo N° 2 : le corps
étranger enlevé

## Cambodian Medicine, Geopolitics, and "International Medical Science"

Reading the *Revue*, we are constantly reminded of the time and place of medicine. The authors carefully enact the particulars of Cambodian medicine through original research and comparison to conditions in other places. Government officials enact another form of medicine in their letters, speeches, and prefaces. Here we read praise for a medicine at once young (with implied reference to colonialism), struggling to develop out of poverty, and vibrant in its growing contribution to the nation's health and to international science. There was impressive government support for the journal. The Minister of Public Health authored the prefaces to each issue. The 1967 and 1968 volumes contain letters from Sihanouk praising the previous issue of the journal and its role in advancing science for the good of the Cambodian medical profession, for Cambodia, and for humanity. In 1967 Sihanouk wrote: "I send my very warm congratulations to you and all the members of the Scientific Committee for this achievement, international in scope, which brings the greatest honor to Cambodia and to the Khmer medical profession."[80] And in 1968 Sihanouk wrote:

> It is with great pleasure that I observe how the Khmer medical profession dedicates itself to scientific research and to making its work known at the international level. This is, for me, a great cause of satisfaction because our superior work shows that Cambodia has taken its place amongst nations that contribute to the progress of humanity.[81]

In the prefaces, Ministers of Health wrote in similarly exuberant terms about the importance of the journal domestically and abroad, linking the journal to science, development, and progress. They note the challenges of pursuing medical science in a newly independent, developing country such as Cambodia, and repeatedly praise the fruitful, selfless collaboration between Soviet and Cambodian teams. Each year we are told how the collaboration advances peace and goodwill among nations, making almost palpable the tensions of the Cold War and threat of regional conflict. Towards the end of the decade, the authors of the prefaces praise the journal for continuing to publish every year on the anniversary of the hospital's construction. In 1971, So Satta, Minister of Health for the new Khmer Republic, explicitly addresses geopolitics when he takes comfort in the journal as a sign of constancy in the face of aggression.

> In this period of enormous difficulty of all kinds caused by the aggression against our country by the North Vietnamese and Vietcong, the persistence of scientific activity is a guarantee of our will to survive the annexationist appetite of the Foreigner.[82]

There is no record of a subsequent issue of the *Revue*. Greatly reduced in content in 1970/71, we can view the demise of the journal as an index of deteriorating conditions for biomedical practice. There was a substantial exodus of trained medical professionals during this period.[83] We can only imagine how the doctors, nurses, and technicians who remained at KSFH became preoccupied by the need to care for increasing numbers of refugees and casualties of war with fewer and fewer resources, and to protect their own self-interest in the face of spiraling economic and political chaos during the Republic.[84]

## Postcolonial Biomedicine and Medical Diplomacy

The Soviet Union's cooperation with economically underdeveloped countries was aimed at a complex development of the national economy and at strengthening the state sector in the economy of these countries. This had a decisive importance in overcoming their backwardness. The chief efforts in this cooperation were aimed at creating a modern industry as the basis for the economic independence of the countries.[85]

Soviet diplomacy in the 1950s and 1960s included economic and technical aid to many new countries in Asia and Africa whose leaders were "national democrats" rather than explicitly communist.[86] Cambodia was a recipient of this "non-capitalist development,"[87] which involved development of the public sector without necessarily having a communist revolution. Part of this aid involved educating foreigners in the USSR, as well as establishing education and training institutions in foreign countries.[88] In the 1960s, Cambodia was one of 16 countries that the USSR targeted for educational and cultural programs in order to counter American and Western European influence.[89] As always, Cambodia was selective. There is evidence that Cambodian students and officials rejected Soviet aid in fields that could be overly ideological, such as education,[90] but welcomed aid in fields that seemed value-free, such as biomedicine and technology, and which furthered Sihanouk's modernist vision for Cambodia. The Institute of Higher Technology, established in Phnom Penh in 1964, was the second major Soviet development project in Cambodia after KSFH.[91] Cambodia also received capitalist development aid, including from the US, where some officials openly advocated "medicine as diplomacy" in the 1960s.[92]

The *Revue* was a dynamic Cambodian-Soviet creation, and an example of how biomedicine is constituted within relations between people, materials, languages, and ideals that extend beyond any one nation. In the 1950s and 1960s, Cambodian public health was taking shape amid the ebb and flow of intervention from different foreign entities—French, Soviet, US, WHO, and others. While it is beyond the scope of this chapter to analyze theories and practices of national medicines, or interrogate the very notion of a national style of medicine, different donors did have different interests. Iliffe notes that in post-independence East Africa, some doctors became "specialists in tailoring plans to the distinctive interests of foreign donors, whether Chinese pride in indigenous medicine, Russian eagerness to display Soviet technology, Scandinavian earnestness about primary health care, or the World Bank's obsession with cost-sharing."[93] One of the relevant features of Soviet medicine for the *Revue* is the priority that medical research be oriented towards practical problems and solutions.[94] In a 1966 article, Mark Field writes that in the USSR, clinical physicians are "constantly urged to engage in research work, and are reminded of the Marxist injunction that theory and practice go together."[95] The *Revue* can be seen as a gesture towards this ideal: research to address practical problems affecting Cambodian health and health care.

It is unclear whether Sihanouk sought Soviet medical aid because he admired the Soviet health system,[96] but his administration did discriminate between donors' priorities, as illustrated by his rejection of an offer from China to build an institute for training "barefoot doctors." Guillou argues this was because the Sangkum favored "the construction of a vast, modern, hospital network."[97] Sihanouk was playing with different models of nation-building and harnessing development resources to achieve modernity. The USSR was promoting its ideal of high-tech, socialized medicine as key to non-capitalist development. The *Revue* was a textual form of these cosmopolitan modernities.

## Conclusion

The *Revue* was an enactment of what modern biomedicine in 1960s Cambodia should want to be, and what a modern doctor should want to do. In the articles, biomedical knowledge and technologies visualize ordinarily unseen processes, and diagnose and treat patients. The authors develop Cambodian norms or compare Cambodian cases to established international ones. In the prefaces, we read about economic challenges and geopolitical pressures against which the Cambodian-Soviet collaboration and the Cambodian medical profession struggle. The advertisements index the growing commercialization of medicine and the centrality of pharmaceuticals in the Sangkum.

A priority of Sangkum nation-building was the improvement of public health and the development of the health system through the construction of hospitals and clinics, training and professionalization of medical practitioners, and creating a body of local biomedical knowledge, in part through the *Revue*. This resembles what Lock and Nguyen describe as a "nationalist" phase of biomedicine, between 1960–80, when "biomedicine began to be used as an emblem of nation-building and modernization by newly independent states in Africa, Asia, and Europe."[98] In post-independence Egypt, a national medical research program was constructed around parasitic illnesses, a pathology defined as specifically Egyptian.[99] In post-independence Uganda, doctors trained at Makerere Medical School published research on the economic and environmental, rather than ethnic or cultural, causes of diseases. Importantly, these included diseases endemic to the "tropics" such as malaria, but also so-called "diseases of civilization" such as cancer and heart disease.[100] The *Revue* points to a similar scope for post-independence biomedicine in Cambodia: recall Figure 4, which illustrates the wide range of conditions covered, not just those deemed "tropical." The *Revue* emphasizes clinical rather than laboratory research, similar to research in 1970s Tanzania.[101] As in Uganda and Tanzania, "hygiene" is central to how *Revue* authors characterize diseases and their prevention, ranging from cancer to parasitic illnesses. But hygiene is not fixed as an essentializing discourse—hygiene related to poverty and environment may imply an economic critique and de-racialization of sickness. In defining the particulars of medical conditions in Cambodia, the *Revue* resembled something of a global ideal practice of decolonizing nations—establishing a domestic, modern program of medical research with foreign scientific mentorship and infrastructural and monetary aid. Future histories of medicine in Southeast Asia would benefit from tracing decolonial ideals and practices across regions; Southeast Asian and African medical histories may have much to tell each other.

In this chapter I have interwoven analysis of the *Revue* texts—visual and written—with analysis of the processes that both created and constrained them. Existing scholarship on biomedicine in the Sangkum pays minimal attention to the *Revue* and as a result, judges efforts for research and knowledge production quite poorly. However, my analysis should not be read as nostalgia for the Sangkum, nor idealization of a medical journal as the marker of progress in education and training. The *Revue* opens up space for a more nuanced conception of Sangkum biomedicine. The biomedicine of the *Revue* is oriented towards knowledge production through research and writing about diseases and treatments relevant to Cambodians; a collaborative enterprise; a commercial enterprise; and part of larger sociopolitical projects. Furthermore, my argument that the *Revue* enacts a particular form of biomedicine during the Sangkum is not an assertion about its impact. I was unable to track whether or not the journal travelled outside of KSFH, the capital, or the country, but the readership was most likely limited. I do not evaluate the journal in terms of its effects on public health policy or population health, in part because it is difficult to measure such effects, but more fundamentally, because my interest here is not in measurement. Just as the presence of the *Revue*—the hundreds of articles, photographs, charts, and tables—tells us about conditions and priorities for biomedicine during the Sangkum, the absence of the *Revue* after 1971 tells us much about conditions and priorities for biomedicine in subsequent years.

Certain features in the *Revue* are unique to the historical moment: self-awareness of the post-independence period; optimism about medical science as a form of national progress; and medical journals as educational forms. This historical moment has long passed. Yet debates about how Cambodia will "modernize" are in vigorous circulation today, now that it is "post-conflict" or "post-socialist" even. Which country, which practices, which ideologies will be Cambodia's model? Cambodia's elites and their networks of foreign investors favor "growth" over equal distribution, yet the government's reliance on development aid and Hun Sen's balancing of China and the United States, as well as domestic and regional forces, evoke some of the diplomatic pressures of the Cold War.

In conclusion, I propose that the *Revue*, an artifact of Cold War diplomacy, has something to tell us today. Whereas some authors within the field of global health advocate adjusting foreign policy to fit health goals, others note that it is global health which often serves foreign policy goals. Cambodia has long been party to these types of aid and humanitarianism, whether funded by the colonial administration, US, Soviet, or other foreign governments, or indeed provided by foreign military.

Key features that distinguish present-day configurations of biomedicine and politics in global health are the number of NGOs, universities, and corporations operating in the health sector, often in archipelago-like "territorial delimitation;"[102] globalized pharmaceutical and clinical research; and the emergent priority of "biosecurity."[103] All of these features apply to global health initiatives in present-day Cambodia, and all signal a fracturing of state control over biomedicine compared to the 1960s and the 1980s. NGOs, which proliferated after 1993 from often contradictory imaginaries of "humanitarian rescue" and "strengthening civil society," are particularly prominent in health-related projects for the poor in Cambodia. These projects tend to provide services or training in the short-term, without claim to knowledge production other than "lessons learned." Signs of renewed interest in research can be seen: medical students again have to fulfill a thesis requirement, and the recent establishment of the National Ethics Committee for Human Research indicates an institutional response to the increase in transnational research. However, the latter does not have a sustained pedagogical aim; training for Cambodian scientists is limited to the scope and time frame of the research project.

The *Revue* enacted a practice of biomedical knowledge production and circulation within collaborative, politically charged, and economically constrained contexts. These contexts are the global norm rather than a temporary stage or exception. Present forms of medical diplomacy are brief interventions, narrowly focused in scope, or a form of top-down technology transfer. With the exception of the Institut Pasteur du Cambodge and projects at the National Institute of Public Health, it does not seem that a collaborative project of knowledge production is under way in Cambodia, despite large amounts of money being spent on diplomatic goals. There is no need to think of such a project as impossible.

## Acknowledgements

This chapter is based on research conducted in Cambodia between 2009 and 2011, as part of a larger project on medical imaging, supported by fellowships from the Center for Khmer Studies and the Wenner-Gren Foundation for Anthropological Research. Revisions were written while I was a fellow at the International Institute for Asian Studies, Leiden University. Trying to locate contributors to the *Revue* was a ritual in which my interlocutor scanned the table of contents, sometimes rapidly, sometimes pausing to think, and recounted which authors had emigrated to France, who had died (of old age, under the Khmer Rouge), and who might still be alive but whose location was unknown. I am grateful to the many people who helped with this often somber accounting. Dr Chan Dara was particularly generous with his time. I thank Rathneary Heang Sokhom, Heang Sokhom, and Y Socheat for help with translation of Khmer speeches and films and for inspired discussion; staff at the National Archives of Cambodia and Bophana Audiovisual Resource Center, particularly Y Dari and Sopheap Chea, for assistance with materials; and Ulvy for patient scanning of documents. Thanks to Laurence Monnais and John DiMoia for initially encouraging the writing of this chapter, and to Sylvia Nam, two anonymous reviewers, and the editors of this volume for their comments which helped me to improve it.

## Notes

1. Bruno Latour, *The Pasteurization of France*, trans. Alan Sheridan and John Law (Cambridge: Harvard University Press, 1988), 94.

2. In 1966, it was renamed the *Annales Médico-Chirurgicales de l'Hôpital de l'Amitié Khméro-Soviétique* [Medical-Surgical Annals of the Khmer-Soviet Friendship Hospital].

3. My methodology follows the analysis of texts and their contexts in Virginia R. Dominguez, "When the Enemy is Unclear: US Censuses and Photographs of Cuba, Puerto Rico, and the Philippines from the Beginning of the 20th Century," *Comparative American Studies* 5, no. 2 (2007): 173–203, and part one of Latour, *Pasteurization of France*.

4. Achille Mbembe, *On the Postcolony* (Berkeley: University of California Press, 2001), 1–23.

5. Conversation with author, Sept. 10, 2009.

6. For Sihanouk's unique merger of his persona with the Cambodian nation, see David P. Chandler, *A History of Cambodia*, 2nd ed. (Boulder: Westview Press, 1992), 191–204, and Ashley Thompson, "'The Suffering of Kings': Substitute Bodies, Healing, and Justice in Cambodia," in *History, Buddhism, and New Religious Movements in Cambodia*, ed. John Marston and Elizabeth Guthrie (Honolulu: University of Hawai'i Press, 2004), 91–112.

7. I utilize periodization based on political change because the lifespan of the *Revue* conforms to this periodization.

8. Margaret Slocomb, "The Nature and Role of Ideology in the Modern Cambodian State," *Journal of Southeast Asian Studies* 37, no. 3 (2006): 375–95.

9. Ibid., 389.

10. Michael Vickery, *Kicking the Vietnam Syndrome in Cambodia: Collected Writings 1975–2010* (2010), 33–7, http://michaelvickery.org/, accessed Jan. 31, 2012.

11. See Ly Daravuth and Ingrid Muan, eds., *Cultures of Independence: An Introduction to Cambodian Arts and Culture in the 1950s and 1960s* (Phnom Penh: Reyum Institute of Arts and Culture, 2001); and Helen Grant Ross and Darryl Collins, *Building Cambodia: "New Khmer Architecture" 1953–1970* (Bangkok: Key Publisher, 2006).

12. Chandler, *A History of Cambodia*, 191–204.

13. Grant Ross and Collins, *Building Cambodia*; Anne Yvonne Guillou, *Les médecins au Cambodge: entre elite sociale traditionnelle et groupe professionnel moderne sous influence etrangère* (PhD diss., École des Hautes Études des Sciences Sociales, 2001), 109–11. During the Sangkum, Guillou estimates the US gave $350 million (from 1955–63); China $25 million; France $25 million (from 1955–62); the USSR $15 million; Japan $4.28 million.

14. Diplomatic relations were re-established between the People's Republic of Kampuchea and the USSR in 1979. Dates from the website of the Embassy of the Russian Federation in Cambodia, http://embrusscambodia.mid.ru/web/cambodia-en/ambassadors-to-cambodia.

15. In this chapter I am concerned with biomedicine, but healing modalities that involve traditional medical practitioners, Buddhist healers, and mediums, were and continue to be prominent in Cambodia. For overviews, see Anne Yvonne Guillou and Évelyne Micollier, "Anthropologie et Santé en Asie du Sud-Est: Dynamiques et Courants de Recherche," in *Moussons* 15: *La santé: miroir des sociétés d'Asie du sud-est*, ed. Laurence Husson (2010): 177–93; and Soizick Crochet, "La santé au Cambodge: histoire et défis," in *Cambodge Contemporain*, ed. Alain Forest (Bangkok and Paris: Irasec and Les Indes Savantes, 2008), 363–418. On medicine during the colonial period, see Sokhieng Au, *Mixed Medicines: Health and Culture in French Colonial Cambodia* (Chicago: University of Chicago Press, 2011) and on pre- and post-independence medical practices, see Anne Yvonne Guillou, *Cambodge, soigner dans les fracas de l'histoire: médecins et société* (Paris: Les Indes savantes, 2009); and Jan Ovesen and Ing-Britt Trankell, *Cambodians and their Doctors: A Medical Anthropology of Colonial and Post-colonial Cambodia* (Copenhagen: NIAS Press, 2010).

16. Figures from Guillou, "Médecines au Cambodge," 119.

17. Au, *Mixed Medicines*, 182.

18. Guillou, *Cambodge, soigner dans les fracas*, 182.

19. Bophana Center, NSI_VI_001568, *La femme Cambodgienne à l'heure du Sangkum, 1960*.

20. Bophana Center, DDC_VI_001282, *Actualités No. 58*, Sangkum (no date).

21. For Khmer Republic newsreels depicting blood donation and military medicine, see (all from Bophana Center), DDC_VI_001299, *Newsreel No. 23 1970*; DDC_VI_001285, *Newsreel No. 55 1970–1975* (no date); DDC_VI_001308, *Newsreel No. 58 1971*; DDC_VI_001281, *Newsreel No. 70 1970–1975* (no date); DDC_VI_ 001290, *Newsreel No. 96 and No. 94 1970–1975* (no date).

22. Health-related aid from other nations such as Poland, China, Japan, and the US also helped break the French monopoly. See Crochet, "La santé au Cambodge," 369–70 and Guillou, "Les médecins au Cambodge," 114–15.

23. It could be said, following Guillou, that up to and including the present day (perhaps with the exception of Democratic Kampuchea), public health has never been entirely in the hands of Cambodian leaders. See Guillou, *Cambodge, soigner dans les fracas*, 186.

24. Ibid, 45.

25. Guillou, "Les médecins au Cambodge," 117. Ovesen and Trankell note that there was no coverage of Calmette Hospital in Sangkum publications, in contrast to extensive coverage of KSFH. Ovesen and Trankell, *Cambodians and Their Doctors*, 80–1.

26. John Iliffe, *East African Doctors: A History of the Modern Profession* (Cambridge: Cambridge University Press, 1998), 4.

27. See Part II, Chapter II of Guillou's thesis, "Les médecins au Cambodge," and 43–50 of her book, *Cambodge, soigner dans les fracas*.

28. Guillou, *Cambodge, soigner dans les fracas*, 43–50.

29. The Royal Society was open to all nationalities, though composed primarily of Cambodian, French, and Soviet physicians. Guillou, *Cambodge, soigner dans les fracas*, 46–8.

30. NAC BOX 284. *La santé publique au Cambodge* (Phnom Penh: Ministre de l'information, 1962 and 1964). It is unclear how many issues were published.

31. For discussion of Jayavaraman VII's *Hospital Edicts* and healing, biopolitics, and sovereign power in different historical moments, see Thompson, "The Suffering of Kings," 91–112.

32. NAC BOX 284. *Bulletin de la Société Royale de Médecine*, Numéro 4, 1er semestre, Séances 19 Déc. 1964 au 29 Mai 1965 (Phnom Penh, 1965) and NAC BOX 284. *Bureau de la Société Royale de Médecine du Cambodge pour l'année 1964–5* (Phnom Penh: EKLIP, 1965). It is unclear how many were published.

33. NAC BOX 284. V.A. Daniline and Kim Vien, *Éléments d'électrocardiographie* (Phnom Penh: Hôpital de l'Amitié Khméro-Soviétique/E.K.L.I.P., Anciennement Albert Portail, 1962). Kim Vien co-authored 27 articles, reviews and foreword in the *Revue* between 1961 and 1969; Daniline co-authored 18 articles between 1961 and 1962.

34. NAC BOX 288. *Tassnavdey nie samakum bokklik sokhaphibal psay chein roal* [*Review of the Association of Health Workers*], Year 2, No. 8, 4th trimester (1968) and Year 3, No. 9, 1st trimester (1969).

35. *Cambodge d'Aujourd'hui* (July–August 1960), 35. This magazine repre-sented the government view and was published monthly starting in 1955 by the Ministry of Information. The website of the Embassy of the Russian Federation in Cambodia has images of the 1957 hospital agreement docu-ment: http://embrusscambodia.mid.ru/web/cambodia-en/documents-and-photos.

36. NAC BOX 315. *Remarks by Secretary of States at the Inauguration Cere-mony of the Khmer-Soviet Friendship Hospital* (Aug. 29, 1960).

37. Ibid., 5.

38. See Grant Ross and Collins, *Building Cambodia*, for a description of the buildings and the construction process.

39. NAC BOX 312. *Dance program 29 Aug 1960 for S.V. Kourachov, Minister of Public Health, USSR.* Original in Khmer, Russian, and French; transla-tion by author.

40. NAC BOX 315. *Remarks by Secretary of States*, 6. The pediatric unit had its own kitchen, and each room had a bed, cabinet, tables, chairs, and toys.

41. Ibid., 14–15.

42. Ibid., 9.

43. Rethy Chhem, personal communication, June 24, 2010.

44. Guillou, "Les médecins au Cambodge," 117.

45. Conversation with the author, Dec. 13, 2010.

46. I write "approximately" because it is not clear whether variations in spel-ling over different years refer to the same person or not. In cases where the differences were slight I counted one person. (Slight differences include a Khmer name which has one "h" in the first instance and two in a second instance, or a Russian name sometimes spelled with a "y" and other times with a "j", but where these authors write on related topics over time.) In other cases, I counted the different spellings as different people.

47. In the *Revue*, Mlle or Mme marked female gender of contributors whereas male gender was usually unmarked. However, this was not consistent; sometimes contributors are cited only by last name and first initial, giving no clue as to their gender.

48. For discussion of the case study in colonial context, see Sokhieng Au, "The King with Hansen's Disease," in *At the Edge of the Forest*, ed. Anne Ruth Hansen and Judy Ledgerwood (Ithaca: Cornell Southeast Asia Pro-gram, 2008), 122–4.

49. Some authors are distinguished as "Mr." or "Mme." and others are "Dr.," suggesting not all are doctors. I refer to the authors as doctors in imperfect shorthand; some may have been nurses, medical or pharmacy students, or technicians.

50. J. Davidson Frame and Mark P. Carpenter, "International Research Collaboration," *Social Studies of Science* 9 (1979): 488.

51. Ibid., 487.

52. Ovesen and Trankell, *Cambodians and Their Doctors*, 127.

53. Crochet writes that consumption of pharmaceutical products increased rapidly in the 1950s and 1960s such that medications "become an independent actor in the health system." According to Crochet, French medications were valued more highly than those from other countries, such that their brands were well known and recalled decades later, in the 1990s, in the remotest villages (*au fin fond des villages*). Crochet, "*La santé au Cambodge*," 373 [French original, my translation].

54. Chimi Khmer (Société Khmer du Industrie Chimique) and its lab, Les Laboratoires Sokeph, placed an ad for various forms of medications (syrup, tablets, powders, ampoules). Entreprise Nationale des Produits Pharmaceutiques (ENAPHAR) placed ads for 11 different medicines and a general ad for its enterprise on the back covers of the 1969 and 1970/71 issues. In 1970/71 Laboratoires Angkor placed an ad for a syrup, and CPC Laboratoires placed five ads for different drugs, including Kinal, which was developed in 1960 and is manufactured again today. See Brayvin, "Government Calls for More Research on Pharmaceuticals on the Occasion of the 50th Anniversary of Kinal," *Rasmei Kampuchea Daily*, Tuesday, Dec. 21, 2010, K1, K5 [Khmer original, my translation].

55. Roche placed ads for Librium (introduced globally in 1960) and Valium (introduced 1963) in each issue of the *Revue* from 1967 to 1970/71. Dates from *Roche from A to Z: Serving Health* (Basel: Hoffman-La Roche Ltd, 2007), http://www.roche.com, accessed Jan. 28, 2012.

56. Tip Mâm, "Preface," *Annales Médico-Chirurgicales de l'Hôpital de l'Amitié Khméro-Soviétique* (1968), ii.

57. I generated a set of terms after reading selected issues for words authors used to talk about medicine and disease in Cambodia and elsewhere. I then searched each issue for the entire set of terms. I searched for variations of words, such as *nation, national, international*. I also searched for different terms used to refer to similar ideas, such as [*pays*] *chaud, froid, tempère, tropical, tropicaux* to refer to the tropics and non-tropics.

58. In Sokan and Bobrovskaia, "Les hémoptysies tuberculeuses," *Revue Médico-Chirurgicale de l'Hôpital de l'Amitié Khméro-Soviétique* (1963): 89–93.

59. J. Guilevitch, Thiounn Thoeun, and Zaitsev, "Certaines questions concernant l'anesthésie combinée effectuée au cours des opérations thoraciques," *Revue Médico-Chirurgicale de l'Hôpital de l'Amitié Khméro-Soviétique* (1961): 8–18, quote on 17.

60. J. Guilevitch, Thiounn Thoeun, and Zaitsev, "Ablation avec succès d'un goitre géant," *Revue Médico-Chirurgicale de l'Hôpital de l'Amitié Khméro-Soviétique* (1961): 146–50.

61. Goueffon, Men Moningam, Tchébourkine, and Or Khèm, "Deux cas d'oc thalassémie," *Annales Médico-Chirurgicales de l'Hôpital de l'Amitié Khméro-Soviétique* (1968): 135–6.

62. Chhéa Thang, "Contribution à l'étude de la poliomyélite antérieur aigue au Cambodge," *Revue Médico-Chirurgicale de l'Hôpital de l'Amitié Khméro-Soviétique* (1963): 80–4.

63. At the time, Kantha Bopha was the pediatric wing of Preah Ket Mealea Hospital.

64. Ibid., 81.

65. Ung Péang, "Aperçu de la Xérophtalmie au Cambodge," *Annales Médico-Chirurgicales de l'Hôpital de l'Amitié Khméro-Soviétique* (1968): 125–8. Xerophthalmia is an eye condition, primarily affecting malnourished young children, where a failure to produce tears results in severe dryness and can lead to blindness.

66. Ibid., 126.

67. Krioutchkov and Tauch Kramam, "La parasitose intestinale," *Annales Médico-Chirurgicales de l'Hôpital de l'Amitié Khméro-Soviétique* (1968): 149–53.

68. Ibid., 151.

69. Latour, *Pasteurization of France*, especially 94–100.

70. Latour has noted that the vagueness of hygiene's boundaries in late nineteenth-century France gave proponents the ability "to express more or less everyone's interests." *Pasteurization of France*, 19.

71. There was a similar focus for medical research in 1960s and 1970s Tanzania. See Iliffe, *East African Doctors*, 215.

72. Peter Stallybrass and Allon White, "The City: The Sewer, the Gaze, and the Contaminating Touch," in *Beyond the Body Proper: Reading the Anthropology of Bacterial Life*, ed. Margaret Lock and Judith Farquhar (Durham: Duke University Press, 2007), 266–85. See also Latour, *Pasteurization of France*, 137–45.

73. See Ovesen and Trankell, *Cambodians and Their Doctors*, 61–5 and Au, *Mixed Medicines*, 103–7.

74. Kim Vien, E.I. Korelova, and S.I. Berezovskaia, "Étude de la cholestérolémie dans l'hypertension artérielle au Cambodge," *Revue Médico-Chirurgicale de l'Hôpital de l'Amitié Khméro-Soviétique* (1965): 43–5.

75. Leao Thean Im, "De l'étiologie et de la prophylaxie des accidents de rupture utérine au cours du travail," *Revue Médico-Chirurgicale de l'Hôpital de l'Amitié Khméro-Soviétique* (1965): 97–100.

76. "Soviet scientists receive fewer citations than one would expect, given the USSR's national research size; this indicates a low usage of Soviet scientific research". Frame and Carpenter, "International Research Collaboration," 490. The authors attribute the isolation of Soviet scientists to linguistic and cultural factors. In their analysis, "science" includes clinical medicine, physics, chemistry, engineering, biology, and other fields.

77. P.N. Kostenko, Nop Puthir, and Khim Kim San, "A propos de l'étiologie du cancer de l'appareil génital masculin au Cambodge," *Annales Médico-Chirurgicales de l'Hôpital de l'Amitié Khméro-Soviétique* (1968): 101–2.

78. Pridvijkine and Heng Kong Kimseng, "Donnes générales des affections dermato-vénériennes au Cambodge, d'après le travail effectue a l'hôpital de l'amitié Khméro-Soviétique," *Revue Médico-Chirurgicale de l'Hôpital de l'Amitié Khméro-Soviétique* (1965): 129–31.

79. My thinking about images in the *Revue* benefited from discussion with Emiko Stock.

80. Norodom Sihanouk, "Cher Sahachivin," *Annales Médico-Chirurgicales de l'Hôpital de l'Amitié Khméro-Soviétique* (1967): v.

81. Sihanouk, "Cher Sahachivin," iii.

82. So Satta, "Preface," *Annales Médico-Chirurgicales de l'Hôpital de l'Amitié Khméro-Soviétique* (1970/71): ii.

83. Crochet writes that up to half of the 450 doctors in the country left during the Republic. Crochet, *La santé*, 374–5.

84. For first-person accounts of medical study and services during the Republic, see Tony Kirby, "Rethy Chhem: From War-torn Cambodia to the IAEA," *The Lancet* 377, no. 9762 (2011): 291, and Haing Ngor, *A Cambodian Odyssey* (New York: Macmillan, 1988).

85. S. Skachkov, "USSR Economic Cooperation with Asian and African Countries," *Current Digest of the Russian Press* 6, no. 12 (1960): 19–20. Originally published in *Pravda*, Feb. 9, 1960, 3–4. http://dlib.eastview.com.proxy.lib.uiowa.edu/browse/doc/13817534.

86. Donald S. Zagoria, "Into the Breach: New Soviet Alliances in the Third World," *Foreign Affairs* 57, no. 4 (1979): 738.

87. Richard W. Franke and Barbara H. Chasin, "Kerala: Radical Reform as Development," *The Anthropology of Development and Globalization: From Classical Political Economy to Contemporary Neoliberalism* (Malden: Blackwell, 2005), 370.

88. Natalia Tsvetkova, "International Education during the Cold War: Soviet Social Transformation and American Social Reproduction," *Comparative Education Review* 52, no. 2 (2008): 199–217.

89. Natalia Tsvetkova, "Penetrated Societies in the Cold War, 1950–1990: Soviet Mode of Influence through Education," unpublished manuscript, 22.

90. Cambodia discontinued participation in education programs in the USSR in 1966 because of the overly ideological content of the curriculum. Tsvetkova, "International Education," 212.

91. The Institute was one of 25 technical schools established by the USSR in foreign countries between 1960 and 1990. Tsvetkova, "Penetrated Societies," 27.

92. See, for example, John S. Badeau, "Diplomacy and Medicine," *Bulletin of the New York Academy of Sciences* 46, no. 5 (1970): 303–12. Global

health programs were also part of US Cold War diplomacy in Latin America. See Marcos Cueto, "International Health, the Early Cold War, and Latin America," *Canadian Bulletin of Medical History/Bulletin canadien d'histoire de la médecine* 25, no. 1 (2008): 17–41.

93. Iliffe, *East African Doctors*, 120.
94. Mark G. Field, "Taming a Profession: Early Phases of Soviet Socialized Medicine," *Bulletin of the New York Academy of Medicine* 48, no. 1 (1972): 83–5.
95. Mark G. Field, "Health Personnel in the Soviet Union: Achievements and Problems," *American Journal of Public Health* 56, no. 11 (1966): 1915.
96. The USSR had made impressive gains. In 1970, life expectancy had increased from pre-Bolshevik levels of 38 years of age for men and 43 for women to 65 and 74 years respectively. Infant mortality decreased from 250 deaths per 1,000 live births in 1917 to 20 per 1,000 in 1970. The USSR had more doctors, nurses, and hospital beds per capita than any other country in the world. Laurie Garrett, *Betrayal of Trust: The Collapse of Global Public Health* (New York: Hyperion, 2000), 121–3.
97. Guillou, "Les médecins au Cambodge," 114–15. Crochet mentions that Sihanouk did later accept US funds to train community health workers, which was a popular feature of WHO programs in the Third World. Crochet, *La santé au Cambodge*, 372.
98. Margaret Lock and Vinh-Kim Nguyen, *An Anthropology of Biomedicine* (Malden: Wiley-Blackwell, 2010), 148.
99. Sylvia Chiffoleau, *Médecines et médecins en Égypte: construction d'une identité professionnelle et projet médical* (Paris: L'Harmattan/Maison de l'Orient Méditerranée, 1997), cited in Guillou, *Soigner dans les fracas*, 46.
100. Iliffe, *East African Doctors*, 140–4 and 177.
101. Ibid., 215.
102. Richard Rottenburg, "Social and Public Experiments and New Figurations of Science and Politics in Postcolonial Africa," *Postcolonial Studies* 12, no. 4 (2009): 426.
103. Vincanne Adams, Thomas E. Novotny, and Hannah Leslie, "Global Health Diplomacy," *Medical Anthropology* 27, no. 4 (2008): 315–23. See also Linsey McGoey, Julian Reiss, and Ayo Wahlberg, "The Global Health Complex," *BioSocieties* 6 (2011): 1–9.

CHAPTER 8

# Epidemics, Empire, and Education: Contested Discourses on the 1918 Influenza Pandemic in the Philippines

*Francis A. Gealogo*

## Introduction

The Philippines was not spared by the influenza pandemic of 1918–19 that reached most parts of the globe. Some analysts have estimated that more than 50 million people died in the pandemic, which affected half of the global population of the time. The pandemic affected mostly the young adult population of the world. Greger noted that "the 1918 virus killed more people in 25 weeks than AIDS has killed in 25 years."[1]

A peculiar feature of the pandemic was that it was experienced by most societies in waves of outbreaks. The first waves occurred from April to July 1918, the second from October to November of the same year, while the last came the following year, in the months of February and March, with the second wave exhibiting the highest mortality and morbidity figures globally.[2] An equally important characteristic of the 1918 influenza pandemic was the trend in mortality figures as experienced by different age groups. Particularly for the second wave, the disease seemed most deadly among the age group between 18 and 40—long considered the age group that constituted the strongest and healthiest of the population. Some countries exhibited extraordinary deaths for this age group compared with the others, with deaths occurring for this population constituting about half of all the victims within the entire population.[3]

In the Philippines, the 1918 pandemic would adversely affect the mortality rates of the archipelago. Data show that from 1904 until the outbreak of the epidemic, the annual death rate would normally occur in the low to middle 20s. But the 1918 outbreak caused a peak annual death rate of 40.79.[4] Most of the provinces proximal to Manila would have the highest death rates with the other large islands also affected by the outbreak.[5] A marked seasonality consistent with the waves of outbreaks that occurred in other countries would also be noted. Moreover, the age groups that exhibited the highest death rates for the year were not confined to the very young and very old. A remarkably high death rate would also appear for the age group between 18–40, indicating the same pattern in other countries affected by the pandemic.[6]

The Philippine experience of the pandemic became a venue for intensification of the implementation of public health information and education campaigns of the American colonial establishment. A number of the information and education campaigns aimed at combatting the disease were, at the same time, also aimed at redirecting Filipino behavior to become consistent with acceptable hygienic patterns that would be cultivated as the new norms of subject peoples. The control of the pandemic also became an appropriate opportunity for the colonial administration to modify Filipino appreciation of health, sanitation, and hygiene in the Western mold. The public information campaigns aimed at combatting influenza became a classic launching pad not only to control the spread of the disease, but also to modify people's perceptions of the epidemic and the supposed benevolent empire that should be assisting people in battling the pandemic.

However, the pandemic itself became a locus for the contestation of ideas between the various modes of appreciating health, epidemics, information, and education, in light of the colonial occupation. While official channels of communication and information dissemination were maximized by the colonial establishment through utilizing newspapers and releasing official reports, local expressions and popular perceptions about the nature of the epidemic and the institutional mechanisms employed by the American colonial administration to combat its spread also became widespread and at times ran counter to the American public health education and information programs.

The efficacy of Western-trained medical professionals, whether American colonial or local Filipino, was judged alongside local traditional practitioners, with the local population becoming the target of both camps to gain popular acceptance and legitimacy. Local sayings, prayers, riddles, poems, and other forms of vernacular expression became current and widespread during the period, reflecting local articulations of the populace on the epidemic itself, and on imperial programs and their health education campaigns. Military-style confinement, limitations on the movement of people, redirection of people's cultural and social practices, as well as information and education campaigns of the colonial administration were adopted as modes of combatting the spread of the disease. But the undercurrent of discourse and reactions to these programs by the local population proved that the campaigns were far from being both effective and acceptable to the local population.

## Public Health Education Campaigns in Confined and Unconfined Populations at the Height of the Pandemic

Public health education campaigns at the height of the outbreak were conditioned by the characteristics of the different target populations at which the efforts were being directed. The military mobilization campaigns of the colonial administration in preparation for an anticipated participation of the Philippines in World War I not only provided a pool for the spread of the disease in the islands, but the military camps also became the major loci of the information campaigns aimed at containing the outbreak. In September 1918, then Governor General Francis Burton Harrison took formal steps to organize the Philippine Council of National Defense aimed at mobilizing military personnel in support of the war efforts in Europe. Troops were mobilized and confined in a big cantonment at Camp Claudio south of Manila by November of 1918 after a three-month training period for officers and troops. The authority to participate in these efforts was received by November 19, at the time when the armistice ending the war had already been signed.[7] The mobilization of troops at the time of the epidemic and the decision to confine them in military camps even before they were deployed for combat to another continent facilitated the spread of disease as the troops were decommissioned later, with most of them being sent to their homes in various islands of the archipelago.

In order to contain the spread of the epidemic, measures were taken for the public in the communities surrounding the camp to moderate the adverse consequences of an epidemic outbreak. An extra cantonment zone within a radius of seven miles from Camp Claudio was established to control the spread of the disease. An official report on the pandemic, as influenced by the military camps, was summarized by Long and de Jesus as follows:

> The district was placed in charge of Senior Surgeon Felino Simpao, and included the towns listed below: Pasay, Parañaque, Las Piñas, Muntinlupa, San Pedro Makati, San Juan del Monte, San Felipe Neri, Pasig, Pateros, and Taguig in Rizal province, Bacoor and Imus in Cavite. The zone included a population estimated to be 107,914.
>
> Six thousand sixty seven cases and 935 deaths from communicable diseases were registered, most of which were due to influenza, the towns of Imus, Pasig and Paranaque being the greatest sufferers thereof....

To check the increase in morbidity and mortality cases in the community due to the pandemic, and in order to ensure that the military camp would be free from the disease, the extra cantonment health service unit listed the following measures to be undertaken in order to combat the spread of the influenza:

a. Lectures on preventive measures against dangerous communicable diseases

b. Influenza campaign. Treatment of cases found and reported by sanitary inspectors and distribution of medicines

c. Distribution of anti-influenza bulletins

d. Inspection of 21,360 houses and sanitary orders issued for general cleaning

e. Weekly inspection of public schools and monthly physical examination of school children

f. Sanitation of populated centers, especially those lying around Camp Claudio

g. Disinfection of houses where cases of dangerous diseases have been registered

h. Disinfection of 40 surface wells

i. Partial vaccination

j. Construction of six public midden sheds

k. Construction of 1,956 closets of the *Antipolo system* (water closet) (italics and translation mine)

l. Sanitation of 486 stables and providing of same with absorbent tanks

m. Inspection of all *tiendas* (local stores), 440 of which were placed in sanitary condition (italics and translation mine)

n. Sanitary supervision of establishments for the sale of candy and ice cream o.　Poisoning of 307 stray dogs

p.　Statistical work in the municipalities of Pasay, Parañaque, Las Piñas, Bacoor, and Imus for automatic sanitary control.[8]

While the list of the anti-influenza activities was relatively long, it must be noted that education and public health information campaigns held the primary spots in the implementation of the program. Lectures on the epidemic, the release of information bulletins to make the people aware of the contagion, and other measures were undertaken to combat the spread of the epidemic. The target of the campaign obviously went beyond the confines of the military camp where the military officers and men were stationed.

Even unconfined communities found beyond the camps became targets of a massive drive to prevent the epidemic from spreading outside the camps. Moreover, authorities attempted to modify some of the social and cultural practices of the local population as these were deemed contributory to the spread of the disease. Inspection, supervision, and education were all undertaken as part of the whole anti-influenza campaign. In order to accomplish these objectives, the population was monitored, constantly inspected, documented, and classified into statistical categories to ensure proper sanitation and disease control. These regulations necessitated limitations on the movement of people and the consumption of certain products, as well as the redirection of social behavior of communities into what the colonial administration deemed essential to controlling the disease. Done under colonial supervision, such programs aimed at controlling the epidemic resulted in furthering the social and cultural reorientation of the subject colonial peoples.

"Aside from military camps, the other notably confined and concentrated populations that exhibited a marked tendency to become centers for the spread of the disease were prisons, leper colonies, and schools."[9] Almost all of the inmates of the national penitentiary at the Bilibid Prison fell ill due to influenza at the height of the epidemic in October and November 1918. Around 50 per cent of those with respiratory complications died during the outbreak.[10] Almost all of the penal colonists of the Iwahig Penal Colony became ill with influenza in 1918, though only 4 per cent of the penal population died as a result of the contagion.[11] A total of 216 patients died of influenza at the Culion Leper Colony, despite its supposedly well quarantined conditions and its relative isolation from the rest of the archipelago.[12] In these cases, the colonists were given leaflets about disease prevention and control, not only for the benefit of the colonists, but, more importantly, for nearby communities as well. Despite the relative isolation of these communities, the epidemic continued to spread beyond the borders of the penal and leper colonies. *The Manila Times* reported that a great number of professors and students were affected by the outbreak at the University of the Philippines, prompting university officials to suspend registration for the second semester of school year 1918–19 due to the outbreak of the epidemic.[13] This was done to control the spread of the disease between students who were coming to Manila from many parts of the country.

Aside from the university, many schoolhouses were also closed and were used as temporary hospitals, with teachers serving as temporary nurses due to a shortage of medical and nursing personnel, who were overwhelmed by the sheer number of patients in the hospitals. These teachers were also mobilized to help in the information and education campaigns to instruct and advise the people on the proper way to contain and combat the disease—similar to what was done near the military camps.[14] The universities, prisons, military camps, and schools therefore became focal points not only in the containment of the disease, but also in the launching of information campaigns to combat its spread to other communities.

The spread of the pandemic notwithstanding, colonial health officials tried to mitigate the spread of the disease by way of the issuance of regular information bulletins to be distributed to university and school students, workers, tradesmen, and householders.[15] These efforts at educating the public were implemented together with other measures taken by the authorities, such as "isolation of the sick whenever possible; disinfection of infected premises, contacts and sputum of the sick; hospitalization, popular lectures, and direct instruction to [sic] the people to escape infection; distribution of pamphlets in Spanish and in the local dialect, etc."[16] All of these efforts would come to naught as the epidemic continued to spread to communities due to what the authorities characterized as the epidemic's high "diffusibility and extreme infectiousness...."[17]

## Newspaper Reports, and Information and Education Campaigns During the Pandemic

One way of looking at how information and public health education were transmitted to the general public was through the newspaper reports of the period. The data generated through reports in *The Manila Times*, though obviously limited in reach due to its English-language format, may provide readers with an idea of how information about the pandemic was being conveyed through print media for a particular reading audience. From June to December of 1918, most of the front pages and the inside local stories carried reports about the contagion.

For the first wave of the pandemic, news reports on the spread of the epidemic were published from June 16 to July 8, 1918. The initial reports detailed the impact of the epidemic as it made its way in the population centers of Manila. Government and business offices were reported to have been affected,[18] with telephone company employees, stevedores from the waterfront, as well as military officers and men in camps and policemen in their stations reported to have been hit by the epidemic. As businesses and offices became affected, *The Manila Times* became more emphatic in reporting the major offices and establishments reputed to be severely affected by the spread, including most public places like the San Andres cockpit, the City engineering office, the Internal Revenue office, and the office of the Manila mayor. Indeed, the mayor himself was a victim of the contagion.[19] Other headlines included reports about sanitary health inspectors themselves falling sick; members of the Congress unable to report to work; and the Board of Health reporting that the "infection is light, mortality is low, and we will rid of it in about six months or so ... if the general public stopped (sic) promiscuous coughing, sneezing and spitting."[20] The latter report noted that those trying to control the disease were experiencing difficulty due to what officials referred to as the "fact that human beings scatter their nose and mouth secretions without any consideration, despite rules and regulations to the contrary."[21] A constant slogan in the newspaper contained the command: "DON'T COUGH, DON'T SPIT, DON'T SNEEZE."[22]

The contagion was so severe that the newspaper reported a plan by the authorities to introduce a card system so that households and families could make sanitation reports to the officials of the health bureau. This plan, though, was not successfully implemented.[23] A sense of panic in the reporting could be gleaned as news reports of the spread of the influenza to the provinces outside of Manila became part of the news thread.

The second wave of the epidemic received even more extensive reporting on the spread of influenza in the country. *The Manila Times* had its first report on the second wave on October 19, 1918, with almost daily reporting beginning on October 27 and lasting up to December 18.

Initial reports on the second wave were rather dismissive in tone, with headlines like "Trancazo[24] is Again Visitor, but Epidemic is not so Severe."[25] But as reports reached the press indicating the problem to be worsening, the reporting became more erratic. Sensational headlines such as "All PI is Hit by Trancazo; Is [sic] Greatest Epidemic in History"[26] were followed by scaled-down, dismissive reports the following day, with headlines such as "Trancazo not Fatal in PI; Only Weaklings Succumb"[27] to counter the possible panic that the earlier report might have created. Premature reports of the epidemic dying down[28] would be countered by numerous reports of prominent personalities being victimized by the contagion. Moreover, as international reports reached the country, the global scope of the contagion was also noted, with reports of the outbreak occurring outside of the country becoming a regular feature of the November–December issues of *The Manila Times*.

Aside from reporting on prominent personalities such as local governors, congressmen, military officers, colonial bureaucrats, and members of the American high society falling prey to the epidemic, *The Manila Times* also carried headlines concerning the social and economic impact of the epidemic, for example, on the production output of workers who were unable to report to work,[29] and on fields being abandoned as agricultural workers became unable to do the harvest work. This prompted landowners to either offer a greater share for workers or higher wages for anyone willing to do the harvest.[30] The University of the Philippines had to postpone the matriculation of students soon after three students died of influenza.[31]

Some interesting features of news reports following this stage were human interest stories that highlighted the preference of the newspaper to report on situations that might catch the attention of prospective readers. The November 16, 1918 issue[32] reported that due to a lack of gravediggers, many of whom had either fallen sick or refused to report to work or simply abandoned work, prisoners were being detailed to the cemetery to help the remaining gravediggers, given the upswing in burials resulting from the high mortality figures caused by the epidemic.

Finally, a number of editorials were written analyzing the inability of health officials to combat the spread of the disease. The November 6, 1918 editorial[33] points to the low nutritional intake of the inhabitants of Manila as one of the reasons the population became vulnerable to the disease. Moreover, it also advanced the idea that the high cost of living, the inability of the government to develop other parts of the city and thus disperse the population, resulting instead in overcrowding of the old districts of Manila and the underdevelopment of the suburbs, created good conditions for the spread of the disease. The November 7, 1918 editorial[34] called for an expansion of the Philippine General Hospital with additional bed capacity and new personnel to attend to incidents such as epidemic outbreaks. Published together with an editorial on World War I, the November 17, 1918 editorial[35] repeated earlier pronouncements regarding the spread of the population, the lowering of prices of foodstuffs, the development of medical facilities, and the hiring of new medical personnel as major proposals so as to prevent future tragedies caused by a possible return of the pandemic. The November 29, 1918 editorial,[36] on the other hand, appealed to the International Red Cross to come to the rescue and aid the Philippines in combating the disease, citing apathy and indifference as major obstacles to the elimination of influenza. The November 30, 1918 editorial[37] was no longer so forgiving of the sectors concerned. It criticized the "negligence and lack of precautions by health officials; the low funding allocated by the government to the health bureau; the indifference among the many illiterate masses—lack of sanitation and use of old remedies and treatment by quack doctors described as both insanitary and foolish."[38] In short, everyone was to be blamed for the outbreak.

Aside from what was being reported daily in *The Manila Times*, one should also note that the newspaper was actually not required to report influenza-related data since influenza was not yet classified as a reportable disease even at the height of the pandemic. Daily health figures found in *The Manila Times* did not manifest any mortality and morbidity figures related to the disease at the height of the pandemic. Figures about reportable diseases and epidemics such as smallpox, cholera, and malaria were regularly featured in the newspaper while influenza mortality and morbidity figures were never part of the daily reportage—figures that would have been crucial for the people to fully grasp the gravity of the situation at a time when the epidemic was raging. The inability of the health authorities to regard influenza as a reportable disease in the immediate period after its initial outbreak made it impossible for the newspapers to report the same, reducing their capacity to inform the public about the gravity of the situation.

## Reporting the Campaigns: Official Reports on, and the Education Drive Against, the Pandemic

One can have a better sense of the information and education campaigns during the period from examining the official reports released by the colonial Bureau of Public Health that highlighted its efforts at combating the outbreak. Leaflets and flyers containing information about the disease were distributed to the population, and were reproduced in the official reports. For example: a bulletin containing prophylactic advice against influenza was profusely distributed [sic] among university and school pupils, shopworkers, tradesmen, laborers and householders. It reads as follows:

PHILIPPINE HEALTH SERVICE

For the information and guidance of all concerned (school teachers, business and working shop managers and foremen, householders and others) the following rules are issued with a view to prevent as much as possible the further spread of the present epidemic influenza (trancazo) in the city of Manila:

HOW TO AVOID TRANCAZO

Personal measures – Immediate contagion can be prevented by a [sic] thorough hygienic care of the mouth and throat; frequent cleanings with a brush and toilet antiseptic (as a weak solution of borax, oxygenated water, etc.), and gargles [sic] several times a day. Avoid also and protect yourself against the tiny drops of saliva or mucus contained in the breath which are expelled on coughing, sneezing or talking excitedly. You should keep a safe distance of four feet or more when talking with other persons and protect your mouth and nose with a handkerchief, so as to prevent danger to others and yourself. You should not spit promiscuously on the floor and other places. The sputum and saliva of the patients should be deposited in spittoons provided with disinfectants.

All the tableware, especially that used by a patient, should be thoroughly scalded (washed with hot water and soap). Also the fingers, when they are used for eating.

It is a vicious and coarse habit at all times, and especially during an epidemic of trancazo, to put the fingers in the nose or in the mouth and then shake hands with friends or infect them with things otherwise clean.

Whether sick or in health everyone should sleep with a mosquito net.

Do not send or permit children or grown persons with an incipient catarrh or malaise with bone-ache to attend the [sic] school, workshop, cine, theater, church or other places of meeting or gathering.

PRECAUTIONS OF A COLLECTIVE NATURE

Daily inspection of all the personnel, excluding all those who present symptoms of catarrh or bone-ache.

Prohibition of the common use of drinking glasses and towels.

MEDICAL ASSISTANCE

Patients need not go to a hospital. They may be attended by their own physician in their homes.

Poor persons may have the services of a health-doctor as soon as the case is reported to the corresponding station.

Anti-influenza vaccination is still in its experimental stage.[39]

The above information campaigns by public health authorities focused on three aspects of influenza control. The first one dealt with the re-orientation of personal habits of the individual; the second dealt with precautions to be handled by the community; while the last focused on medical interventions to be given to patients believed to have fallen ill from influenza. All three focused on the reorientation of Filipino habits concerning health, sanitation, and perceived well-being. The reduction of exposure by limiting public gatherings, constant hand washing and washing of dinnerware, prohibition of common drinking glasses and towels, and especially the use of handkerchiefs and prohibition of spitting in public—while measures to combat the spread of disease, were also measures adopted to bring about change in the personal and community habits of the Filipinos that were related to health and sanitation.

The official reports are also somber reminders that after all was said and done, the anti-influenza campaigns were only partially successful, to say the least. The radical measures undertaken, such as limiting public gatherings, massive information campaigns, forced isolation of victims, and medical intervention, all failed to contain the spread of the disease. Ultimately, nature would take its course and define the outcome of the pandemic cycle.[40]

## Contesting Discourses on the Outbreak

A more tangential way of providing a narrative report of the contagion is through the use of folk and popular literature that became widespread during the height of the epidemic. This not only reflected a form of popular perception about the disease, but also explained, in the popular mind, the causation of the illness and the local population's discomfort with it. Some of the pieces of literature were in the form of satirical prayers patterned along Catholic ones and modified to provide a critical perspective on the crisis of the day. Others were repetitions of the earlier *oraciones*[41] and prayers that had been popular during earlier outbreaks of other epidemics, more specifically the cholera epidemic of 1902–05. One example of this was the series of *oraciones* that became popular during the height of the cholera epidemic of 1904.

| | |
|---|---|
| *Sa sakit na kolera* | *Iligtas mo po kami* |
| *Sa mga sanitaryong sikulate* | *Iligtas mo po kami* |
| *Sa mga nakakagulat na vagon* | *Iligtas mo po kami* |
| *Sa mga inspektor na abusado* | *Iligtas mo po kami* |
| *Sa mga medikong walang muwang* | *Iligtas mo po kami* |
| *Sa mga hirap at sakit sa San Lazaro* | *Iligtas mo po kami* |
| *Sa mga Amerikanong lasing* | *Iligtas mo po kami* |
| *Sa mga Amerikanong abusado* | *Iligtas mo po kami* |
| *Sa mga mandudukot* | *Iligtas mo po kami* |
| *Sa mga mandarambong* | *Iligtas mo po kami* |
| *Sa mga hingoista* | *Iligtas mo po kami* |
| *Sa mga mag-aapi...* | *Iligtas mo po kami* |
| *Ibigay sa atin ang independensiya* | *Siyang dapat* |
| *Magkaroon ng pagpapapantay pantay* | *Siyang dapat* |
| *Siya na ang pag iiringan* | *Siyang dapat* |
| *Ihalal ang mga Pilipino ng mangatuto* | *Siyang dapat* |
| *Magkaisa tayong lahat* | *Siyang dapat* |
| *Ora pro novis celerastis politcitis sanitariarum* | *Siyang dapat* |
| *Oh diene ofeciamos permacionem amen* | *Siyang dapat* |

*OREMUS*
*Lahatur nang mga bagay bagayatur sa letaniaturm ay siyang larawatum ng bayanang Pilipinarum per kahirapan rebentatum.*

English translation:

| | |
|---|---|
| From the disease of cholera | Save us |
| From the sanitary guards | Save us |
| From the alarming wagons | Save us |
| From the abusive inspectors | Save us |
| From the unknowing medical practitioners | Save us |
| From the hardships and pains of San Lazaro (hospital) | Save us |
| From the drunken Americans | Save us |
| From the abusive Americans | Save us |
| From the pickpockets | Save us |

| | |
|---|---|
| From the highwayman | Save us |
| From the jingoists | Save us |
| From the oppressors… | Save us |
| | |
| Give us independence | Let it be/Amen |
| To have equality | Let it be/Amen |
| Enough of the infighting | Let it be/Amen |
| Elect the Filipino who will learn | Let it be/Amen |
| Let us be united | Let it be/Amen |
| | (translation mine) |

*Ora pro novis celerastis politcitis sanitariarum*
*Oh diene ofeciamos permacionem amen*
*OREMUS*
*Lahatur nang mga bagay bagayatur sa letaniaturm ay siyang larawatum*
*ng bayanang Pilipinarum per kahirapan rebentatum.*[42]

It should be noted that the last stanza "*Lahatur nang mga bagay bagayatur sa letaniaturm ay siyang larawatum ng bayanang Pilipinarum per kahirapan rebentatum*" is a combination of Tagalog and Latin-sounding terms which were unintelligible even to the local population. This combination is usually resorted to in order to invoke the *oracion* tradition of Latin-based prayers. The popular belief is that the more unintelligible and Latin-sounding a phrase is, the greater the efficacy of the prayer. In this case, the phrase is a satirical interpretation of the Philippine condition. Stripped of its Latinized rendering, the phrase may be read as "*Lahat nang mga bagay bagay ay siyang larawan ng bayang Pilipinas na nasa kahirapan*," which roughly translates into "Everything reflects the picture of the Philippine nation under poverty."

It is apparent in the preceding satirical prayers that popular perceptions about disease and its spread were not related at all to the notion of spread of bacteria or any other 'scientific' propositions. The popular perception was that the epidemic occurred as a result of colonial occupation and the inability of the Filipinos to unite against the perceived oppressor. In this regard, an absence of wellness was indicated as a matter of socio-political conditions that resulted from colonialism and internal strife. Local notions of disease and suffering, all interchangeably meant the same, and terms like *kahirapan* (poverty/suffering), *sakit*, (disease/illness/suffering), and *dusa* (sorrow/suffering) were not presented as mere medical conditions but socioeconomic and political conditions brought about by historical circumstances resulting from colonial occupation and elite collaboration with the colonizers. The colonial preference for the hegemony of science and bureaucratic efficiency was regarded as essentially oppressive and tyrannical. The modern medical profession brought by American colonialism was viewed as unable to address the suffering of the people and, rather, was perceived to be the cause of suffering. The sanitary guards, alarming wagons, abusive inspectors, unknowing medical practitioners, drunken and abusive Americans, were lumped together with the jingoists, pickpockets, and highwaymen as harbingers and heralds of suffering that the people must be saved from. The education and health campaigns of the Americans, far from being benevolent and magnanimous, were regarded as the cause of the suffering of the people.

The answer to all of these, as the prayer went, would not be found in the scientific journals or in the medical books promoted by American medicine. The answer would come by way of independence, equality, and the unity of the people. Here, the reception of American medical and sanitary order would become a site of political contestation. Health and wellness were both presented as related to the assumption of freedom from the 'malpractices' committed by American military and medical campaigns.

Knowledge production and transmission, particularly on disease and wellness, need not come from the formal education and training of practitioners. Indeed, some of those who were presented as knowledgeable about health and wellness were actually causing death and destruction for the population, while those presented by the colonial establishment as representatives of the old, unsanitary, superstitious ways, were actually the ones who were perceived as being able to heal the sick.[43]

Some health officials used the same mode of employing popular religious literature to advance medical explanations of the phenomenon of the disease. They utilized popular publications such as the almanacs that adopted religious tones in order to transmit messages regarding the spread of the disease. An example was the *Almanake* officially published by the Sanitation Commission in the aftermath of the influenza pandemic, which stated:

*SAMPUNG UTOS UPANG WALANG MAGKASAKIT*

   *I. Papurihan ninyo ang inyong bayan at sundin ang mga kautusan niya ukol sa kalinisan.*

   *II. Huwag ninyong kaligtaan ang araw ng paglilinis, at tuparing tibobos.*

III.  *Mahalin ninyo ang inyong mga anak at bigyan sila ng maayos na tahanan, mabuting pagkain at laruan.*

IV.  *Palagiin ninyo ang dalisay na hangin gabi't araw sa inyong bahay.*

V.  *Linisin at iayos ninyo ang inyong mga daana, looban, buluwagan (salas) at hagdanan.*

VI.  *Huwag kayong magpahamak ng inyong katawan o ng inyong mga kalapit bahay, sa pamamagitan ng hanging nakalalason o mga duming binubukalan ng sakit.*

VII.  *Huwag ninyong pabayaan mabuhay ang salaulang langaw.*

VIII.  *Huwag kayong magpahamak umimbot ng kaligayahan ng inyong mga anak sa pagpapabaya ng kanilang kalusugan.*

IX.  *Huwag kayong magpabayang mabulok o dumumi ang inyong ngipin o magkagayon sa bibig ng mga nasasakupan ninyo.*

X.  *Huwag kayong lulura sa mga daan, sa sahig, sa mga sasakyan, sa alin mang pook na pinagkakatipunan ng mga tao.*

## TEN COMMANDMENTS IN ORDER NOT TO BE SICK

I.  Praise your nation and obey its order about cleanliness.

II.  Do not forget the day assigned for cleaning, and fully follow this.

III.  Love your children and give them an orderly home, good food, and toys.

IV.  Always keep the air pure, night and day, inside your house.

V.  Clean and put in order all of your pathways, yard, living area, and stairs.

VI.  Do not put to harm your own body or your neighbor's by allowing toxic air to circulate from the garbage where disease originates.

VII.  Do not let the filthy housefly live.

VIII.  Do not restrain the happiness of your children by neglecting their state of health.

IX.  Do not let tooth decay or having a dirty mouth be the case for you or those under your care.

X.  Do not spit on the road, on the floor, on vehicles or on any other places where people congregate.[44] (translation mine)

The above commandments, created by health officials, show the bureaucracy's appreciation of folk and popular discourses to address issues that reflect their orientation. This indicated that even the very mediums reflecting folk perceptions became arenas of contestation for other forces to challenge. The campaign focused on the means to combat the 'dirty,' 'filthy,' and unsanitary habits of the Filipino, especially pertaining to spitting in public, poor dental hygiene, and the presence of the common housefly in Filipino households. These 'commandments' of healthy living were presented as part and parcel of developing good citizenship, fostering obedience and subservience to the colonial public health system as part of developing one's loyalty to the country, and imploring the reordering of the physical environment of the Filipino to be made orderly, sanitary, and clean and thus suitable for modern living. Thus, the medium found in popular, folk discourse was appropriated and brought in line with the colonial campaigns of public health and sanitation.

## Some Concluding Remarks

The spread of the influenza pandemic not only highlighted the public health challenges faced by medical officials in combating the disease, it also became an arena for cultural contestation and the politicization of the public health delivery system. This included the system of implementing sound information and education drives about the health campaign, with American health officials lamenting the propensity of the local population to believe more in local healers and herbalists than in the Western-oriented medical practitioners. There was also a powerful economic and financial dimension to this—as Western medical practitioners proved to be beyond the financial capacity of the ordinary masses, the people relied heavily on the less costly local healers. To wit, the Census report (Census, 1918 v.2, 1028) stated

> …Another serious aspect of the medical problem in the Islands is the belief, now happily on the wane, of the lower masses of the people in the healing power of certain *curanderos* [local healers] who, claiming to have received a supernatural gift from above, exploit the sick under the guise of charity. To these charlatans the sick often apply, seeking the services of physicians only in extreme cases. When they are sick, they are loath to call a physician that can cure them for one or two pesos; on the other hand, when summoned to appear in court they tremble in fear, and lose no time

in selling the house in which they live, the only *carabao* they use in their work, and the last piece of land they have, which they had inherited from their forefathers, to pay for the services of an '*abogadillo*', a pettifogging (sic) who can do nothing for their defense.[45] (italics mine)

In another part of the report, it is stated that

...Epidemics were usually regarded by the common people as 'the visitations of providence' or the 'scourge of God' and no efforts were made to combat them except by means of supplication and prayer. It used to be a popular belief that the devil in person was the forerunner of the epidemic.... Hospitalization was bitterly opposed, as they looked upon it with horror. Physicians were and still are scarce, and if any are available, they are not usually called to the bedside of the patient until he is actually in extremis hence the popular couplet

*Guinamot ng ulol*
*Pinatay ng marunong*

(Cured by the fool
Killed by the intelligent one)....[46] (translation mine)

The above maxim may very well represent the prevailing multi-level and multi-layered tensions in Philippine colonial public health policy as viewed by the local population. On the one hand, there was this perceived tension between what colonial public health would like to project as 'modern, Western, and scientific' medicine, represented by the medical doctor and projected as the able wise man, and the 'backward, local, and non-scientific' represented by local healers and herbalists. To the dismay of the colonial public health officials, the local population tended to rely more on the services of local healers and herbalists and to shy away from Westernized medical doctors. As a matter of fact, the above dictum would suggest that to the local mind, local herbalists and healers, though projected as fools, had greater efficacy in terms of providing wellness and healing than the medical doctors trained by Western medicine, who would simply bring death to the community.

The other tension stems from within the medical community of professionals trained along the lines of Western medicine. As early as the late nineteenth century, there was already a growing number of Filipino doctors, pharmacists, and other medical practitioners trained in the Western mode who presented themselves to the local population as the modern and Westernized equivalent of the local healers. While the public health bureaucracy under the Americans was heralded as harbingers of modernity and wellness to the Filipino population, the role of Filipino doctors in this new scheme of things in the American colonial public health bureaucracy remained precarious. After two decades of American occupation, the colonial bureaucracy allowed Filipino doctors to head the public health bureau, beginning with the appointment of Dr. Vicente de Jesus as bureau head, despite opposition from some camps about the program of Filipinization of public health administration in the country. The opposition to the Filipinization of the public health bureaucracy also brought to the fore the challenges faced by Filipino medical practitioners in combating public health problems such as epidemic outbreaks. The relative success of the campaigns against the cholera epidemic of 1902–05 under American leaders would be compared with the relative failures of the campaigns against influenza in the 1918–19 pandemic under Filipino leadership.

In conclusion, the 1918–19 influenza pandemic in the Philippines presented different levels of the impact of health education when confronted with challenges. On one level, the different impact on the sick employing local healing practices compared with those accessing Western medicine was being brought to the fore in the above aphorism. The supposed 'fool's medicine' of local healers were curing the sick, while 'intelligent medicine' represented by Western practice was bringing death to the afflicted. On the other hand, one can also sense the tension within the Filipino medical community, for both the Western-oriented medical practitioners and the local healers. By 1918, there were already a sufficient number of Filipino medical practitioners who were trained along Western lines, and who looked differently on the practices of local healers, more often viewing them as ineffective.

It must also be stated that the influenza pandemic occurred at a time of great contestation between Filipino and American colonial officials in general, and health officials in particular, especially in the light of debates on independence and autonomy. The development of a public health situation reminiscent of the political and social problems experienced when public health control measures were implemented to contain the cholera epidemic a decade earlier were enough for the Americans to be wary of the possible panic and unnecessary problems that a sensationalized reporting of the influenza outbreak might create for the people. Moreover, Filipino preference for local healers might be an indication of the more pragmatic approach that the subject peoples might have adopted in addressing their health needs, and a clear indication of the multiplicity of possible modes of addressing such needs outside of the colonial state health programs. The 1918 influenza pandemic highlighted and made more pronounced and apparent the different perceptions of the people, the public health officials, and the medical community regarding medical and public health education, wellness, and disease control in a colonial setting like the Philippines.

## Notes

1. Michael Greger, *Bird Flu: A Virus of Our Own Hatching* (New York: Lantern Books 2006), 6.
2. R. Edgar Hope-Simpson, *The Transmission of Epidemic Influenza* (New York: Plenum Press, 1992), 26–7.
3. Gerald Pyle, *The Diffusion of Influenza: Patterns and Paradigms* (New York: Rowman and Littlefield, 1986), 40. See also Arthur Silverstein, *Pure Politics and Impure Science: The Swine Flu Affair* (Baltimore: The Johns Hopkins University Press, 1981), 17.
4. Philippine Islands Census Office, *Census of the Philippine Islands* (Manila: Bureau of Printing, 1920–21), 1046.
5. Francis A. Gealogo, "The Philippines in the World of the Influenza Pandemic of 1918–19," *Philippine Studies* 57, no. 2 (2009): 261–92.
6. Ibid. For the actual mortality and morbidity figures, see Philippine Islands Census Office, op cit.
7. "The Philippines and their part in the great war," *Manila Daily Bulletin Anniversary Number* (Feb. 1919): 81ff.
8. John D. Long and Vicente de Jesus, *Report of the Philippine Public Health Service Fiscal Year 1918* (Manila: Bureau of Printing, 1919), 19–20.
9. Gealogo, "The Philippines in the World of the Influenza Pandemic," 284.
10. Ibid., 14–15, 32.
11. Ibid., 52–3.
12. Ibid., 45.
13. *Manila Times*, Nov. 12, 1918.
14. Bureau of Insular Affairs, Record Group 350, Entry 5, Box 422, General Classified Files 1898–1945, United States National Archives and Records Administration, College Park, Md.
15. Long and de Jesus, *Report of the Philippine Public Health Service*, 63.
16. Ibid., 119.
17. Ibid.
18. *Manila Times*, June 18, 1918.
19. *Manila Times*, June 17, 1918.

20. *Manila Times*, June 16, 1918.
21. Ibid.
22. Ibid.
23. *Manila Times*, July 8, 1918.
24. *Trancazo* is the local term for influenza.
25. *Manila Times*, Oct. 27, 1918.
26. *Manila Times*, Nov. 1, 1918.
27. *Manila Times*, Nov. 2, 1918.
28. *Manila Times*, Nov. 5, 1918.
29. *Manila Times*, Nov. 17, 1918.
30. *Manila Times*, Nov. 27, 1918.
31. *Manila Times*, Nov. 12, 1918.
32. *Manila Times*, Nov. 16, 1918.
33. *Manila Times*, Nov. 6, 1918.
34. *Manila Times*, Nov. 7, 1918.
35. *Manila Times*, Nov. 17, 1918.
36. *Manila Times*, Nov. 29, 1918.
37. *Manila Times*, Nov. 30, 1918.
38. Ibid.
39. Long and de Jesus, *Report of the Philippine Public Health Service*, 63.
40. Ibid., 119–20.
41. Prayers.
42. "Luhod Kayo't Mamumuno Ako," Bulalakaw, *Muling Pagsilang*, 21 Hulyo 1906, in *Ang Dagling Tagalog, 1903–1936*, ed. Rolando Tolentino and Aristotle J. Atienza (Quezon City: Ateneo de Manila University Press, 2007), 93–5.
43. Philippine Islands Census Office, Census of the Philippine Islands in the Year 1918, 1060.
44. Mamerto Tiangco, *Almanake at Kalendario ukol sa Kalusugan sa mga taong 1919, 1920 at 1921 ng Kagawaran ng Sanidad ng Pilipinas*, 1918 (Manila: Bureau of Printing, 1921), 2.
45. Census, 1918 v. 2, 1028.
46. Ibid., 1059–60.

CHAPTER 9

# Medical Education "from Below": Self-medication, Medical Pluralism, and Therapeutic Citizenship in Colonial Vietnam

*Laurence Monnais*

## Introduction

In the early twentieth century, French doctors posted in Vietnam described—and condemned—in their monthly reports to their superiors acts of refusal by indigenous people to consume medicines given to them. For these doctors, this refusal was an expression of both mistrust and deep ignorance as to the benefits of modern medicine. In the interwar period, however, these same doctors, as well as their Vietnamese colleagues, reported a certain amount of enthusiasm among their patients for some Western (French) pharmaceuticals. They presented this enthusiasm as undeniable proof of success in their mission to civilize, and its growing popularity. What can one make of this dual discourse? Surely, the key factor cannot simply be the passage of time.

The hypothesis of this chapter can be described thus: that the Vietnamese made complex individual choices in their recourse to "colonial medicines."[1] Some therapeutic products were accepted, often with surprising ease and speed, while others were rejected, at times quite forcefully so. This chapter focuses on this process of selection by first describing its patterns, and then seeking to identify the reasons behind it. Even heavily biased sources—administrative and medical—that essentially neglect the voices of the sick and consumers of therapeutic services give us a starting point for discovering these reasons. Besides

250

drawing on this first set of sources, we will also draw on additional, seldom used sources, in particular Vietnam's popular press and health magazines, published in the 1920s and 1930s. Three broad aspects of local therapeutic practices will be discussed: the gap in the colonial health care system between the actual and idealized provision of medicines, the weight of local medical culture(s), and the nature of the therapeutic relationship that was imposed on the Vietnamese population by the colonizer. It will be argued that the Vietnamese tendency to select medications reveals unexpected and hybrid forms of lay medical education that account for early forms of "therapeutic citizenship" in a colonial context.

## Colonization, Colonial Medicines, and Health Education

The modern history of medicine in Vietnam is tightly linked to the French domination of Indochina (1858–1954) and the attempts at medicalization with which it was associated.[2] Indeed, the association between medicalization and colonization is a powerful one: scientific medicine[3] that emerged in the nineteenth century became a "tool of empire," that is, a political, economic, and humanitarian instrument that was dedicated to the cause of pacification and then of exploitation and of *mise en valeur*—the rational development of human and natural resources[4]— of the region. By 1905, this endeavor was structured within a formal health care system under the generic heading of *Assistance Médicale Indigène* (Indigenous Medical Assistance) or AMI. The AMI was founded on a desire to demonstrate the alleged scientific nature of European medicine and the power of public health and its promoters. Among its core priorities, one could find mass vaccination campaigns (with an emphasis on smallpox prevention), a process that could be seen as a continuation of previous interventions that began as early as the 1860s with the conquest of Cochinchina, and, to a lesser extent, the provision of hospital care, for which a network of institutions was built. By 1936, there were over 600 health facilities in Indochina, of which at least two-thirds were small clinics, dispensaries, and infirmaries.[5]

The system was founded on the idea of free health care for the needy (*indigents*), with needy, in this case, meaning most of the Vietnamese population. It placed special emphasis on the two-pronged objective of mass prevention (through vaccination and sanitation) and the transmission of basic hygiene through education (in elementary schools and through public conferences and the distribution of pamphlets, for instance). These two elements were used to justify attempts to transform local norms and intrusions into people's intimate lives. Indeed, metropolitan legislative frameworks dealing with public health were quickly imposed, particularly in urban areas, to regulate a wide range of domains, from the appropriate supply of drinking water to the cleanliness of buildings, funeral rites, and the control and surveillance of prostitutes and the contagiously ill. During the interwar period, signs of an adapting colonial health system began to appear, as colonial medical agents were better able to grasp the geographic and pathological—and to a lesser extent sociocultural—environments in which they worked. This willingness to adapt was made most concrete through qualitative as well as quantitative shifts: institutional care was provided for several *maladies sociales* or social diseases, including venereal, pulmonary, and ocular infections, cancer, leprosy at the time; sanitary protection was extended to mothers and children; the diffusion of "essential care" into rural areas was prioritized; and the number of medical, especially subaltern, personnel was increased considerably, primarily through a process of "Vietnamization." By 1939, some 3,500 indigenous nurses and midwives worked for the AMI. These transformations can thus be seen as a polymorphous movement of indigenization.[6]

What was the importance of medication in this system, at a time when the Western pharmaceutical industry was rapidly growing? What functions were attributed to medicines, and did these functions change over time? The fact that, consistently, medical and administrative sources barely touch upon this issue is in itself revealing. Originally, it seems that medication was relegated to a secondary role, and was tacitly assimilated with other minor medical tools and techniques in the provision of hospital care. Only vaccines—promoted by followers of Pasteur, whose heavy presence in Indochina was unrivalled in any other colonial territory[7]—were put at the forefront of health policy. In contrast, starting in 1905, the legislative and institutional framework of AMI had strictly defined the contours of the population's access to Western drugs. It regulated imports of pharmaceutical substances, particularly those containing toxic substances,[8] the conditions for obtaining some medicine—such as those medical specialties requiring a prescription—and the distribution of free medicines to the poor, government agents, and several groups deemed to be "at risk."

As of 1909, a state quinine service (*Service de Quinine d'État,* SQ) was meant to provide inhabitants of areas with a high prevalence of malaria with opportunities to obtain free or subsidized quinine to prevent the disease—not to cure it.[9] Most notably, however, was the creation, authorized by a law passed on April 18, 1920, of basic medicine stores (*dépôts de médicaments*). As an upshot of the interwar reorientation of health policies, these stores launched a broader diffusion of essential medicines in communities further than 10 kilometers from an AMI facility or a private pharmacy. These products, according to the 1920 text, were "ready to use," in that they should not require any manipulation or preparation on the part of the distributor,[10] as well as being non-toxic and could be sold without a prescription. It was required only that they be accompanied by a notice describing their therapeutic indications. However, consumers had to pay for these medicines. To some extent, these medicine stores existed outside of the free public health care system, just like the SQ, since in both cases distribution occurred through stores managed by non-medical providers. The discourse on the value of pharmaceuticals in the attempt to medicalize Vietnam would, in the later half of the 1930s with the introduction of the antibacterial sulfonamides, gather some steam, as these new wonder drugs would show encouraging results in the fight against several infectious diseases such as gonorrhea and pneumonia.[11]

The fact that medicines were given very little importance in French Vietnam for several decades can be explained by a combination of factors both general and specifically colonial. Firstly, Western doctors adopted a position of therapeutic skepticism, both in the metropole and the colonies,[12] out of an awareness of the limits of their therapeutic arsenal—at least until the introduction of arsenobenzols and the first "magic bullet," Salvarsan (Compound 606), in 1910.[13] Second, colonial doctors put priority on mass prevention over individualized treatments when faced with endemic and epidemic tropical diseases that were not only devastating, but about which, in some cases, they knew very little. Mass prevention was not only a necessity of which most colonial doctors and their Western-trained Vietnamese colleagues[14] were convinced: it was an absolute priority in their attempts to civilize the "natives." In contrast, drugs could not be civilizing tools as they were too often seen as unreliable, ineffective, or too toxic; they would not be proper tools of education since they might induce negative side effects, and did not require the expertise or even the presence of a doctor to be ingested.[15] Some doctors also perceived the promotion of the consumption of pharmaceuticals as a path that might lead to giving some legitimacy to "traditional" Sino-Vietnamese medicine—heavily based on therapeutics —and to native "bad habits" in terms of health practices.

## Manifestations of Therapeutic Selection

To what extent did the Vietnamese people comply with the rules imposed by the colonizer upon (limited) access to pharmaceuticals and accept this supremacy of mass prevention over personal care? Colonial and medical sources reveal wide contrasts in reactions to therapy ranging from categorical rejection to expressions of enthusiasm that were virtually instant and unconditional. One of the most striking features of medical discourses dating from the early years of the AMI is the expression of a particularly vehement refusal, or at least an obvious recalcitrance, by the Vietnamese in response to the first colonial medicines diffused in this region: vaccines.

### Rejecting Medicines

As of 1871, smallpox vaccination became compulsory for the population of Cochinchina—an obligation that was extended to the rest of Vietnam (and the whole of Indochina) in the late 1880s.[16] Vaccines would soon come to be produced by several local *Instituts Pasteur*, and would become the nucleus of a massive prevention campaign that seems to have produced a rather one-sided reaction from the Vietnamese. At the turn of the twentieth century, in one village, those with a little spare money would pay to be replaced by poorer neighbors during the campaign's visit through their hometown; in another village, mothers sucked on their babies' arms to extract the noxious substance from their child's body.[17] Similarly, plague and, later, anti-cholera vaccination campaigns gave rise to varied expressions of discontent, some even escalating into large-scale anti-French protests.[18] Introduced in some Saigon schools in 1921, the anti-tuberculosis vaccine BCG was perhaps the first vaccine to arouse more interest than dissension; however, its use would remain circumscribed and was accompanied by the distribution of information about the procedure, as well as social and financial support to families affected by pulmonary tuberculosis.[19]

Colonial doctors also decried the rejection of quinine in the prevention of malaria; with the prime cause of morbidity in Indochina throughout the period of domination being malaria, the disease was seen as a major public health issue, especially since it affected, among others, portions of the population that had been put to work in the colonial economic development plans.[20] Not only did the Vietnamese seem reluctant to consume medicines as preventative measures, they seemed to reject medicines that induced side effects (gastric intolerance, buzzing noise in consumers' ears, extreme fatigue, and sometimes nervous reactions in the case of quinine), or at least perceptible bodily reactions. Thus, the use of copper sulfate to treat trachoma, "the application of which, in addition to being very painful, often provokes an intense reaction of the conjunctiva," would also be massively vetoed by sufferers in the 1920s.[21] During the same period, leprosy treatments consisting of chaulmoogra oil injections, known to be very painful and to provoke nausea and high fever, probably boosted leprosaria escape rates.[22] Similarly, patients reportedly rejected the dairy diet prescribed for dysentery; they complained about the discomfort it caused—probably as a consequence of lactose intolerance in many cases—or categorically refused to consume foods which were completely absent from their usual diets.[23]

In addition, some AMI doctors complained that Western medicine and its agents were being sought out as a "last resort," that is, after trying to obtain relief from local therapists and druggists and the consumption of Sino-Vietnamese remedies. Colonial practitioners attributed this tendency to a preference for a "crude empiricism" rooted in ignorance and fear.[24] They saw it as an obstacle to their own therapeutic interventions, producing conditions under which their treatments became more difficult and less effective. One might suggest, however, that this tendency was actually the manifestation not so much of a refusal of modern therapies but of mutating practices of medical pluralism.

### Demanding Medicines

After World War I, a change seems to occur and a number of medical reports begin to draw attention to successes encountered in offering some Western cures. Other sources confirm this enthusiasm, perhaps less directly, but also more convincingly (the truthfulness of reports that government-employed doctors were forced to submit to the administration to which they were accountable is open to question). Among these are documents issued by judiciary and customs services, in which one finds statements of violations of laws regulating the practice of medicine or pharmacy, reports of cases of theft of medicines from AMI hospitals and of lucrative black market trading of certain substances,[25] as well as a plethora of advertisements for patent medicines in the local press, published in French and in *quốc ngữ*.[26]

More specifically, the most prominent feature of this enthusiasm was the popularity of dozens of commercial specialties in urban environments. Upon consulting several contemporary magazines and newspapers,[27] one is struck by the strong presence of French private pharmacies in this media landscape and by the efforts their owners deployed to praise, often in Vietnamese, the merits of a plethora of products that were allegedly highly popular in colonial society and, for the most part, in metropolitan society as well.[28] While making a direct link between the advertisement and the consumption of featured products would certainly be problematic, the Vietnamization of trademark names —for example, Gastrol (for stomach pains) was referred to as *Ga-tò-rôn*, while Morrhuol (a cod liver oil-based remedy for colds and bronchitis) as *Mo-ru-ôn*—does seem to indicate a certain level of local familiarity with some of the remedies being advertised. Additional evidence for this interpretation is provided by a growing number of seizures of counterfeit French products, produced locally or in China,[29] and by the local manufacture, by French pharmacists in small laboratories adjacent to their shops, of products destined for the Vietnamese market. For example, the Pharmacie Montès in Hanoi marketed its own "cachets antiseptiques" (antiseptic tablets), while the Pharmacie Chassagne produced a "collyre jaune selon la formule du Dr Casaux" (yellow eye drops based on the formula of Dr. Casaux, a colonial ophthalmologist who was the director of the Hanoi ophthalmological institute in the 1920s), which was allegedly tailored for the "native constitution."[30] These "local specialties" and the "hybrid specialties"[31] that mixed "Western" and "Sino-Vietnamese" elements (combining a synthetic component and local plants, for example, or a "traditional" product revamped with Western-style packaging) are clear markers of medical pluralism embodied at the level of the pill or the spoonful of syrup. It is significant that Pharmacie Chassagne published a health magazine, the *Vệ Sinh Báo: Journal de vulgarisation d'hygiène* (VSB). With a monthly circulation of 13,000 copies from 1926 to 1933, the publication was used by Chassagne's successors, Mr. Lafon and Mr. Lacaze, as an advertising platform, but also as a channel to diffuse knowledge and basic principles concerning matters of health, prevention, and self-care.

Advertised remedies were indicated for a variety of conditions. These medicines were often portrayed as panaceas and sometimes as cures for specific ailments.[32] They usually promised relief for various symptoms: cough, pains, "generalized weakness," anemia, anxiety, insomnia, digestive discomfort, fever and dermatological affections. In terms of pricing, some evidence seems to show that they were relatively inexpensive (0.30 piaster for eye drops; 0.40 for a bottle of Gastrol) and thus accessible to a relatively high proportion of households.[33] On the other hand, the modest cost of this type of product does not, in and of itself, constitute an argument "for" or "against" extensive recourse to Western medicines: while the high cost of French medicines was often brought up by associations of traditional therapists in the 1930s as an argument against restricting their practice, other sources convey the idea that Vietnamese were accustomed to paying a high price for some "very efficient" Chinese medicines.

Outside urban areas, enthusiasm for colonial medicines would be directed towards some of the products distributed through the *dépôts de médicaments*, which would rapidly suffer chronic shortages across the country.[34] Among the medicines found in these stores were quinine, purgatives (sodium sulfate), analgesics, and antipyretics (sodium salicylate, pyramidon, antipyrin, Aspirin), ointment for scabies (Pommade d'Hélmerich), pills for diarrhea (Pilules de Second), emetine hydrochloride for dysentery, several types of eye drops, copper sulfate, two or three antiseptics and anthelminthics (santonin, thymol), as well as a few syrups and expectorants. As with the advertised specialties, these essential medicines were for the most part indicated for the treatment of common symptoms—fevers, diarrheas—and of minor but recurring infections—worms, parasites, benign eye infections—and meant to be sold at very low cost: a dose of antipyrin, for example, cost 0.10 to 0.20 piaster in 1930.

Finally, some pharmaceuticals, in the 1930s, seem to have elicited immediate and widespread enthusiasm. Unlike most advertised remedies and the basic medicines sold in rural stores, these products could only be legally obtained with a prescription; they were considered to be highly toxic and to carry a risk of therapeutic accidents when used without medical guidance. The local introduction of Salvarsan in 1911 seems to have instigated a growing recognition of the efficacy of specific chemical treatments against several devastating or previously incurable afflictions. The class of medicines that exemplified this third movement of enthusiasm for Western medical specialties were sulfonamides, especially Dagénan, which was used in Tonkin from 1938 onwards to treat gonorrhea, pneumonia, as well as some forms of urinary infections and meningitis. A large black market bloomed around the supply of this class of drugs, reaching epidemic proportions during World War II, during which time it implicated French military personnel and employees in pharmacies and hospitals who had access to their employers' prescription pads.[35]

These three aspects of pharmaceutical enthusiasm clearly indicate that the therapeutic choices made by Vietnamese people did not easily cohabit with, and often sought to bypass, the rules governing the distribution of medicines promoted by colonial doctors. An analysis of the potential determinants of this selection, taking into account divergent opinions and interpretations of medicines' functions and of the conditions under which they could be obtained, helps to better understand its basis and confirms its political, economic, and cultural dimensions.

## Choosing Medicines: Reasons Behind Therapeutic Selection

The seemingly contradictory attitudes elicited by quinine offer us keys for understanding the factors that came into play in processes of therapeutic selection. While colonial doctors remarked on stubborn resistance against its ingestion for preventive purposes they suggested was triggered by "fear of lethal suffocation,"[36] they also observed a growing tendency for it to be sought out as a treatment for bouts of fever. In some areas, SQ stores could not meet the popular demand in the 1920s and 1930s, whereas in other areas, stallholders did not know what to do with their unsold stock. These apparent inconsistencies may in fact be symptomatic of a set of factors shaping therapeutic choices: the influence of pre-colonial representations and therapeutic practices, the challenges experienced by doctors in getting their patients to comply with the therapeutic rules they sought to impose, and most importantly, the issue of accessibility (both in terms of price and geography—quinine was not offered as a gratuity in every location, and quite often stores were far apart). These factors represent concrete conditions arising from a considerable gap between the ideals and realities of therapeutic provision in colonial Vietnam.

### Provision of Therapeutic Care: From Theory to Reality

Before the start of World War I, Vietnam became the destination for an ever-increasing transfer of pharmaceuticals exported from France and other Western countries.[37] In response to this movement, colonial authorities sought to impose increasingly strict rules on the importation and distribution of these products. Guided by clearly protectionist interests, but also by concerns for public health, they searched for ways to drastically limit access to a growing number of toxic substances.[38] These restrictions must have clashed with the lively atmosphere of rapid therapeutic expansion and diversification, in which a growing number of protagonists and their varied logics were colliding. One might think, in particular, of the frustrated objectives of French pharmaceutical manufacturers, such as Spécia Rhône-Poulenc, which, at the time, were seeking to take advantage of overseas markets while at the same time hoping to eliminate foreign competition.[39]

Nor did this increasing rigidity function within the budgetary realities and chronic personnel shortages that plagued AMI, and which may have created a mismatch between what Vietnamese patients sought to obtain and what could realistically be offered to them. What might be perceived here is that medical authorities' condemnation of a Vietnamese refusal of pharmaceuticals might, in some cases, have masked a lack of accessibility. Colonial medicines were thus probably often "not consumed" because of *imposed* barriers rather than rejected out of *conviction*. Some doctors were remarkably frank about the shortcomings of the AMI. They noted that many of their colleagues were overworked and unable to offer proper care. Practitioners admitted to turning patients away without treatment on account of shortages—pharmaceutical supplies were mainly imported from the metropole, a system that saved money but was often unreliable—or because the appropriate treatment was too costly and therefore not provided by the AMI.[40] Others reported that they had to "dilute" certain products in order to preserve stocks, even if they risked weakening the effectiveness of their treatment.[41] Others still deplored their own inability to personally follow up on their patients' care; they were constantly being reassigned to new posts in an ultra-bureaucratized system and could therefore hardly become familiar with the inhabitants of a particular district, nor provide them with any kind of extensive knowledge about Western therapeutics even if they expressed a willingness to do so.[42]

In contrast, Sino-Vietnamese therapists were more numerous, certainly more available, and perhaps also better supplied in drugs than AMI doctors. In 1931, a commission for the inspection of Indochina's pharmacies estimated that at least 1,700 medicine resellers were practicing in Tonkin, not including itinerant vendors whose numbers were impossible to estimate. In the same year, there were only 65 Western-style (private) pharmacies and basic medicine stores according to the official estimate of the Inspection of Health Services and about 100 prescribing doctors affiliated with AMI, amounting to about 1 doctor for 100,000 potential patients, that is, proportionally, 45 times fewer than in metropolitan France in 1911.[43] The obvious persistence of popular recourse to Sino-Vietnamese drugs and the undeniable gap between colonial intentions concerning the distribution of medicines and its realities (illicit networks, shortages, costs that were beyond AMI's means) would eventually lead, in the 1930s, to legislative amendments as well as some improvements in the health care system. There were increases in the training and appointment of Vietnamese medical personnel; nurses and midwives were granted limited rights to prescribe; Vietnamese doctors obtained the right to enter private practice; and rural stores of commercial specialties managed by traditional druggists were authorized —at least for a few years.[44]

Just before World War II, a habit of condemning the rejection of colonial medicines morphed into a genuine reflection on how, given Vietnam's political, economic, and cultural realities, to best carry on diffusing the benefits of modern Western medicine. And some doctors, mainly Western-trained Vietnamese practitioners but also a few French colonial ones, were even ready to accept therapeutic pluralism as a necessary path towards achieving this diffusion.[45]

### Dealing with Health the Confucian Way

The continuous supply and use of Sino-Vietnamese medicine by the Vietnamese population can be seen as the product of necessity: indeed, it served to address the limitations of a public health care system that ultimately never had the means, financial or ideological, to match its ambitions. It can also be seen as the product of enduring representations and practices regarding one's own health and management. In this context, therapeutics became absolutely central.

Vietnam is the only country in Southeast Asia to be part of the Confucian world—a consequence of nearly 1,000 years of colonization by its powerful neighbor. It has developed rich and complex medical traditions, within which a distinction is usually made between "Northern medicine" (*Thuốc Bắc*) or Chinese medicine and "Southern medicine" (*Thuốc Nam*) or Vietnamese medicine, the latter referring to a more popular tradition of healing that draws on a rich local biodiversity.[46] *Thuốc* translates as tobacco, remedy, as well as medicine or healing;

its multiple meanings illustrate the centrality of medicinal substances in the double-stranded medical heritage it designates, in which drug therapies are indistinguishable from the art of healing and have long constituted the core of actions on illness and sick individuals. In this context, it seems reasonable to believe that Western pharmaceuticals might have been rapidly adopted by the population, at least more so than other kinds of interventions into health that were less familiar in terms of local cultural references. Some colonial doctors were quick to declare that the Vietnamese customarily view them as a mere "automatic distributor of medicines."[47]

This is not to say, as mentioned earlier, that all Western pharmaceuticals received the native population's approval. Consumption practices reflected popular representations of illness, health, and the body. Local explanatory models of illnesses seem to have influenced patterns of recourse to therapy. For example, some diseases categorized by biomedicine as diagnosable pathologies did not figure in similar nosological terms within local popular conceptions. Cholera, which was traditionally seen as a manifestation of revenge by an evil spirit, was interpreted as having supernatural origins; in this case, purely medical interventions were considered to be ineffective. Smallpox, on the other hand, was frequently viewed as a necessary rite of passage: according to a Vietnamese proverb, the child who has not yet had smallpox has not yet been born. In the case of both these conditions, the conversion to biomedical interpretations took place only slowly and partially, especially because many colonial doctors played down the significance of such beliefs in approaching local people. This was especially the case when populations were to be intervened upon collectively and anonymously, as in vaccination campaigns.

In the same vein, one can suppose that some pharmaceuticals, whether patent or "ethical," may have been more easily rejected or integrated into therapeutic practices on the basis of their therapeutic indications. When a therapy's promised or actual effects were translatable into terms that resonated with familiar notions, such as the hot/cold dichotomy or the principle of balance, that were fundamental in Confucian medical culture, they became likelier to be accepted by the Vietnamese. A clear example of this can be found in recourse to tonics, which remain to this day the class of drugs with the highest consumption in Vietnam.[48] The impact of other types of analogies merit closer attention, such as the possible rejection (or acceptance) of medicines on the basis of prior familiarity with their active substances, meaning whether their components were customarily included in the Sino-Vietnamese pharmacopoeia or local diets. In this respect, the popularity of opotherapeutic products (or organotherapeutic products derived from animal products) is a fascinating example.[49] Rejection or acceptance may also have been influenced by an experience of the shape, packaging, or even color or taste[50] of a product, although probably not independently of its effects. Along these lines, the diffusion of pills and tablets that, from the seventeenth century onward were exported from China to Vietnam, both legally and illegally, and continued to be exported throughout the colonial period,[51] may have played a significant role in the diffusion of certain products as well as in the instigation of a movement of commodification of health.[52] In these forms, medicines were also more easily transported, consumed, and preserved, which reduced the risk of their being altered and losing their effectiveness.

The Vietnamese nevertheless seemed to have a clear preference for curative treatments. This is not to say that prevention did not exist in Vietnamese culture. However, rejection of preventive therapies may have arisen from a dissonance between the intentions of those who provided them, that is, to prevent a targeted disease, most often a contagious one, and the conceptions of disease causation and prevention by those who were meant to take these medicines. For the latter, diseases were an imbalance; their origins, precipitating factors, and manifestations could not necessarily be predicted or identified precisely, and yet they might be avoided through healthy eating. There are also indications that the Vietnamese were not keen adopters of the idea of long-term therapies and medication for chronic diseases. Indeed, preferred remedies were those with rapid and measurable effects that occurred within hours —might this account for the tremendous enthusiasm for anthelmintic medications repeatedly reported by AMI doctors?[53]—or, at most, within days.[54] Such beliefs may, in any case, account for the frequent complaints on the part of medical authorities about patients' behaviors of non-compliance and therapeutic pluralism (some "traditional" drugs were also used on occasion to counter the perceived toxic effects of some Western pharmaceuticals).[55]

## The Therapeutic Relationship as Confrontation

In the colonial context, the provision of health care was particularly authoritarian. Compulsory vaccination, intrusions into private life and into public spaces in the name of reducing risks of contagion, reinforced an inextricable link between colonialism, medicine, and social control.[56] Yet, one often forgets a colonial encounter that may, in and of itself, have seriously hampered the development of an indigenous affinity for biomedicine and its therapies, and thus have constituted a major obstacle for the colonial enterprise of medicalization: the therapeutic relationship.

With the establishment of the AMI, access to medicines was codified and obligations were imposed, as we mentioned earlier: individuals wanting to obtain a medicine that either contained toxic substances or was free of cost were forced to submit to the biomedical framework of the therapeutic relationship. It is not difficult to see the authoritarianism and rigid standardization entailed by this framework, which permeated both the procedure of the medical consultation and the resulting treatment. First there was an obligation to abide by the doctor's availability and respect the consultation schedule. Most dispensaries and hospitals were open to the public only a few hours each day, sometimes only a few hours per week. From rural areas, it was often necessary to travel long distances at dawn in order to be sure not to find a closed door. After having their name inscribed in a register, which provided permission to wait in line, patients were granted access into an aseptic but often archaic, and certainly impersonal consultation space. When the size of the building allowed for it, this space was separated into rooms dedicated to surgery and bandaging; the latter room, when there was one, was usually where medicines were dispensed.[57] Following the shock of entering such a space—something that had to be done unaccompanied,[58] often without knowing who or what to expect—patients had to submit to the diagnostic ritual (undressing and physical examination, which was perceived as humiliating) and to the eventual, unilateral suggestion of a treatment.[59] In addition, the patient was often not even entrusted with the prescribed medicine: they were made to consume it right there, in front of a nurse or even a warden.[60] There are several explanations for this desire to maintain a close watch on medicine-taking: a concern not to waste medication (clinics' supplies were often meager and not easily renewed) but especially, worries about inappropriate usage. As such, the largest dispensed dose (of toxic medicines) was a 24-hour prescription. Underlying this practice was a perception of the patient as ignorant, untrustworthy, and incapable of managing his or her own health. Regardless of the reasons behind it, it is not difficult to imagine that this tight control may have been poorly received by patients, particularly when they were required to return over and over again for successive doses.

Here, again, we are a long way from local references. In pre-colonial Vietnam, there was such a thing as a therapeutic relationship, but it was optional; self-information and self-care were seen as essential in therapeutic behaviors and a Confucian duty. One's health was to be promoted at home and on a daily basis; this could include following a balanced diet, exercising daily, avoiding stressful events, and so on.[61] Nor was the therapeutic relationship highly formal; it might be with some kind of dispenser of remedies who had different possible functions and forms of training[62] that would vary according to clients' financial means but also according to their expectations and interpretations of a condition (particularly whether an illness was deemed to have natural or supernatural causes). It was a relationship initiated by a patient's desire rather than imposed by a therapist, which unfolded on the basis of a shared conviction that each case was unique and required a treatment tailored to the patient. The patient was trusted by his therapist, in the sense that his knowledge of and expertise with his own body were taken into account. The belief in the uniqueness of every case inevitably widened the gap between traditional and biomedical care, which was increasingly moving towards a standardization of treatment for duly diagnosed pathologies or symptoms.

In its aspiration to "convert" its participants to a "superior" form of medicine and its expectations of an immediate allegiance from an ignorant patient (twice ignorant: once as a patient, once as a colonial subject), the highly formatted colonial clinical encounter may have produced the opposite effect. It may have contributed to maintaining parallel recourse to traditional therapists, particularly among those who lacked the means to call upon private physicians and thereby consult in a more convivial experience. And the question of whether AMI doctors refused patients who confessed to first having tried several local reme-dies has yet to be answered—that is, when the consultation took place in a language spoken by both doctor and patient.[63] In contrast, some Sino-Vietnamese therapists were quick to appropriate biomedical tech-niques in order to respond to their clients' demands. Although they were deemed to be acting illegally, since they sometimes injected toxic remedies and dispensed pills that looked remarkably similar to French drugs, they proved themselves to be much more flexible than colonial services in their provision of health care.[64]

## By Way of Conclusion: Therapeutic Education "from Below"

The flexibility observed in some traditional therapists as well as lay practices of medical pluralism force us to consider bottom-up health care demand and the importance of "colonized (patient) agency" in the process of colonial medicalization. In the late colonial period, self-medication and therapeutic pluralism were still at the core of local health practices for various reasons, ranging from simple lack of accessibility to efficient medicines to a popular distrust of colonial hospitals. However, these practices had been "modernized," in particular in urban areas where the supply of care was diversifying the most. These therapeutic behaviors may even be indicative of a complex set of adaptations to Western pharmaceuticals and their functions, as well as to Western medicine more broadly, within and beyond the context of the formal public health care system promoted by the AMI.

In the 1930s, part of the Vietnamese population read health magazines such as the VSB (owned by a private French pharmacy) and then the *Bao An Y Báo: Revue de vulgarisation médicale* (BAYB, 1934–38) owned by a Western-trained private doctor, Dr. Nguyễn Văn Luyện, who had previously published several papers in the VSB on prevention, pediatrics, and maternal care. The latter offered virtual medical consultations through its "letters from readers." The simple fact of this column's existence (which could account for as much as a quarter of each issue of the journal) would be a symbol for the syncretism between the Confucian duty to be self-informed and the importance of a biomedical opinion when making therapeutic choices.[65] It also demonstrates the evolution of attitudes towards certain toxic pharmaceuticals and prescription-only drugs (sulfonamides, synthetic derivatives of quinine that were in high demand and short supply during the 1930s), as well as of methods of administration that accelerated or intensified their effects, such as the intravenous injections introduced with arsenobenzols and increasingly used to administer a wide range of tonics.[66] By ingesting a pill—and the experience of toxicity and/or efficacy—Vietnamese came to think differently of their body, their health, and access to health care and Western medicine.

Vietnamese cities in the 1930s were, moreover, the location of a flowering private medical sector.[67] Private practices, whether of general or specialized medicine (Luyện was himself a well-known pediatrician in Hanoi), were held by Vietnamese and French doctors; they offered proximate personalized care, in the context of which patients would not hesitate to ask for a particular medication they had heard good things of. Some private doctors went as far as to consider the possibility of establishing "partnerships" with traditional therapists, or agreed to provide their patients with local remedies in order to avoid losing them to competitors—they were "educated" by their patients to a certain extent.[68] These behaviors constitute unexpected evidence of a process of vernacularization of the colonial health care system as well as of the emergence of early forms of therapeutic citizenship. According to medical anthropologist Vinh-Kim Nguyen, therapeutic citizenship is both a political act of belonging to a global community that offers access to treatment for the ill, as well as a personal engagement that requires self-transformation. The concept thus allows the possibility of understanding how being treated in a specific way embodies the historical process by which local ideas and practices relating to health and the body are articulated with the global political economy of pharmaceuticals and disease relief.[69] In the case of colonial Vietnam, the "old" individual duty of self-transformation and education met with a "new" collective right to health and to efficient, safe, and free medication—claimed by various Vietnamese newspapers and by Dr. Nguyễn Văn Luyện himself in the 1930s[70]—to become essential components of belonging to a rapidly changing society.

## Notes

1.  "Colonial medicines" mean here modern medicines (or at least those labeled as such) available imported from the West or manufactured on site by Western(ized) pharmacists. "Modern medicine" means any pharmaceutical product, whether made up of synthetic or natural components, that is industrially produced. This includes "commercial specialties" (modernized patent medicines sold without a prescription and profusely advertised directly to the consumer) and "medical specialties" or "ethical" medicines (produced and experimentally tested according to scientific principles and usually requiring a medical prescription). See Sophie Chauveau, *L'invention pharmaceutique: la pharmacie Française entre l'état et la société au XXe siècle* (Paris: Sonéfi-Synthélabo, 1999), 19–21.

2.  Indochina was a territory made up of five countries (Cochinchina, Annam, and Tonkin, which comprise Vietnam, Cambodia, and Laos). Its domination by France begun with the conquest of Saigon (1858), and ended with their defeat at Dien Bien Phu (1954). Naming it French Indochina formalized its administrative and political foundation in 1887, which conferred extensive powers to the Governor General at its head. On the general history

of French Indochina, see Pierre Brocheux and Daniel Hémery, *Indochine: la colonisation ambigüe, 1858–1954* (Paris: La Découverte, 2001).

3. The terms "scientific medicine," "modern medicine," and "biomedicine," although not synonymous, are used interchangeably here; the chapter's purpose is not to revisit their respective meanings or to discuss their equivalence.

4. Alice Conklin, *A Mission to Civilize: The Republican Idea of Empire in France and West Africa, 1895–1930* (Stanford: Stanford University Press, 1997).

5. Laurence Monnais-Rousselot, *Médecine et colonisation: l'aventure Indochinoise, 1860–1939* (Paris: CNRS Editions, 1999), 177–225.

6. Laurence Monnais, "De la reproduction d'une idéologie à la naturalisation d'un système: essai sur la médecine 'moderne' au Viêt nam avant la Deuxième Guerre Mondiale," *Outre-mers: Cahiers d'Histoire* 53, no. 352 (2006): 171–208.

7. Monnais-Rousselot, *Médecine et colonisation*, 400–40.

8. Based on the metropolitan model, the legislation on toxic substances would determine the conditions under which a certain number of pharmaceuticals containing them could be stocked, manipulated, and distributed—under medical prescription only—by qualified pharmacists as defined by the French law (April 11, 1803). In order to apply this legislation, the Governor General decreed the creation in October 1908 of a commission for the inspection of pharmacies that was entrusted with the task of verifying the conditions under which medicines were sold in all pharmacies and drugstores, both French and indigenous (Vietnam National Archives I, Hà Nội [hereafter VNA-I], RST 48339).

9. Malarial zones were classified according to their rate of malaria prevalence; this rate then determined whether quinine was distributed free of charge or sold at low cost.

10. The manager of each store was authorized by the administration after having produced a certificate of good morals and followed some minimal training on the art of dispensing medicines (Archives Nationales d'Outre-Mer [hereafter ANOM], Fonds du Gouvernement général [Gougal] 6530).

11. Sulfonamides prefigured antibiotics. On their history, see John Lesch, *The First Miracle Drugs: How the Sulfa Drugs Transformed Medicine* (Oxford & New York: Oxford University Press, 2007). They were introduced from the second half of the 1930s in the West and in the colonies, including Vietnam.

12. Olivier Faure, *Les Français et leur médecine au XIXe siècle* (Paris: Belin, 1993), 221.

13. Replacing mercury in the treatment of syphilis, Salvarsan was the first anti-infectious drug to be extensively tested in Vietnam beginning in 1911.

14. A school of medicine opened its doors in Hanoi in 1902, and the first class graduated in 1905, the year the AMI was inaugurated.

15. On pharmaceuticals "autonomy," see Sjaak van der Geest and Susan Whyte, "The Charm of Medicines: Metaphors and Metonyms," *Medical Anthropology Quarterly* 3, no. 4 (1989): 357–60.

16. Monnais-Rousselot, *Médecine et colonisation*, 121–38. It is relevant to note that compulsory vaccination was imposed in metropolitan France in 1902, more than 30 years later.

17. Dr. Mougeot, *La vaccine en Cochinchine et les idées Chinoises sur la variole et la variolisation* (Saigon: Imprimerie L. Ménard, 1901), 20–4.

18. ANOM, Gougal 6738–9.

19. François Guérin, Paul Lalung-Bonnaire, and Michel Advier, "Premiers résultats de l'enquête sociale sur la tuberculose dans les écoles de Cholon," *Archives des Instituts Pasteur d'Indochine* 1 (1925): 189–212.

20. Monnais-Rousselot, *Médecine et colonisation*, 51–4.

21. ANOM, Fonds de la Résidence Supérieure du Tonkin Nouveau Fonds [hereafter RST NF] 4007.

22. ANOM, RST NF 3823.

23. ANOM, RST NF 4024.

24. Medical officers reported that a number of traditional therapists circulated counter advertisements, telling their patients that French medicines were harmful for their constitutions and that French doctors performed surgery "just for the pleasure of cutting into human flesh" (ANOM, RST NF 4014).

25. ANOM, RST NF 3710; Nouveau Fonds Indochine [hereafter NFI] 2298; Gougal Service économique [hereafter Gougal SE] 219.

26. *Quốc ngữ* is the romanized version of the Vietnamese language that was imposed as the written language of the colonial administration and education system. One of the known consequences of this imposition was the rise in rates of literacy and, with it, of written media including the press. See Shawn McHale, *Print and Power: Confucianism, Communism, and Buddhism in the Making of Modern Vietnam* (Honolulu: University of Hawaii Press, 2004), 28.

27. The systematic consultation of these sources concerned a dozen serials dealing with matters of health and science, both for general and specialized readership, that were published in Vietnam both in French and *quốc ngữ* between 1914 and 1945. These periodicals were chosen on the basis of their period of publication and the extensiveness of their circulation.

28. On the sidelines of the public health care system, Vietnamese could visit a private doctor or pharmacist as long as they were able to pay.

29. ANOM, Gougal 18751; ANVN, Centre no. 2 (Ho Chi Minh Ville), Fonds du Gouvernement de la Cochinchine IA-8/237 (4).

30. The fact that about 85 French and Vietnamese Western-trained pharmacists were established in Hanoi and Saigon in 1940, while only a few thousand

Europeans were settled in these cities, indicates that they must have had a growing Vietnamese clientele.

31. These hybrid specialties are quite similar to the "new medicines" being disseminated at the same time in neighboring China. See Sherman G. Cochran, *Chinese Medicine Men: Consumer Culture in China and Southeast Asia* (Cambridge: Harvard University Press, 2006), 38–63.

32. The term "specific" designates a substance with a targeted action on a specific disease or symptom. Conversely, a panacea promises to heal multiple ills and symptoms, most often those neglected by official medicine or which its treatments fail to relieve.

33. In the 1930s, a syrup made up of local plants was priced at 0.50 piaster, while a dose of a sulfonamide such as Dagénan (Spécia Rhône-Poulenc) could cost up to 30 piasters on the black market. At that time, a Vietnamese secretary was paid between 40 and 60 piasters per month.

34. ANOM, RST NF 4024.

35. "Correctionnelle indigène: le boy docteur," *La Dépêche d'Indochine*, July 2, 1942.

36. ANOM, Gougal 65324.

37. Laurence Monnais, *Médicaments coloniaux: l'expérience Vietnamienne, 1905–40* (Paris: Les Indes Savantes, 2014), 63–71.

38. A December 27, 1916 decree modeled on the metropolitan law of July 1916, ratified the rules on access to substances figuring in tables A (toxic substances), B (narcotics), and C (dangerous substances) for the French colonies. Through this decree, the authorities in Hanoi restricted the freedom of Sino-Vietnamese medicine, forcing its therapists to give up any preparation that figured on one of these lists. Despite the fact that this law could never be truly enforced, it nevertheless represents a step towards relegating traditional medicine to a secondary role, redefining it as limited to inoffensive or "gentle" interventions on minor ills.

39. Monnais, *Médicaments coloniaux*, 64–7.

40. In 1915, only 6 per cent of the budget of a provincial hospital was dedicated to purchasing medicines (ANOM, RST NF 4003). Although this percentage reached 25 per cent of the budget of a rural dispensary around 1930, this amount would barely cover the cost of a single aspirin pill per patient (ANOM, NFI 2303).

41. ANOM, RST NF 3683, 4003, 4014.

42. Van Thê Hoi, "La valse des médecins auxiliaires indigènes," *L'Echo Annamite*, Sept. 11, 1920.

43. Faure, *Les Français et leur médecine*, 187.

44. Between 1927 and 1936 (Monnais, *Médicaments coloniaux*, 139).

45. Colonial authorities never directly legislated on Sino-Vietnamese medicine, for reasons ranging from the highly pragmatic—how could they regulate something they knew so little about?—to the highly political: fear

of uprisings fuelled by demands for the right to choose one's own medicine according to one's convictions and means (ANOM, Gougal SE 213;
NFI 2298).

46.  The boundaries between these two "bodies" of medicine are neither clear
     nor fixed, and both follow similar rules and therapeutic formulae. On
     the identity of Vietnamese medicine, see Laurence Monnais, C. Michele
     Thompson, and Ayo Wahlberg, eds, *Southern Medicine for Southern
     People: Vietnamese Medicine in the Making* (Newcastle upon Tyne:
     Cambridge Scholars Publishing, 2012).

47.  ANOM, RST NF 4014.

48.  David Craig, *Familiar Medicine: Everyday Health Knowledge and Practice
     in Today's Vietnam* (Honolulu: University of Hawaii Press, 2002), 47–9;
     David Marr, "Vietnamese Attitudes Regarding Illness and Healing," in
     *Death and Disease in Southeast Asia: Explorations in Social, Medical and
     Demographic History*, ed. Norman G. Owen (Oxford: Oxford University
     Press, 1987), 163–77.

49.  Opotherapeutic drugs were made up of substances extracted from animal
     organs and blurred the boundary between medicine and food. They were
     most often presented as fortifying substances for the restoration of the
     human organism within an openly holistic and global approach to health.
     Abundant advertisements for these products are to be found in the Viet-
     namese press at the time.

50.  In 1930, for instance, Dr. Massias was in contact with the French drug
     company Laboratoire Byla and sought to obtain a preparation containing
     vitamin B (Vitaminol), which apparently had a taste reminiscent of Viet-
     namese flavors and would enable him to treat beriberi. Charles Massias,
     "Le traitement du béribéri par une préparation contenant vitamine B et
     acides aminés (vitaminol)," *Bulletin de la Société Médico-Chirurgicale
     de l'Indochine* 11 (1933): 389–91.

51.  Monnais, *Médicaments coloniaux*, 183. There was no such familiarity with
     the hypodermic syringe, which was introduced in Indochina by the French
     in the last quarter of the nineteenth century.

52.  Sjaak van der Geest, Susan Whyte, and Anita Hardon, "The Anthropology
     of Pharmaceuticals: A Biographical Approach," *American Review of
     Anthropology* 25 (1996): 163–4.

53.  ANOM, RST NF 3682, 4003, 4007, 4014, 4019.

54.  It should be specified that traditionally, the payment of Chinese or Viet-
     namese therapists was due only once the patient was cured, and was
     generally calculated according to the difference between the predicted and
     actual duration of treatment.

55.  However, although several medical reports describe popular fears of overly
     "strong" therapies and beliefs according to which these were not adapted

to Vietnamese bodies and "temperaments," one must not forget the long-standing tradition of recourse to products containing mercury, arsenic, or *nux vomica* that were imported from China and known to be particularly toxic (Albert Sallet, *L'officine Sino-annamite: la médecine Annamite et la préparation des remèdes* [Paris: Imprimerie Nationale, 1931].)

56. Biswamoy Pati and Mark Harrison, eds, *Health, Medicine, and Empire: Perspectives on Colonial India* (Hyderabad: Orient Longman, 2001), 3–4.

57. ANOM, RST NF 4014.

58. The notion of a one-on-one relationship between patient and doctor is assumed in the West at the time, but goes against Vietnamese customs in which social networks play a valued part in the management of episodes of illness. Several medical reports complained about the challenge of making hospitalized patients and their families understand the concept of limited and regulated visiting hours.

59. Robert Debusmann describes similar attitudes of resistance to medical consultation, and particularly to hospitalization, synonymous with discipline and rules that were often very different from Camerounian references. See Robert Debusmann, "Médicalisation et pluralisme au Cameroun Allemand: autorité médicale et stratégies profanes," *Outre-mers. Revue d'Histoire* 90, no. 1 (2003): 225–45.

60. ANOM, RST NF 4003.

61. Craig, *Familiar Medicine*, 49–52, 88–93.

62. Historically, in Vietnam, the boundaries between the roles of therapists, prescribers, and sellers of remedies are easily blurred. See Sallet, *L'officine sino-annamite*, 10–30.

63. The colonial administration did attempt to make the ability to speak an "Indochinese" language a requirement for its agents, but this failed. Training "Vietnamese auxiliary doctors" from 1902 was meant, among other things, to provide a solution to this doctor-patient communication issue.

64. ANOM, Gougal SE 219.

65. Today the Vietnamese press still plays an important role in informing its readership about health and promoting self-medication. See David Finer, Torsten Thuren, and Goran Tomson, "Tet Offensive, Winning Hearts and Minds for Prevention: Discourse and Ideology in Vietnam's 'Health' Newspaper," *Social Science and Medicine* 47, no. 1 (1998): 133–45. Health education with as objective the enforcement of mass prevention of infectious diseases and hygiene has in fact been an important part of Vietnam's construction as an independent communist country since the advent of the Democratic Republic in September 1945, in clear continuity with Western/colonial principles. See Shaun K. Malarney, "Germ Theory, Hygiene and the Transcendence of Backwardness in Revolutionary Vietnam (1954–60)," in *Southern Medicine*, ed. Monnais, Thompson, and Wahlberg, 107–32.

66. This may be one of the reasons for the current popularity of injections that constitutes a major public health problem in various developing countries including Vietnam.

67. Evaluated to be around 100. See Monnais, *Médicaments coloniaux*, 281.

68. Monnais, *Médicaments coloniaux*, 294–5.

69. Vinh-Kim Nguyen, "Antiretroviral Globalism, Biopolitics, and Therapeutic Citizenship," in *Global Assemblages: Technology, Politics, and Ethics as Anthropological Problems*, ed. Aihwa Ong and Stephen J. Collier (Oxford: Blackwell Publishing, 2005), 124–43.

70. See, for instance, Luyện's editorials in the BAYB in Oct.–Nov. 1936 (no. 28) and Dec. 1936 (no. 29). The right to free, safe, and efficacious medications also appears in the answers given by the colonized to a questionnaire drawn up in the context of the Guernut Commission (1937), which was supposed to evaluate the needs of the colonized and understand the global impact of the colonial enterprise in terms of health care. See ANOM, Fonds de la Commission Guernut, carton 107, dossier 18.

## CHAPTER 10

# The Invention of Medical Tradition in Thailand: Thai Traditional Medicine and Thai Massage

*Junko Iida*

The exploration of the history of Thai traditional medicine overlaps with an examination of both the processes of nation-state building and of the medicalization[1] of Thailand, as well as, more recently, the process of the commercialization of Thai traditional medicine. Developing and becoming established quickly, these processes combined are thought of as the process of the "invention of medical tradition"[2] in Thailand. Within these combined processes, the standards of Thai traditional medicine and Thai massage have been constructed. This paper discusses the knowledge that has been chosen as the standard, in which context, by whom, and why.

In what follows, by examining the textual materials often referred to as evidence of the historical legitimacy of Thai traditional medicine and Thai massage, I first reveal that the "traditional" healing art emerged alongside the region's encounter with the West and within the process of nation-building. Next, I describe the process of the institutional marginalization of traditional medicine and the utilization of "traditional massage" in tourism and the sex industry in Thailand. Following this, I examine the domestic traditional medicine revivalist movements and the recent policy of the Ministry of Public Health which demonstrates that the standardization of traditional medicine in Thailand has been conducted on the basis of nation-state ideology and biomedicine. Finally, I mention local healing practices to demonstrate the variety of knowledge concerning health and healing that exists in contemporary Thai society.

## Encounter with the West and the Compilation of
## Medical Texts

While popular discourse presents Thai traditional medicine as an ancient therapeutic art dating from the time of the historical Buddha, little is known about medicine in the region that now constitutes the territory of Thailand until the seventeenth century AD. The earliest textual material found so far is a record of *Sakdina* (a social hierarchy system in pre-modern Thailand) dating from the mid-fifteenth century. This record contains a ranking of royal physicians (*mo luang*), including massage practitioners (*mo nuat*),[3] and suggests the existence of more or less institutionalized medical professions in this period.

The historical material referred to by researchers today as the oldest canonical text of Thai traditional medicine found thus far is *Tamra Phra Osot Phra Narai* (*The Pharmacopoeia of King Narai*). It was compiled in 1661 during the reign of King Narai (1656–88). During this period, trade among Asian and European countries flourished in Ayutthaya and there was a significant influence of the West in Ayutthaya, which led to the construction of churches, schools, and clinics by French missionaries.[4] Chinese, Indian, and French physicians joined Siamese physicians at the court of King Narai, according to *Tamra Phra Osot Phra Narai*.[5] The presence of these physicians from outside the region is also confirmed in *The Kingdom of Siam*, written by Simon de la Loubère, the third French envoy sent to Siam by King Louis XIV, who stayed in Ayutthaya from 1687 to 1688.[6] Compiled in this multicultural environment, *Tamra Phra Osot Phra Narai* is thought to be a response to foreign influence, especially to influence from the West.

*Tamra Phra Osot Phra Narai* consists of descriptions of drug prescriptions for particular symptoms and ailments. The basic principle that this text follows later becomes what is commonly referred to the "theory of Thai traditional medicine."[7] The principle is outlined as follows. A human body consists of Four Elements (*that thang si*): Earth (*din*), Water (*nam*), Air (*lom*), and Fire (*fai*). Imbalance and disharmony between the Four Body Elements are the causes of various diseases.[8] Factors that influence and can be related to the fluctuation of the condition of the Four Body Elements are the seasons in which a patient's disease occurs, the age of the patient, his or her birthplace, and place of residence.[9] The apparent similarity between the principle above and that of Ayurveda might have been the result of the multicultural environment at the royal court, although the extent to which South Asian medicine influenced Thai traditional medicine has been the subject of debate.[10] It is thought that there is a consistency between this principle and the principle in the medical texts compiled in the Rattanakosin period, as described later.[11]

This text also contains the description of massage (*nuat*) as a therapy. It says that massage is applied to body lines called *sen* to relieve the tension and constriction of those same lines. *Sen* are considered to be the fibrous bands in ethno-anatomy that cause pain or stiffness when they are tensed or shifted out of alignment. Similar to the inscriptions at Wat Pho described in the following section, several names of *sen* are referred to in *Tamra Phra Osot Phra Narai*.[12]

The most famous historical sources of instruction for Thai traditional medicine and Thai massage are the inscriptions and statues that still exist today in Wat Pho, the royal temple in Bangkok. These inscriptions and statues were constructed under the supervision of royal physicians in 1832 as part of King Rama III's project to assemble knowledge concerning medicine, art, literature, and history at *Wat Pho*. The purpose of this project was to make this knowledge accessible to all classes of people.[13] In doing so, King Rama III created a shared common knowledge base which can be considered as a step towards the development of the nation-state. This project was also an effort to conserve "Siamese knowledge," viewed as threatened by Western imperialism, which included the work of the Protestant missionaries who were actively introducing Western medicine to Siam.[14] "Thai traditional medicine" thus emerged alongside the region's encounter with the West and within the process of nation-state building.

The inscriptions on the walls of Wat Pho describe remedies based on the principle of the Four Body Elements and depict the location of pressure points for massage along *sen* on the body (see Figure 1). Statues of hermits are posed in postures of therapeutic exercises called *ruesi datton* (see Figure 2). There are 60 inscriptions about the human body with reference to pressure points and 80 statues of hermits' exercise.[15] The inscriptions and statues are said to be the result of the collection and examination of the knowledge of royal physicians, monk doctors, and folk healers.[16] As the first systematic and encyclopedic collection of medical knowledge in Thailand, these inscriptions and statues became one of the most important sources of Thai traditional medicine in the revivalist movement and standardization of knowledge in the late twentieth century.

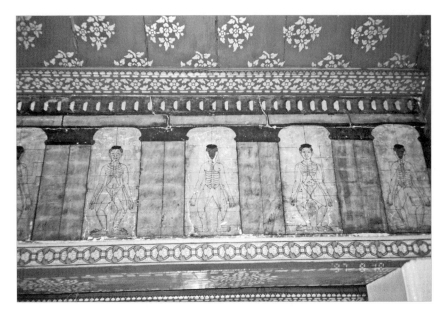

**Figure 1.** Inscriptions on the walls at Wat Pho.

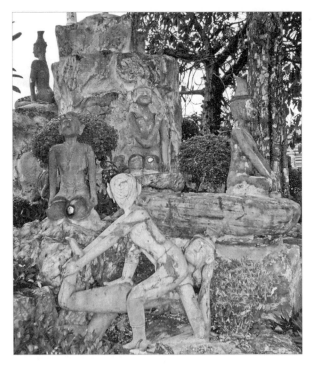

**Figure 2.** Statues of hermits at Wat Pho.

With the introduction of Western medicine and Western-style medical education, beginning at the Siriraj Hospital in 1887, the knowledge preserved at Wat Pho was put into text and published. The Siriraj Hospital, opened during the reign of King Rama V, was the first hospital to adopt Western medicine in Thailand. At first, both Western medicine, practiced by American physicians, and conventional medicine practiced by Thai royal physicians were adopted at this hospital and at Siriraj Medical School. This was because very few people accepted Western medicine and there was a limited number of Western physicians. In records written by students at that time, the word "modern medicine" (*kanphaet phaen patjuban*) was used for Western medicine, and "traditional medicine" (*kanphaet phaen boran*) was used for the conventional medicine practiced by royal physicians.[17] This suggests that the conventional mode of medicine came to be called "traditional medicine" as Western medicine was introduced into Thai society.

After the Siriraj Medical School was established, several textbooks were published. Among them, *Tamra Wetchasat Wannana* (*Textbook of Medical Description*) and *Tamra Phaetthayasat Songkhroh Chabap Luang* (*Collective Textbook of Medicine Royal Edition*), were compiled by the royal physicians at Siriraj Medical School and were published in 1907. These were the first publications about traditional medicine in Thailand. The contents of these textbooks overlap with *Wetchasat Chabap Luang* (*Royal Edition of Medicine*), compiled by royal physicians in 1870. They include etiology based on the principle of the Four Body Elements, diagnosis, therapies including massage, prescriptions and effects of drugs, as well as ritual procedures and ethics. *Tamra Phaetthayasat Songkhroh Chabap Luang* and its digest version published in 1908 were later adopted as the standard textbooks at traditional medical schools sanctioned by the Ministry of Public Health.[18]

The knowledge materialized at Wat Pho and published as textbooks in this period thus became the sources for the standard of "Thai traditional medicine" thereafter. This period is therefore viewed as the beginning of the invention of medical tradition in Thailand. Many authors point out the consistency between the knowledge in this period and that in the Ayutthaya period,[19] due apparently to an effort by rulers in the beginning of the Rattanakosin period to repeatedly compile medical knowledge as part of the revival of the political, social, and cultural aspects of Ayutthaya tradition lost in wartime. However, several authors have argued that the principle of the Four Body Elements, for example, is not integrated within the rest of the texts nor within practice.[20]

## The Marginalization of Traditional Medicine

At the end of the nineteenth century, witnessing the overwhelming effectiveness of Western medicine, especially against infectious diseases such as smallpox and malaria, Thai people gradually came to accept Western medicine. As the influence of Western medicine increased, traditional medicine became institutionally marginalized. Siriraj Hospital and Siriraj Medical School discontinued their use of traditional medicine in 1915,[21] and Thai government organizations did not readopt traditional medicine until the 1980s.

Two factors that led to the marginalization of traditional medicine in Thailand have been pointed out. One of them is the disorganization of traditional doctors, especially the lack of cooperation between court doctors and people's doctors. The other factor is the Westernization of medical education, which intensified with the support of the Rockefeller Foundation in 1922.[22]

The law that first defined "traditional medicine" in Thailand was the Act for the Control of the Practice of the Healing Art (*Phraracha-banyat Khuapkhum Kanprakop Rok Sinlapa 2479 B.E.*), implemented by the government in 1936. In this law, traditional medicine was defined as "a medical practice by using textbooks or whatever that has been passed down before, without scientific foundation." With this definition, practitioners of traditional medicine were prohibited from using scientific medical knowledge and technology, and medicinal herbal products tested in a laboratory and manufactured by modern technology were categorized as modern medicine.[23] The activists of the traditional medical revivalist movement later criticized this law as it prevented the development of the knowledge of traditional medicine.

In the licensing system for traditional doctors legislated in 1953, there were three types of licences available, namely, medicine (*wetcha-kam*), pharmacy (*phesatchakam*), and midwifery (*phadungkhan*). The training period required was three years for medicine and one year each for pharmacy and midwifery.[24] This system was later criticized during the traditional medicine revivalist movements for its lack of licensing for massage practitioners, making it difficult, some argued, to professionalize the practice.[25]

With the development of the sex and tourism industries in Thailand in the 1960s, "Thai traditional massage" began to be perceived as a tourist-oriented service and was often used as a cover for prostitution.[26] Although prostitution was outlawed in 1960, the sex industry in Thailand developed significantly throughout the 1960s, when Thailand became the principal destination for American soldiers' "Rest & Recuperation" (R&R) during the Vietnam War. After the war, investors tried to expand R&R into the global market. With the increase in male tourists from Europe, North America, Asia, and the Middle East, as well as an increase in domestic demand, the sex industry continued to expand. From the 1980s onwards, the tourist authority began to combat the sexual imagery associated with the country by emphasizing other aspects including Thailand's nature, history, ethnicity, and culture. Regulations against prostitution have been put in place to some extent. However, since the tourist industry is one of the primary means of acquiring foreign currency, and because of the cozy relationship between police and shops, the attempted crackdown on prostitution has had little effect.[27]

Among the various forms the sex industry takes, it is massage parlors that utilize "Thai traditional massage" as a cover for sexual services. They display signs advertising "traditional massage" (*nuat phaen boran*), pretending to provide traditional massage as traditional medicine or simply as relaxation. While some parlors provide sexual services in addition to traditional massage, others let the customers go out with masseuses for sexual services after a traditional massage. Yet others provide only sexual services in spite of the "traditional massage" signs.

Shops actually providing Thai traditional massage and not sexual services, primarily for foreign tourists, also increased. Thai traditional massage as relaxation or as an "exotic experience" became very popular among tourists. Originally a therapeutic form of bodywork indicated for specific ailments, Thai massage became a whole-body technique in the last decades of the twentieth century, with an additional, sometimes dominant, emphasis on relaxation, following a step-by-step routine from foot to head. The need to satisfy tourists without specific ailments and/ or symptoms was one of the factors in the production of the whole-body style of massage.[28] Famous shops were presented in guidebooks, and package tours included Thai traditional massage. Among foreigners it became popular not only to experience Thai massage but also to learn how to conduct it. As a result, Thai massage schools increased in number in the 1980s and 1990s. The popularity of Thai traditional massage can be seen in the results of the research conducted by the Ministry of Commerce in 1998. The results revealed that the most impressive service according to tourists in Thailand was Thai traditional massage.[29]

The flourishing of Thai traditional massage in the sex and tourism industries was the result of various factors including a wealth gap in the global economy, the sexualized image of "oriental women," corruption within Thai society, and the vague legal status of Thai massage. Because of these factors, as well as the marginalization of traditional medicine, the phrase "Thai massage" has ambiguous overtones relating to relaxation, tourism, and sexual services.

## Traditional Medicine Revivalist Movement

In contrast, a number of private traditional medicine organizations have been founded primarily at Buddhist temples in urban areas since the 1930s. The activities of these organizations include education surrounding the use of traditional medicine and treatment using herbal remedies and traditional massage. Many of the organizations offer weekend courses on medicine (three years) and pharmacy (one year) as preparation for the national licence examination.

The most authoritative organization among them is the School and Association of Traditional Medicine in Thailand (*Ronrgian lae Samakhom Phaet Phaen Boran Haeng Prathet Thai*) established in 1957 at Wat Pho. At this school, the old texts of the royal doctors mentioned earlier, *Tamra Phaetthayasat Songkhroh Chabap Luang* and its digest version, have been republished and used in classes.[30] In 1962, the school also published a printed textbook version of the inscriptions and statues made in Wat Pho in the period of King Rama III. Thai massage today is a combination of point pressing along *sen*, as inscribed on the walls at Wat Pho, and stretching techniques thought to be based on the postures of the hermits' statues at the same temple. Some of the graduates of this school have further established traditional medicine organizations in Bangkok and other regions.

In his work, Irvine points out the influence of nation-state ideology, "Nation (*chat*), Religion (*satsana*), and Monarch (*phramahakasat*)," on Thai traditional medicine.[31] This ideology was first developed by King Rama VI (1910–25), when Thailand was threatened by European colonialists, and became the central ideology for nation-building from the 1950s onward, when the Thai government was challenged by communism. As Irvine suggests, the status of traditional medical practitioners was, and continues to be, legitimated and elevated by their articulation of monarchist allegiance and Buddhist loyalty. That is, at least partly, the reason why these private traditional medicine organizations are based at Buddhist temples and use textbooks said to be founded on the knowledge of royal doctors.

The Alma-Ata Declaration, accepted at the international conference on primary health care held by the WHO and UNICEF in 1978, identified primary health care as the key to the attainment of the goal of "Health for All." It states that primary health care relies, at local and referral levels, on health workers including traditional practitioners. Since the Alma-Ata Declaration was accepted, many countries, especially "developing countries," have been promoting the use of traditional medicine in primary health care.[32] Influenced by this WHO policy, traditional medicine revivalist movements, led primarily by medical professionals, have developed in Thailand since the late 1970s.

One of the most influential organizations of these revivalist movements was Ayurawet College (*Rongrian Ayurawet Witthayalai*). It was founded in 1982 by Dr. Uai Ketusing, a professor at the Faculty of Medicine, Siriraj Hospital, Mahidol University. With the permission of the Ministry of Education and the Thai Buddhist sangha, this organization renovated the school and printing office of the royal temple Wat Bowonniwetwihan and established the college and the attached clinic.[33] This college was supported by the royal family, the Ministry of Public Health, and Mahidol University.

The aim of Ayurawet College was to develop personnel with a basic knowledge of biomedicine as well as the practical skills of traditional medicine including herbal and massage remedies. It was illegal until 1999, however, for traditional medical practitioners to use scientific medical knowledge and technology as described earlier. In order for the graduates of this college to practice lawfully, a new category of traditional medicine was created in 1987. Called "applied traditional medicine" (*kanphaet phaen boran baep prayuk*), this category incorporated basic scientific knowledge with traditional medicine. The graduates of this college became certified "practitioners of applied traditional medicine" (*phu prakop roksinlapa phaen boran baep prayuk*)[34] and were generally called "Ayurawet doctor" (*mo ayurawet*). While they were not allowed to conduct operations or prescribe biomedical drugs, they were permitted to use simple medical instruments including sphygmomanometers, thermometers, and stethoscopes.[35] Other practitioners became "practitioners of general traditional medicine" (*phu prakop roksinlapa phaen boran baep thua pai*).[36]

The massage adopted by Ayurawet College is called "royal style massage" (*kannuat baep rachasamnak*). The practice of this style of massage is governed by a number of rules regarding politeness, as it is a method developed for use with the royal family and is applied with only finger and palm pressing. This is in contrast to "folk/general style massage" (*kannuat baep chaloeysak/thua pai*), which uses various techniques including stretching, employing not only the hands but also the elbows, knees, and feet of the practitioner.[37] The Ministry of Public Health explains that folk style massage is practiced among families and friends while royal style massage is used for the treatment of certain ailments.[38] It explains the efficacy of royal style massage anatomically. For example, royal style massage practitioners stimulate blood circulation and the nervous system to affect organs and tissues deep inside the body.[39] At Ayurawet College, they do not teach the folk concept *sen* but they use anatomy while teaching massage.

Many graduates of this college became public health personnel in government agencies including local hospitals and public health offices. Chantana therefore categorizes the activity of this college as a "bureaucratic (traditional medicine revivalist) movement."[40] The college was incorporated into the Faculty of Medicine, Siriraj Hospital, Mahidol University in the mid-2000s.

In contrast to the work of Ayurawet College, the "Thai Massage Revival Project" (*Khrongkan Fuenfu Kannuat Thai*), which began in 1985, is categorized by Chantana as a "democratic movement."[41] Among the founders of this project is Dr. Prawet Wasi. A professor at Mahidol University and the winner of the Ramon Magsaysay Award for his research in hematology in 1981, Dr. Prawet is one of the most famous physicians and intellectuals in Thailand. He has influenced civil society and government policy in Thailand, not only with this project but also with various other activities including initiatives in primary health care, social development, and democratic movements. He has also effected change as an organizer of NGOs, as a member of several committees of the WHO and several government bodies, and as a writer. He has criticized Western-orientated, capitalist medicine in Thailand and insisted that self-reliance in health care, including freedom from a dependence on doctors and expensive overseas drugs, should be promoted. He has argued that self-reliance should be based on a "community culture" (*watthanatham chumchon*) philosophy.[42] "Community culture" was a popular discourse among Thai intellectuals and activists of the urban middle class in the late 1980s and 1990s. These intellectuals and activists criticized and fought against industrialization and urbanization, working to make traditional local culture a valued basis for rural development. The Thai Massage Revival Project is thus a part of this idealistic enlightenment activity.

Before the development of the Thai Massage Revival Project, Dr. Prawet and his colleagues addressed problems caused by the over-consumption of painkillers throughout the country, including inflammation of the stomach. They tried to find a substitute for painkillers and felt that the alternative therapy should be something indigenous. However, herbal remedies were not considered a suitable alternative because they were slower in taking effect than painkillers. It was also unlikely, they thought, that rural people would do exercise to relieve pain caused by physical labor. They thus turned to Thai massage as a possible substitute for painkillers.[43]

Members of the Thai Massage Revival Project had a wide range of occupations, including traditional and modern practitioners of medicine in governmental and non-governmental organizations.[44] Practitioners and teachers from traditional medicine organizations and Ayurawet College mentioned in the previous sections also participated in this project.[45]

First, the participants in the project worked to standardize knowledge concerning Thai massage in order to construct teaching and learning manuals. Initially they gathered the old textbooks on massage and traditional medicine mentioned earlier, but the information in such texts was difficult to understand, especially for biomedical professionals. Therefore, traditional practitioners were invited to demonstrate their techniques and massage points.[46] In my interview in 1999 with him, Mr. Yongsak Tantipidoke, then head of the Foundation for Public Health and Development, the nucleus of this project, revealed that the standardization of massage skills was hard work, because different schools and practitioners had different techniques. In this process of standardization, they focused on how to persuade biomedical professionals to accept Thai massage as a viable therapy. They thus eliminated from the standard some techniques including stretching methods likely to be regarded by biomedical doctors as dangerous. They accepted, on the other hand, techniques with effects that could be scientifically explained so that biomedical professionals might acknowledge the benefit of the practice. Therefore, while the techniques were standardized on the basis of the knowledge of practitioners from traditional medicine organizations, biomedicine was the standard with which the safety and effects of the techniques were evaluated.[47]

The knowledge standardized by this project was not only massage techniques but also the ethics, rules, and rituals of massage practitioners. These ethics and rules were stipulated apparently in order to counteract the negative image of traditional massage in Thailand described earlier.

The procedure of "*wai khru*" (worship teachers) ritual was also standardized. In Thailand, those who learn traditional knowledge must worship "*khru*," the aggregate of teachers that include not only the living teachers from whom they learn directly, but also all teachers since ancient times who have passed down their knowledge. It is believed that the founder of Thai traditional medicine was the legendary Chiwakakomaraphat, the personal physician of the historical Buddha over 2,500 years ago.[48] Traditional practitioners periodically conduct a *wai khru* ritual to pay respect to these teachers. A manual regarding the instruments used, procedure of, and words recited in this ritual was published by the Thai Massage Revival Project in 1999.[49]

The second activity of the Thai Massage Revival Project was to spread the standardized knowledge throughout the country. It provided a three-level training course: a three-day basic course for the general public, a three-month intermediate course for those who wished to become practitioners at biomedical hospitals and public health centers, and a five-day advanced course for massage practitioners who wanted to acquire knowledge about anatomy and diagnosis.[50]

The third objective of the Project was to create an association of massage practitioners and to institutionalize Thai massage. Holding seminars and conferences, as well as publishing newsletters, it promoted networking between practitioners and organizations. It was not easy to organize the association of massage practitioners because of the differences among the members, however, and some organizations, including Wat Pho and Ayurawet College, stopped participating in the project. The Project also insisted that the government amend the Act for the Control of the Practice of the Healing Art in order to legitimize Thai massage as a therapy and one of the established subjects of traditional medicine.[51]

While differences existed between the Ayurawet College and the Thai Massage Revival Project, they also shared similarities. First, they were both developed by biomedical doctors, and evaluated the efficacy and safety of Thai massage from a biomedical point of view. Second, both adopted the knowledge of practitioners who were said to be the successors of the royal doctors. Third, the relationship between their activities and Buddhism was emphasized. As a result, while these movements emerged as criticisms of the medicalization of Thai society, and the Thai Massage Revival Project aimed at self-reliance based on "community culture," these movements ultimately contributed to the medicalization of Thai society and the reproduction of its nation-state ideology, "Nation, Religion, and Monarch."[52]

## The Institutionalization of Thai Traditional Medicine

Stimulated by both the policies of the WHO and domestic traditional medicine revivalist movements described in the previous section, the Thai government began to institutionalize "Thai Traditional Medicine" (TTM) in the 1990s. The Seventh National Economic and Social Development Plan, 1992–96, included the statement: "national health promotion involves the development of local wisdom regarding health care, such as Thai traditional medicine, herbal remedies and massage, in coordination with modern health care services." The Ministry of Public Health explained the reasons for the decision as follows. First, national expenses for medical care had increased, and the modern medical system relied too heavily on imported medicine and medical supplies. Second, dangerous illegal drugs had become widely available in the domestic market. Traditional medicine was adopted as a response and a possible solution to these problems.[53] This was also influenced by the popular discourse on "local wisdom" (*phum panya*), a successor of "community culture" in the 1990s. The new constitution established in 1997 included the statement that "Persons so assembling as to be a traditional community shall have the right to conserve or restore their customs, local knowledge, arts or good culture of their community and of the nation…."[54]

In 1993, the National Institute of Thai Traditional Medicine (NITTM, *Sathaban Kanphaet Phaen Thai*) was established at the Department of Medical Service,[55] Ministry of Public Health, and became the administrative center of TTM. The decade from 1994 to 2003 was designated the "Decade of Thai Traditional Medicine." The phrase "Thai Traditional Medicine" is the official English translation for the Thai phrase "*kanphaet phaen thai*," which literally means "Thai-style medicine." The latter has been in use since the 1990s, replacing the old-fashioned term "*kanphaet phaen boran*" (old/traditional style medicine). "Thai Traditional Medicine" (*kanphaet phaen thai*) is a newly created concept defined as the medical system that systematized (*tham pen rabop*) and developed (*phatthana*) the folk medicine (*kanphaet baep phuen ban*) as practiced in different areas in Thailand.[56] The meaning of the words "systematize" and "develop" will be examined in the following description.

The NITTM aims to systematize and standardize the knowledge of TTM to make the practice of TTM "safe, effective, and convenient."[57] It conducts and coordinates and supports research on traditional medicine, and produces texts, manuals, books, videotapes, CD-ROMs, and

DVDs. Publications include texts and books on the history and theory of TTM, diagnosis, and the effects of herbal remedies, massage, and the Hermits' Exercise. The history of TTM was reconstructed on the basis of the historical materials concerning the royal courts.[58] The theory and diagnosis concerns the etiology based on the principle of Four Body Elements interpreted in terms of biomedicine.[59] The effects of herbal remedies are explained in terms of the Four Body Elements as well as through biomedical experiments using rats.[60] The manuals of Thai massage show pressure points along "Ten Primary *Sen*" depicted on the wall of Wat Pho and methods of massage for various types of symptoms with anatomical explanations.[61] It is thus suggested that the "systematization" and "development" of TTM means verifying and standardizing the knowledge represented in the texts of royal physicians from a biomedical viewpoint. The NITTM has also conducted research on local healers, probably due to the influence of the popular discourse of "local wisdom" and the decentralization policy. While local knowledge is not excluded from TTM, it is not the standard of TTM but rather a local variation of TTM.[62]

The NITTM has been trying to spread TTM to medical professionals, local practitioners, and the general public.[63] First, it holds seminars and training courses for medical and public health professionals. It also promotes education about TTM at faculties of medicine and pharmacy throughout the country. In the 2000s, several universities established undergraduate and graduate programs in TTM.

Second, local practitioners include both "traditional practitioners" who study or have studied at schools of traditional medicine and "folk healers" who practice without licences. The NITTM has been promoting local public health offices and TTM Coordination Centers (*Sun Prasanngan Kanphaet Phaen Thai*) to develop networks of folk healers and to bring the quality of their services and education up to standard. For example, they hold training programs to teach local practitioners how to produce herbal medicines in a hygienic environment.

Third, for the general public, the NITTM has been introducing TTM into local hospitals and public health centers, providing a budget for TTM at each health institution. According to the Chiang Mai Provincial Public Health Office, all of the 25 district hospitals and 271 subdistrict health centers in the province provided Thai massage services in 2009. It also holds various events including exhibitions, sales, demonstrations, and seminars to promote TTM to the general public.

Based on the criticisms of the Act for the Control of the Practice of the Healing Art described earlier, the Ministry of Public Health legislated a new law in 1999. Under the new law, the phrase "Thai Traditional Medicine" (*kanphaet phaen thai*) is used instead of "traditional medicine" (*kanphaet phaen boran*) and practitioners were permitted to use scientific knowledge and technology. New rules for massage were also enforced in 2001, requiring 2 years or 800 hours of training for certification, which is in turn necessary for the opening of a Thai massage clinic. Three hundred and thirty hours are required for those wishing to become assistants to traditional Thai doctors and 372 hours for those practicing in hospitals. During the course, students learn anatomy as well as the practical skills of massage. This increase of requirements in the training of massage practitioners is partly an effort to differentiate therapeutic massage from tourist and sexual services.

## The Commercialization of Thai Traditional Medicine

The traditional medicine revivalist movement criticized excessive health care costs and changes were made to health policy in an attempt to address the issue. These processes went, however, hand in hand with the commercialization of TTM on a wider scale. Since the 1980s, Thai massage has become increasingly popular with foreign tourists as described earlier. As the Thai urban middle class—oriented towards health and nature—increased in the late 1990s, the market for TTM also grew. This change has also been brought about by the transnational circulation of the culture of "healthism," as well as by a shift in the main causes of death in the urban areas of Thailand. From the causes associated by the WHO with "low income countries" (malnutrition and infectious diseases), the pathological landscape in Thailand has changed and now increasingly involves what are called lifestyle diseases, such as cancer, cardiovascular disorders, and diabetes.[64] As a "natural therapy," TTM has gained popularity among Thai urbanites as well as foreigners, and has become one of the growing areas in the health industry, which includes herbal remedies, massage, spas, herbal cosmetics and health foods.[65]

This process of the commercialization of traditional medicine is not only a domestic phenomenon but also a global one. Pharmaceutical companies from Europe, North America, and Japan searched for natural resources for health products in Thailand, and an increasing number of foreign companies monopolized the production rights of some of the products in the 1990s. The Thai government was obliged to control the quality of health products and services provided by Thai producers, so that they could compete with these transnational companies. For example, while in the past people who were prescribed herbs had to decoct them by themselves, or had to put up with the bitterness of herbal remedies, the Ministry of Public Health has started to support institutions and groups of TTM in buying instruments to powder and encapsulate the herbs so consumers can take them more easily.[66]

## Variety of Knowledge

In contrast to this spreading commercialization and institutionalization, a wide variety of forms and practices of healing, including herbal remedies, massage, and magical healing, continues to exist across each region in Thailand. Each local practitioner has inherited his or her knowledge from his or her family, relatives, and neighbors. For example, in northern Thailand, there are local healers called *mo mueang*, spirit mediums called *mae ti nang*, and massage practitioners called *mae jang*. *Mo mueang* is a man who uses herbal remedies and magic to practice healing; *mae ti nang* is an elderly woman possessed by a spirit who reveals the cause and solution of an illness; and *mae jang* is often a former midwife before most Thai women started to deliver their children in hospitals. Much about the history of such local healing is unknown, as written materials concerning these practices have rarely been found.

As described earlier, the knowledge of local healers has not been excluded, but it rarely appears within the standard knowledge of TTM. Local healers in different areas use different kinds of herbs because of the variety of vegetation in each region and this is not dealt with in the national examination for practitioners' licences. The national examination focuses on the 'naturalistic' aspect of traditional medicine such as the etiology based on the principle of Four Body Elements; magical healing along with regional variation has been eliminated from the examination as well as from the texts used by organizations of traditional medicine in urban areas.[67]

Today, these local healers have been influenced by the revivalist movement, as well as the institutionalization and commercialization of traditional medicine. While local healers usually practice individually, groups of practitioners have been organized throughout the country so TTM can be spread. Although the control and regulation is soft because of the political and social trends to revalue local culture and traditional medicine, people's practices have become more thoroughly controlled than previously, when they were ignored. Training programs to teach "safe and effective ways of practice" are held for local healers at local hospitals and health centers. These programs and projects sometimes provide new opportunities, especially for young practitioners to work with biomedical professionals. However, they sometimes cause problems as they often contradict what elderly healers have been doing in local contexts. For example, the massage technique standardized in Bangkok did not fit with the body technique of the elderly village women in the northern region who never wear pants.[68] Elderly local healers sometimes feel excluded from the licensing system, as less experienced younger people tend to pass the national exam more easily than elderly healers.[69]

## Conclusion

Hsu suggests that Traditional Chinese Medicine as taught and practiced in government-run institutions of the People's Republic of China appears to fit the definition of "invented tradition" by Eric Hobsbawm perfectly "because it was constructed and formally instituted within a brief and dateable time period and established itself with great rapidity."[70] Thai Traditional Medicine can also be one of these "invented medical traditions." As shown elsewhere by studies on Traditional Chinese Medicine in China[71] and Ayurveda in India,[72] the standardization of traditional medicine in Thailand has been conducted on the basis of nation-state ideology and was modeled after biomedicine. The making of this "tradition" followed the official monarchy-centered national history, and its efficacy and safety were, and still are, subject to biomedical scrutiny. This "tradition," efficacy, and safety have also become important resources in the context of the commercialization of traditional medicine today.

## Notes

1.  Medicalization is defined as "the way in which the jurisdiction of modern medicine has expanded in recent years and now encompasses many problems that formerly were not defined as medical entities." See Jonathan Gabe and Michael Calnan, "The Limits of Medicine: Women's Perception of Medical Technology," *Social Science and Medicine* 28 (1989): 223–31.

2.  Elisabeth Hsu, "The History of Chinese Medicine in the People's Republic of China and Its Globalization," *East Asia Science, Technology and Society: An International Journal* 2, no. 4 (2009): 465–84.

3.  Prathip Chumphon, *Prawattisat Kanphaet Phaen Thai: Kansyksa jak Ekasan Tamra Ya* [A History of Thai Traditional Medicine: A Study from the Texts of Pharmacopoeia] (Bangkok: Akhithai, 1998), 28–9. As in conventional usage, Thai authors are referred to by their first names in the text and are listed in the references by their first names, followed by their surnames.

4.  Prathip, *Prawattisat Kanphaet Phaen Thai*, 48.

5.  Ibid., 35.

6.  Simon de la Loubère, *The Kingdom of Siam* (reprint of 1691 edition) (Oxford: Oxford University Press, 1969), 62.

7.  For example, see Sathaban Kanphaet Phaen Thai, *Kanphaet Phaen Thai: Kanphaet Baep Ong Ruam* [Thai Traditional Medicine: Holistic Medicine] (Bangkok: Rongphim Ongkan Songkhro Thahan Phan Suek, 1996).

8.  Somchintana Thongthew Ratarasarn, "The Principles and Concepts of Thai Classical Medicine" (PhD diss., University of Wisconsin, Madison, 1986), 63.

9.  Somchintana, "The Principles," 115.

10. Junko Iida, "Holism as a Whole-body Treatment: The Transnational Production of Thai Massage," *European Journal of Transnational Studies* 5, no. 1 (2013): 93–4.

11. Somchintana, "The Principles," 59.

12. Ibid., 251–3.

13. Dhani Nivat, "The Inscriptions of Wat Phra Jetubon," in *Collected Articles by H.H. Prince Dhani Nivat* (Bangkok: Siam Society, 1969 [1933]), 5.

14. Benja Yoddumnern, *The Role of Thai Traditional Doctors* (Bangkok: Institute for Population and Social Research, Mahidol University, 1974), 9; Stanley J. Tambiah, *World Conqueror and World Renouncer: A Study of Buddhism and Polity in Thailand against a Historical Background* (Cambridge: Cambridge University Press, 1976), 204–13; Walter Irvine, "The Thai-Yuan 'Madman' and the 'Modernizing, Developing Thai Nation' as Bounded Entities under Threat: A Study in the Replication of a Single Image" (PhD diss., School of Oriental and African Studies, London, 1982), 39; Prathip, *Prawattisat Kanphaet Phaen Thai*, 91.

15. Prathip, *Prawattisat Kanphaet Phaen Thai*, 64–5.

16. Rongrian Phaet Phaen Boran, *Tamra Ya Sila Jaruek nai Wat Phrachetuphonwimonmangkhlaram (Wat Pho) Phranakhon* [Pharmacopoeia on the Inscription at Wat Pho] (Nonthaburi: Khrongkan Prasanngan Phatthana Khrueakhai Samunphrai (Herbal Network Development Coordination Project), 1994 [1962]).

17. Sut Saengwichian, "Jut Jop khong Phaet Phaen Boran lae Kanroemton khong Kanphaet Phaen Patjuban khong Thai [The End of Traditional Medicine and the Beginning of Modern Medicine in Thailand]," *Warasan*

*Sangkhomsat Kanphaet* [Journal of Social Science of Medicine] 1, no. 2 (1978): 20–8.

18. Benja, *The Role of Thai Traditional Doctors*, 7–11; Chaninthon Rattana-sakon et al., "Phatthanakan khong Kanbanthuek lae Kanthaithot Khwamru thang Kanphaet Phaen Thai" [The Development of the Record and the Inheritance of the Knowledge of Thai Medicine], in *Kanbantuek lae Kanthaithot Khwamru thang Kanphaet Phaen Thai* [The Record and the Inheritance of the Knowledge of Thai Medicine], ed. Saowapha Phonsiri-phong and Phonthip Usurat (Bangkok: NITTM and Institute of Language and Culture for Rural Development, Mahidol University, 1994), 49–50; Prathip, *Prawattisat Kanphaet Phaen Thai*, 100, 102.

19. Yuwadi Tapaniyakon, "Wiwatthanakan thang Kanphaet Thai tangtae Samai Roemton jon thueng Sinsut Ratchakan Phrabatsomdetphrajunlajomklaojao-yuhua" [Development of Thai Medicine from the Beginning until the End of the Era of King Chulalongkorn] (MA Thesis, Chulalongkorn Univer-sity, Bangkok, 1979), 52–5; Somchintana, "The Principles," 59; Chaninthon et al., "Phatthanakan," 26–8; Prathip, *Prawattisat Kanphaet Phaen Thai*, 123.

20. Jean Mulholland, "Ayurveda, Congenital Disease and Birthdays in Thai Traditional Medicine," *Journal of the Siam Society* 76 (1988): 175; and Viggo Brun and Trond Schumacher, *Traditional Herbal Medicine in Northern Thailand* (Bangkok: White Lotus, 1994), 30–3.

21. Benja, *The Role of Thai Traditional Doctors*, 40, and Prathiip, *Prawattisat Kanphaet Phaen Thai*, 119.

22. Kenneth P. Landon, *Siam in Transition: A Brief Survey of Cultural Trends in the Five Years since the Revolution of 1932*, 1939 reprint (New York: Greenwood Press, 1968), 118; Suchai Trirat, "Itthiphon Munlanithi Rokkifenloe to Rongrian Phaet Thai" [The Influences of the Rockefeller Foundation on the Thai Medical School], *Warasan Sangkhomsat Kanphaet* [Journal of Social Science of Medicine] 1, no. 2 (1978): 40–55; Chantana Banpasirichote, "The Indigenization of Development Process in Thailand: A Case Study of the Traditional Medical Revivalist Movement (Thai Mas-sage)" (PhD diss., University of Waterloo, 1989), 63–70.

23. Chantana, "The Indigenization," 59.

24. Benja, *The Role of Thai Traditional Doctors*, 43, 61–4.

25. Ministry of Public Health, Thailand, *Proceedings of the National Seminar on the Development of Thai Traditional Medicine* (S.l.: S.n., 1987), 13. Chantana, "The Indigenization," 59–60, 79.

26. Chantana, "The Indigenization," 59–70.

27. Pasuk Phongphaichit, *Massage garu: Thai no Keizai Kaihatsu to Shakai Henka* [From Peasant Girls to Bangkok Masseuses] (Geneva: International Labour Office, 1980), trans. Noriko Tanaka (Tokyo: Dobunkan, 1990), 26–30; Thanh-Dam Truong, *Baishun: Sei Rodo no Shakai Kozo to Kokusai*

*Keizai* [Sex, Money and Morality: Prostitution and Tourism in Southeast Asia] (London and New Jersey: Zed Books, 1990), trans. Noriko Tanaka and Akiko Yamashita (Tokyo: Akashi Shoten, 1993), 292–347; and Erik Cohen, *Thai Tourism: Hill Tribes, Islands and Open-Ended Prostitution* (Bangkok: White Lotus, 1996), 2–12.

28. Iida, "Holism."

29. Krasuang Phanit (Ministry of Commerce), "Kanchai Borikan Thurakit Borikan khong Thai khong Nakthongthiao Chao Tang Prathet" [The Usage of Thai Business Services by Foreign Tourists] (survey report submitted to the meeting set up by the Department of Export Promotion, Nonthaburi, Ministry of Commerce, 1998).

30. Benja, *The Role of Thai Traditional Doctors*, 43–4; Jean Mulholland, "Thai Traditional Medicine: Ancient Thought and Practice in a Thai Context," *Journal of the Siam Society* 67, no. 2 (1979): 83.

31. Irvine, "The Thai-Yuan 'Madman'," 61–82.

32. Robert H. Bannerman, John Burton, and Wen-Chieh Chen, eds, *Traditional Medicine and Health Care Coverage: A Reader for Health Administrators and Practitioners* (Geneva: World Health Organization, 1983).

33. Rongrian Ayurawet Witthayalai, *Rabiap Kan Sop Khao pen Naksueksa Ayurawet Witthayalai (Chiwakakomaraphat)* [Regulations of Entrance Examination for Ayurawet College] (Bangkok: Rongrian Ayurawet Witthayalai, 1997), 1.

34. Rongrian Ayurawet Witthayalai, *Rabiap Kan Sop Khao*, 3.

35. Pennapa Subcharoen and Daroon Pechprai, "Present Status of Traditional Medicine in Thailand," in *Proceedings of International Seminar on Traditional Medicine* (S.l.: S.n., 1995), 5–6.

36. Ibid.

37. Pennapa Subcharoen, *Sen Jut lae Rok nai Thritsadi Kannuat Thai* [Lines, Points and Diseases in the Theory of Thai Massage] (Bangkok: Rongphim Ongkan Songkhro Thahan Phan Suek, 1995), 9.

38. Sathaban Kanphaet Phaen Thai, *Kannuat Thai phuea Sukkhaphap* [Thai Massage for Health] (Bangkok: Loef and Lip Press, 1997), 4.

39. Pennapa, *Sen Jut lae Rok*, 9.

40. Chantana, "The Indigenization," 85.

41. Ibid., 87.

42. Paul T. Cohen, "Buddhism, Health & Development in Thailand from the Reformist Perspective of Dr. Prawase Wasi," in *Health & Development in Southeast Asia*, ed. Paul T. Cohen and John Purcal (Canberra: Australian Development Studies Network, 1995).

43. Junko Iida, *Tai Massaji no Minzokushi: "Tai-shiki Iryo" Seisei Katei ni okeru Shintai to Jissen* [Ethnography of Thai Massage: Body and Practice in the Process of the Creation of "Thai Traditional Medicine"] (Tokyo: Akashi Shoten, 2006), 72.

44. Chantana, "The Indigenization," 87.

45. Klum Sueksa Panha Ya/Munlanithi Satharanasuk kap Kanphatthana (Drug Problem Study Group/Foundation for Public Health and Development, KSPY/MSKK), *Rangkai khong Rao: Phuenthan Kannuat Thai* [Our Body: The Basics of Thai Massage] (Bangkok: KSPY/MSKK, 1986), 5.

46. Chantana, "The Indigenization," 89.

47. Iida, *Tai Massaji no Minzokushi*, 73.

48. Dr. Dan Beach Bradley, a missionary and one of the most important figures who introduced Western medicine to Thailand, mentioned in his record in 1865 that Siamese doctors believe 'KOMARA-P'AT' to be the founder of medicine. See Dan Beach Bradley, "Siamese Theory and Practice of Medicine," *Sangkhomsat Parithat* [Social Science Review] 5, no. 2 (1967 [1865]): 117. Chiwakakomaraphat is an important source of legitimacy of Thai traditional medicine and is often mentioned to explain its long history. In several old texts on traditional medicine, it is written that these texts were originally told by Dr. Komarapatt. See Benja Yoddumnern, *The Role of Thai Traditional Doctors* (Bangkok: Institute for Population and Social Research, Mahidol University, 1974), 9. The formal name of Ayurawet College is Ayurawet College (Chiwakakomaraphat).

49. Munlanithi Satharanasuk kap Kanphatthana and Samaphan Phaet Phaen Thai Haeng Prathet Thai (Foundation for Public Health and Development and the Federation of Thai Traditional Doctors in Thailand), *Khumue Kanprakop Phithi Wai Khru Phaet Phaen Thai* [Manual of Wai Khru Ceremony for Thai Traditional Doctors] (S.l.: S.n., 1999).

50. Iida, *Tai Massaji no Minzokushi*, 75–6.

51. Chantana, "The Indigenization," 94.

52. Iida, *Tai Massaji no Minzokushi*, 77–9.

53. Sathaban Kanphaet Phaen Thai, *Sathaban Kanphaet Phaen Thai* [National Institute of Thai Traditional Medicine] (Nonthaburi: Ministry of Public Health, 1994), 2–6.

54. Section 46, the Constitution of the Kingdom of Thailand, 1997.

55. The NITTM was incorporated in the Department for Development of Thai Traditional and Alternative Medicine established by the Ministry of Public Health in 2005.

56. Iida, *Tai Massaji no Minzokushi*, 80–1.

57. Sathaban Kanphaet Phaen Thai, *Sathaban Kanphaet Phaen Thai*, 16–17.

58. Pennapa Subcharoen, *Prawat lae Wiwatthanakan Kanphaet Phaen Thai* [The History and Development of Thai Traditional Medicine] (Bangkok: Chi Hua Printing, 1995).

59. Sathaban Kanphaet Phaen Thai, *Kanphaet Phaen Thai: Kanphaet Baep Ong Ruam* [Thai Traditional Medicine: Holistic Medicine] (Bangkok: Rongphim Ongkan Songkhro Thahan Phan Suek, 1996).

60.  Sathaban Kanphaet Phaen Thai, *Chut Nithatsakan Kanphaet Phaen Thai* [Program of the Exhibition of Thai Traditional Medicine] (Bangkok: Rongphim Ongkan Songkhro Thahan Phan Suek, 1999.

61.  Pennapa, *Sen Jut lae Rok*. Sathaban Kanphaet Phaen Thai, *Kannuat Thai phuea Sukkhaphap*, 1997.

62.  Iida, *Tai Massaji no Minzokushi*, 84–5.

63.  Ibid., 85–9.

64.  Komatra Chuengsatiansup, "Alternative Health, Alternative Sphere of Autonomy: Cheewajit and the Emergence of a Critical Public of Thailand," (paper submitted to the 7th International Conference on Thai Studies, Amsterdam, 1999), 8–9.

65.  Iida, *Tai Massaji no Minzokushi*, 80.

66.  Ibid., 86.

67.  Irvine, "The Thai-Yuan 'Madman,'" 46–7.

68.  Junko Iida, "The 'Revival' of Thai Traditional Medicine and Local Practice: Villagers' Reaction to the Promotion of Thai Massage in Northern Thailand" (paper presented at the 9th International Conference on Thai Studies, Northern Illinois University, DeKalb, Illinois, 2005).

69.  Iida, *Tai Massaji no Minzokushi*, 86.

70.  Hsu, "The History of Chinese Medicine," 468. Eric Hobsbawm, Introduction to *The Invention of Tradition*, ed. Eric Hobsbawm and Terence Ranger (Cambridge: Cambridge University Press, 1983), 3.

71.  Elisabeth Hsu, *The Transmission of Chinese Medicine* (Cambridge: Cambridge University Press, 1999).

72.  Jean M. Langford, *Fluent Bodies: Ayurvedic Remedies for Postcolonial Imbalance* (Durham, NC: Duke University Press, 2002).

CHAPTER 11

# Honoring the Teachers, Constructing the Lineage: A *Wai Khru* Ritual among Healers in Chiang Mai, Thailand

*C. Pierce Salguero*

This chapter discusses a major public celebration held at a Traditional Thai Medicine school in Chiang Mai, Thailand, in the summer of 2012.[1] Organized in honor of the fiftieth anniversary of the founding of the institution, the event was an especially elaborate version of the annual ceremony for "honoring the teachers" (*wai khru*), through which healers renew their connection with their living teachers, Buddhist figures of authority, and spiritual guides. This paper provides a description of the setting and layout of the celebration, as well as of the specific rituals, Buddhist and otherwise, that were undertaken that morning. While I am primarily concerned with understanding the event's logic and significance for the participants and organizers, I also analyze its social function. Examining the ceremony through both emic and etic perspectives leads to an understanding of how Buddhist rituals work to unite a disparate group of healers behind the leadership of the current director of the school, and how a notion of lineage is built and maintained among members of this community.

## The Setting

Like other "traditional" medicines of contemporary Asia, Traditional Thai Medicine or Thai Traditional Medicine (*phaet phaen thai*, commonly abbreviated TTM) is a product of the confluence of ancient medical ideas, modern sensibilities, and contemporary global capitalism.[2] Practitioners and teachers commonly say that TTM originates in the teachings of ancient Indian sages, and many of the doctrines that inform its contemporary practice clearly derive in some way or another from ancient Buddhist and Ayurvedic ideas.[3] However, the corpus of TTM texts considered canonical today was compiled only in the 1870s, and little is known about the history of Thai (i.e., Siamese) medicine before the nineteenth century.[4] Despite royal support for the codification of its central texts in the nineteenth century and their subsequent publication in the early twentieth, TTM enjoyed only sporadic support from the Thai government prior to the late 1970s.[5] Following the 1978 decision by the World Health Organization to promote indigenous medicine as part of its global primary health care initiative, however, particular government offices became increasingly involved in the promotion of TTM and regulation of its training curricula and licensing standards. Today, both the Ministry of Education and the Ministry of Public Health play an important role in the administration of TTM at the national level, although direct royal patronage and private initiatives have also been influential.

The most iconic practitioner of modern TTM is the *mo boran* (i.e., "traditional doctor"). The *mo boran* earns his or her status by holding the highest degree of formalized training in Thai medical theory, herbal medicines, diet, regimen, and other therapies, and by being examined and licensed by the national government. Aside from the *mo boran*, the range of other types of clinicians rounding out the TTM spectrum include pharmacists, midwives, and therapists with various levels of training in *nuat boran* (a hybrid of massage, chiropractics, and yoga-like stretching).

Despite their less-than-prestigious position in the TTM hierarchy, the latter category of practitioners have been instrumental in shaping the economics and urban life of the northern Thai city of Chiang Mai. The city has long supported a thriving tourism industry, but it emerged in the 1980s and 1990s as an especially popular destination for Western travelers interested in experiencing or learning how to do *nuat boran*.[6] With the explosion of demand, the pace of development of spas, massage clinics, and schools became feverish by the mid-2000s. I personally have been conducting training and field study among *mo nuat* (literally, "massage doctors") and other healers in Chiang Mai since 1997, and have watched as enthusiasm for *nuat boran* has completely transformed life in the city. Today, massage clinics, foot massage stations, and spas are dominant features of the urban landscape.

No doubt sparked by the success of *nuat boran*, Chiang Mai and the surrounding region has in recent years begun to see a surge in tourist interest in other facets of TTM, as well as healing practices that are tangentially (if at all) associated with that tradition. Today, the city is the scene of a competitive massage industry that pits practitioners of *nuat boran* against therapists who practice any number of Lanna, Hill-tribe, Chinese, Indian, and Western massage styles. These practitioners are both licensed and unlicensed, and operate both inside and outside of national regulatory frameworks. The city is additionally home to a wide range of herbalists (*mo ya*), spirit healers (*mo song*), exorcists (*mo phi*), seers or diviners (*mo du*), magicians (*mo saiyasat*), soul-doctors (*mo sukhwan*), specialists in protective tattoos (*mo sak yan*), and many other providers of health-related services and education catering to the local and tourist markets alike.[7]

Located just outside the southwestern corner of the old city moat, the Shivagakomarpaj Traditional Thai Medicine School (*Rongrian phaet phaen thai Chiwakakomaraphat*), more widely known in English by the mistranslation "Old Medicine Hospital," is an institution that has in many ways been at the heart of the development in TTM in Chiang Mai.[8] Founded in 1962 by the late Sintorn Chaichakan, the school became the first in Chiang Mai to teach *nuat boran* in English in the 1980s. Since that time, it has pursued the multiple missions of providing TTM training in Thai for locals, running short (2–10 days) massage courses for tourists in English, and offering a range of massage, herbal, and other therapies to a mixed clientele.

Having weathered vicissitudes in the popularity of TTM in the earlier decades of its existence, the intensive commercialization of *nuat boran* beginning in the mid-1980s, and the increasingly competitive environment and government regulatory regime that have characterized the massage industry more recently, the facility continues to grow. It has supported two generations of the Chaichakan family, who make up the major proportion of the administrative staff. Another measure of the influence of the Old Medicine Hospital on the development of the massage industry in Chiang Mai is the number of similar training programs that have cropped up all around the city. Though lacking statistics to quantify the phenomenon, I have noted that many of the competing programs that have emerged in the city over the last three decades are directed or staffed by graduates of the Old Medicine Hospital's training programs, by previous employees of the school, or even by members of the Chaichakan family.

At the time of this writing (late 2013), the school itself is run by the eldest son of the founder, Wasan Chaichakan, who is a *mo boran* and who long taught under his father's direction. Since the father's passing away in 2005, the training available at the school under this new *achan* (literally, "master" or "teacher") has been diversified with the addition of courses on Chinese- and Western-style massage, in order to better compete with other local institutions. The Old Medicine Hospital has also launched an English-language website, received accreditation from several American professional bodies, and engaged in other novel promotional campaigns.[9] Notably, the facility has also undergone dramatic expansion and development over the years, including a major reconstruction in the early 2000s. The school today consists of two large multi-storied buildings for classroom and clinical space, with a multi-purpose central courtyard in between that houses a large altar and open space for public functions.

## Daily *Wai Khru*

The courtyard altar just mentioned is the setting for the Old Medicine Hospital's twice-daily *wai khru*, a brief ceremony that honors the lineage of teachers of the school. Literally meaning "paying respect to the guru(s)," *wai khru* is a normal part of everyday life in Thai culture. Children in school honor their teachers at certain times of the year by giving them gifts and singing songs, muay thai boxers perform a dance to honor their teachers before a fight, traditional musicians do so before a performance, and practitioners of virtually all other Thai cultural arts have developed ritualized ways of honoring their teachers as well.[10] Daily *wai khru* in these different settings might involve paying respects to living teachers through prostrations, gifts, and other gestures of devotion. They may also involve lighting candles and incense before a picture of the practitioner's departed teacher(s), as well as offerings to deities or spirits that are considered patrons of the particular art form in question.

*Wai khru* is widely considered a daily obligation for Thai healers. In Chiang Mai's TTM schools and *nuat boran* clinics, *wai khru* typically involves venerating Chiwakakomaraphat (often transcribed as Shivagakomarpaj or Shivago Komaraphat) as the principal guru. This figure, whose name appears in the formal name of the Old Medicine Hospital, is a legendary hero from Buddhist scriptures. Known as Jīvaka Komārabhacca in Pāli and Jīvaka Kumārabhṛta in Sanskrit, this idealized

Indian physician is the hero of a biography that is extant in multiple versions across the Buddhist world, including in Pāli, Sanskrit, Chinese, and Tibetan translations.[11] Ostensibly, the authoritative version of the story for Theravada Buddhists is found in the eighth chapter of the *Mahāvagga* section of the Pāli Vinaya (i.e., the monastic disciplinary code). The narrative introduces Jīvaka as the orphaned son of a local courtesan who was abandoned on a trash heap, but is found and adopted by the royal family. Upon reaching adulthood, he travels to Taxila, the ancient north Indian center of medical learning, to study with a renowned physician. Returning home after his training, he treats a series of patients suffering from various diseases using abdominal and cranial surgery, nasal irrigation, medicated ghee, and other Indian therapies. The sequence of cures climaxes in Jīvaka's treatment of the Buddha, who is said to have been suffering from a case of the *doṣa* (conventionally translated as "peccant humors"), with a mild inhaled purgative.[12]

In Thailand, however, a thick layer of local lore has arisen around "Mo Chiwok" (that is, "Dr Jīvaka"), which greatly extends his activities and healing exploits beyond the above account from the scriptural source. He is, for example, often said to have visited Thailand and to have taught the Thai people various TTM therapies. He is even officially attributed with the authorship of two TTM texts on general medical theory.[13] Statues of Jīvaka are objects of cultic devotion at numerous temples around Thailand, including at the central temple Wat Phra Singh in Chiang Mai and at Wat Phra Kaew, the national temple in Bangkok. Devotional statues or images of Jīvaka are also commonplace in TTM schools and clinics, where they serve as focal points for daily *wai khru* ceremonies. Teachers, employees, students, and sometimes patients at these institutions come together to make offerings and chant homages to Jīvaka in mixtures of Pāli, Thai, and Sanskrit.

Other spiritual patrons are usually present on the altar alongside Jīvaka during a typical Chiang Mai medical practitioner's *wai khru*, though exactly which ones tends to vary depending on the particular lineages, traditions, or conventions of individual schools and practitioners. It is routine, for example, to include an image of a departed teacher or family member. The devas (*tewada*), Hindu deities adopted into Thai popular religion as divine protectors, are commonly included as well—most often Brahmā, Gaṇeś, and Śiva. The Chinese Buddhist bodhisattva Guanyin (Th. Kuan Im) is also sometimes included on the altar, particularly if the practitioner is of Chinese-Thai heritage. In addition to these deities, a whole spectrum of angelic beings and demon-like guardian spirits can also be incorporated, as can various quasi-divine rishis (Th. *ruesi*; Skt. *rṣi*) famed for their medical wisdom, past and present Thai kings, and any number of famous monks noted for magical powers.[14]

Given this diverse range of divine figures, cultural heroes, and other beings that can be considered teachers, it is not surprising that there is a wide range of possibilities for designing *wai khru* ceremonies.[15] In my field study in Chiang Mai, I have found *wai khru* practice to differ between each school or teacher I have visited in the city, often significantly. However, one constant feature is the framing of the ceremony through Buddhist symbolism and ritual. Altars constructed to house the images or statues of the teachers virtually always contain an image of the Buddha in the most significant location. Also, the chants honoring the teachers always begin with at least a few lines of Pāli paying homage to the Buddha, Dhamma, and Sangha. When I have asked for clarification on the structure of the *wai khru*, I have almost always been told that the Buddha should be honored as the chief among teachers, as the teacher of the highest truths.

The principal purpose of the *wai khru*, however, is not to honor the Buddha, but rather the lineage of divine and human teachers that have more directly contributed to one's healing practice. There is a general consensus among those I have spoken with that doing so is necessary to their safety, efficacy, and success as healers. When properly honored, the teachers provide protection against nefarious spirits (*phi*), negative energies (*lom*), and other potential dangers the healer faces daily in interacting with sick patients. Many practitioners additionally use ritual chants (*mon*) or sacred diagrams (*yan*) during their *wai khru* to empower their medicines or the tools of their trade.[16] It is also fairly common to integrate various types of attraction magic—for example, chants, *yan*, or statues of the prosperity goddess Nang Kwak—in order to attract clients.

The chief sign of a successful *wai khru* is that the presence of the teachers is felt by the practitioner. For certain types of healers, such as exorcists and spirit mediums, venerating the teachers likely means allowing their spirits to possess the practitioner's body.[17] However, most practitioners of TTM and *nuat boran* are likely to seek more subtle signs of the presence of the spirits. For example, one explanation I have heard from more than one *nuat boran* practitioner is that, because of their practice of daily *wai khru*, they can sense Jīvaka sitting behind or above their heads during treatments, both protecting them and providing guidance or flashes of intuition that help shape the therapeutic session. In any event, whether invoking spirit possession or a more subtle presence, *wai khru* generally involves a three-step process: (1) the practitioner invites the spirit teachers to be present, (2) he or she honors them with offerings and praise, and (3) the teachers in return protect and empower the practitioner.

## Preparing for a Special *Wai Khru*

In addition to daily *wai khru* ceremonies lasting anywhere from 5 to 30 minutes, some schools in Chiang Mai hold a more elaborate annual *wai khru* (also called *liang khru*, i.e., "caring for the teachers") that brings together current students and staff, alumni, family, friends, and members of the community. The Old Medicine Hospital holds such an annual event, as do several of its offshoots in and outside of Chiang Mai. In the summer of 2012, the Old Medicine Hospital's annual ceremony was even more elaborate than usual, as it was also the celebration of the fiftieth anniversary of the founding of the institution. This public event was held in the courtyard of the school around the central altar, under an overhang of one of the buildings, and under makeshift tents erected for the occasion (see Figure 1 for the layout of the courtyard). In my estimation, the total attendance appeared to be around 100 people.

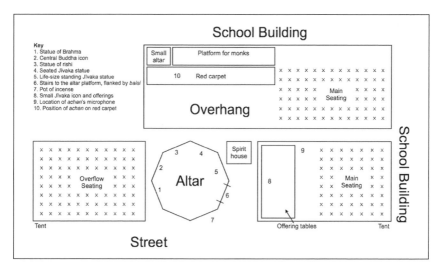

**Figure 1.** Layout of courtyard on the day of the celebration (author's personal collection).

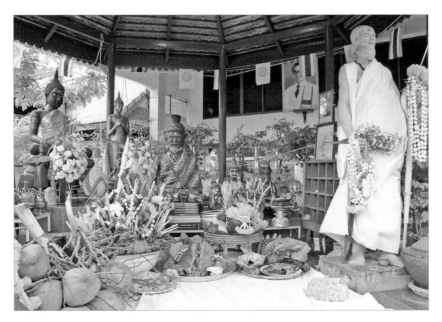

**Figure 2.** View of altar pagoda, with main icons, offerings, and *khan khru* (the white bowl at left) (author's personal collection). Note the hog's head in the center and the *sai sin* under the eaves.

Surprisingly to me, I recognized among the group several previous employees of the Old Medicine Hospital who had left to start their own massage practices and schools in direct competition with the institution. Somewhat less surprising was the fact that only a half-dozen or so of the school's current cohort of Western students were present.[18]

The ceremony took place on a Thursday, the auspicious day for teachers. A great deal of work had obviously been done by the school staff in the days leading up to the event and that morning in order to prepare ornate offerings around the courtyard. The school's altar is an elevated octagonal platform covered by a pagoda perhaps 3 meters in diameter and 5 meters in height to the top of the roof. Inside the pagoda, a large seated statue of the Buddha is permanently installed, flanked by statues of Jīvaka, a rishi, Brahmā, and various other divine protectors (see Figure 2). All of these statues were adorned with cloth, rosary beads, and flower garlands for the celebration. On stage left, a life-size standing statue of Jīvaka towers over the other figures, on this day fittingly draped in even more garlands than the rest. In front of the statue of the rishi (who, I have been told, is a generic statue representing

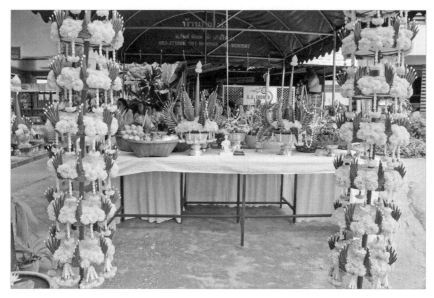

**Figure 3.** *Bai si* and other items on the offering table (author's personal collection). Note the *sai sin* descending to the small white statue of Jīvaka.

all of the 108 great rishis of Thai tradition), a stack of TTM and *nuat boran* texts new and old are placed on an elevated platform, symbols of the wisdom of the founders of the tradition and the continuity of that wisdom through the succeeding generations up to the present day.

In front of the deities on the altar platform and spilling over onto a series of tables set up under a tent adjacent to the pagoda (Figure 3), a rich display of offerings was arranged by participants as they arrived for the ceremony. These included heaping baskets of fruit and flowers, massive clusters of green coconuts and ripe bananas, and a pot stuffed full of burning incense sticks.[19] Platters were piled with sweets, steamed rice in banana leaves, cups of water and whiskey, cigarettes, and an array of medicinal herbs and herbal preparations. One centrally-located platter displayed a whole hog's head, a particularly auspicious offering. *Bai si*, decorative arrangements meticulously made of folded banana leaves and flowers, were placed all around as well.[20]

Adjacent to the altar was the *san phraphum*, a dollhouse-sized construction in the shape of a temple that is used to house tutelary spirits (see Figure 4).[21] These "spirit houses" are commonly established and cared for by homeowners and proprietors of businesses in order to contain potentially dangerous spirits (e.g., spirits of the land or spirits

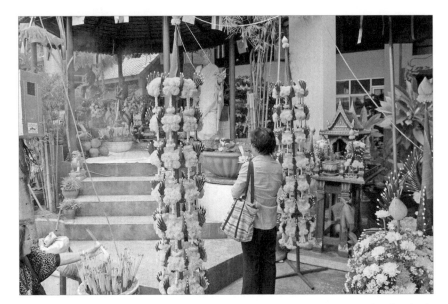

**Figure 4.** Devotional activities around the pagoda (author's personal collection). Note the spirit house at center right, and *sai sin* connecting different objects.

of the dead that have not been cared for properly) and to prevent them from meddling in human affairs. Though normally kept at a location that is removed from the comings and goings of a home or business, the spirit house occupied a more prominent location in this ceremony. As part of the preparations for the *wai khru*, the spirit house was earlier in the morning supplied with fresh offerings of incense, garlands, food, and water in order to pacify its potentially unpredictable inhabitants in advance of the events to come.

In the midst of this resplendent display of colors and rich aromas, the most elaborate offering of all was the *khan khru*, a large white bowl loaded with layers of folded banana leaves, incense, candles, flowers, spools of white cotton string, and other offerings placed directly in front of the central Buddha image (see Figure 2).[22] While the other gifts presented on this day would either be consumed, recycled, or disposed of after the ceremony, this particular offering would be hung in a place of honor within the altar pagoda, suspended from the ceiling for one whole year. At the annual *wai khru* next year, it will be taken down, its contents will be distributed among the participants, and it will be replaced with a fresh bowl. Receiving part of the previous year's *khan khru* offerings is considered to be very auspicious, and many practitioners will take that home to place on their own altars and integrate it into their own daily *wai khru* rites.

An important part of the preparations for the ceremony was that sacred objects throughout the ritual space had been connected with lengths of *sai sin* (also *sai sincana*).[23] This nine-stranded, white cotton cord encircled the ceiling of the altar pagoda, marking off a ritual perimeter. From there, lengths of string descended to the statues on the altar platform, wrapping around each one. Another length extended toward the offering tables, where it wrapped around a small Jīvaka statue and connected to the items placed there (see Figure 3). *Sai sin* is a common feature in Thai rituals, but its use is taken especially seriously among healers in Chiang Mai. It has multiple functions that are directly relevant to controlling spirits and energies: it can be used to delineate a protected space, as an implement for binding beneficial influences to the patient's body, as a vehicle for trapping and removing evil influences, or as a conduit to direct or channel the powers generated through rituals (*palang*).

As more people continued arriving, the courtyard gradually filled with guests. Participants with closer connections to the school or the family sat themselves under the overhang or in the main seating area by the offering tables, while others sat in the overflow area behind the altar platform. As each guest arrived, they arranged their offerings on one of the tables and placed lit sticks of incense in the ceramic pot by the entrance to the pagoda. They removed their shoes and climbed the steps up to the altar platform in order to bow to the various statues there (Figure 4). They then milled about chatting or fussed with the displays of offerings, waiting for the ceremony to begin.

## The Ceremony

About an hour after our arrival, a group of five monks clad in bright orange arrived, and the ceremony got underway. The director of the school (whom I will refer to as "the *achan*" from this point forward) led the monks through the crowd to take their seats on a long platform that had been set up under the overhang (Figure 5). The monks seated themselves on ornate golden cushions that had been laid out for them. At the end closest to the most senior monk was a small, though ornate, altar with a single golden statue of the Buddha, a pot with a few sticks of incense, and some candles.

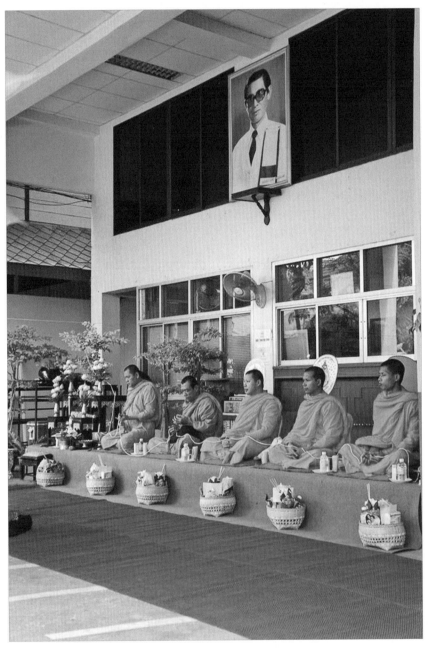

**Figure 5.** Monks seated under the overhang for the *paritta* ritual (author's personal collection). Note the portrait of the founder of the school above, and *sai sin* connecting the monks with the small altar at left.

After the monks settled into their seats and arranged their robes, the *achan* lit the candles and incense on the small altar to signal the beginning of the ceremony. He then assumed a kneeling position on a long red carpet directly in front of the monks, alongside some other senior members of his family. What followed was a typical Theravada Buddhist protection rite. The monks led the audience in taking Refuge, as well as other basic chants of homage that are a familiar part of any formal Thai Buddhist ceremony. After these preliminaries, the laity fell silent while the monks began chanting *paritta* (Th. *parit*) scriptures in the monotonous and nasal style of Thai monastics. Their sonorous voices reverberated against the sides of the buildings surrounding the courtyard, ostensibly clearing the physical space of any negativities, extending the power of the Buddha's protection and blessings to the area and all of those in it, and establishing an auspicious and sanctified zone in which further ritual activities could take place. The guests, sitting in rows of chairs and benches by the monks' platform and in the other seating areas, held their palms together in a gesture of respect (the *wai* that gives the *wai khru* its name), kept their eyes closed, and concentrated on absorbing the power of the chanting into their minds and bodies.

Routine in Theravada societies, protection scriptures and their rituals have been discussed in detail by other scholars, and I do not need to elaborate further upon this part of the morning here.[24] However, the role of the *sai sin* in this particular rite is worth mentioning. Before the chanting, the head monk had taken up a spool and had passed it down the line so that all of the monks were holding it (Figure 5). From their hands, this string extended to the smaller altar, where it wrapped around the golden Buddha. It then ascended the wall of the building, stretched across to the ceiling of the pagoda about 7 or 8 meters away, and tied into the *sai sin* that united the images and offerings throughout the courtyard. By holding one end of this extensive network in their hands, the monks thus could channel the power of their chanting to all of the objects within the ritual space.

After chanting for about half an hour, the lead monk took up a golden bowl of water that had been placed near his seat. He wrapped the *sai sin* around a bamboo whisk, and began slowly stirring the water with it while the monks chanted the *Jayaparittam* ("Victory Paritta"). This incantation called upon the blessings of the Buddha, Dharma, Sangha, and all the devas, which the monk transferred into the water.

After a few minutes, he rose from his seat and walked around the court-yard, dipping the whisk into the bowl and shaking it into the air, in the process sprinkling the ground, the altar, the offerings, and the assembled guests with the enchanted water (*nam mon*, literally "mantra-water").

The purification of the space, the sacred objects, and the partici-pants having been completed, the monks rose and retired into one of the buildings. This next part of the ceremony was private, but we were told that the monks were being given food and other offerings on behalf of the entire assembly. Feeding monks and taking care of their other daily needs is a gesture of devotion and an opportunity to earn meritorious karma (*tambun*) that is routine in many Buddhist cultures throughout the world and that is especially important in Thailand.[25] Some guests had contributed to the Old Medicine Hospital in advance in order to fund this meal, and a donations box was made available in an unobtru-sive corner of the courtyard for anyone else who wished to contribute and share in the merit. (Participation in the *wai khru*, I should note, was completely free of charge, and I saw no visible pressure to contri-bute to this box nor guidance on how much should be given.)

When the *achan* returned from serving the monks, the second half of the morning's ceremonial activities began. Now, the focal point shifted from the overhang in the rear of the courtyard to the altar in the center. The *achan* now entered the pagoda, bowed several times to the various statues, and began to chant in a distinctive high-pitched and melodious voice that was quite different from the tone of the monks. This was not a protection chant, but a gentle call to the devas, rishis, departed teachers, and other beneficial spirits to become present in order to be honored and receive the group's offerings.[26] This special chant is only performed by the *achan* once per year during the annual *wai khru*, and he follows a written manuscript that only his closest students or lineage heirs are allowed to see.

When this opening chant was completed, the *achan* then led the group in chanting an invocation specifically addressed to Jīvaka. This section of the liturgy was familiar to everyone from the daily *wai khru* ceremony, and the entire crowd recited it with gusto. The chant opened with the standard homage to the Buddha, Dhamma, and Sangha in Pāli. Then came a set of two verses in Pāli honoring Jīvaka, the first of which was repeated several times:

> OM. I bow my head in homage to Jīvaka. With compassion for all
> sentient beings he has brought divine medicine. Shining bright as

the sun and moon, luminous Komārabhacca. I pay my adoration to the Teacher, the wise one. May I be free from disease and happy.

[To he whom is] beloved by deities and humans, beloved by Brahma, I pay the highest homage. [To he whom is] beloved by *nāgas* and heavenly beings, of pure faculties, I pay homage.[27]

The chants to Jīvaka were then followed by a series of short incantations for health, effectiveness, prosperity, and success in business.

Now that the spirit teachers had been invited and had been suitably honored, the *achan* descended from the altar and moved to a position near the altar tables where he took up a microphone. He gave a short speech thanking the guests for attending. Singling out newly graduated advanced students for special recognition, he invited them up to receive diplomas that had been sitting on one of the offering tables. He then received one by one all of the other guests, who formed a line stretching across the courtyard.

As the participants approached the *achan* individually, they each *wai*-ed him deeply in a gesture of respect and held out their left arm. Taking a short length of the *sai sin* string that had been used in the ceremony, he tied it around each person's wrist. As he did so, he gave each guest a personalized blessing. The binding of the wrist as a form of blessing is a very common feature of Chiang Mai ceremonies of all kinds.[28] As the *achan* has explained to me on another occasion, its use in the *wai khru* ceremony derives from the belief that the guardian spirits that reside in the participant's body (*khwan*) have been nourished through participation in the auspicious rituals of the day. The string now binds the merits and blessings accumulated in the *wai khru* to the body, helping to keep the *khwan* content and secure in their proper place.

After tying the string to each guest's wrist, the *achan* then dipped a finger into a small pot of white paste, and applied a *choem*, or auspicious marking, to the participant's forehead. The gesture is symbolic of the teacher opening the student's "third eye" (*ta thisam*)—in other words, opening up the student's capacity to receive the wisdom and learning of the lineage. Finally, as each individual took their leave of the *achan*, they reached into a large basket on the nearby offering table to retrieve a small amulet (*phra khreuang*).[29] These thumb-sized clay tablets, stamped with the image of Jīvaka in bas-relief, were especially commissioned by the *achan* to be given away in commemoration of the fiftieth anniversary celebration. Having been empowered during the ceremony via a length of *sai sin*, they are now sacred objects that can be placed on the practitioner's altar, or encased in clear plastic to be worn around the neck for protection while working with patients.

Once guests had paid their respects to the *achan* and received his blessings, they began taking apart the offerings. Collectively, the group began the day by caring for the spirit house; then they fed the monks, made offerings to the spiritual teachers, and paid their respects to the *achan*. Having taken care of the entire range of teachers and spiritually significant beings, it was now time to share the food among the community, who had not yet eaten. The offerings had been filled up with powers of protection, blessings, healing, and prosperity conducted to them via the *sai sin* throughout the morning, and everyone in attendance was now invited to partake in the auspicious food. The fruit was cut and placed into bowls, sweets and cakes were passed around, rice and curries were revealed inside of banana leaves, and coconuts were opened up for drinking.

Pieces of fruit and other treats were also packaged up to take home for family and friends who could not attend the celebration. Many of us were given containers of herbal balm, massage oil, or other medicinal preparations to take home too, which, thanks to the ritual, were now empowered with particularly efficacious healing qualities.[30] While the consecrated food and medicines would be consumed or used, after a week or so, the *sai sin* around the participants' wrist would be respectfully removed and then placed in a special container reserved for storage of such sacred objects. Pieces of the *khan khru* offerings would be kept on altars until the next major ceremony, and amulets would be displayed or worn for many years to come.

The ceremony was now over, and the atmosphere was jubilant and social. While some people took their leave, many stayed behind for the rest of the afternoon, enjoying each other's company and helping to dismantle the tables and clean up the courtyard.

## Analysis

In many ways, the fiftieth-anniversary *wai khru* at the Old Medicine Hospital was a typical Thai ceremony. Unique features that differentiated it as a celebration by and for healers included the ubiquitousness of Jīvaka throughout the morning and the prominence of medicinals and medical textbooks among the offerings on the altar. The other elements of the ceremony—the visiting monks, enchanted water, and *sai sin*; offerings of fruit, garlands, and *bai si*; the binding of the wrists, application of *choem*, and distribution of amulets—all are common features of the popular Thai ritual repertoire. Individually or in combination, I have seen these at graduations, weddings, funerals, and other rites of passage in Chiang Mai quite regularly. While the ritual's contents may be somewhat conventional, however, the specific ways familiar ingredients were brought together for this event are worth analyzing a bit further for what they can tell us about the social functions of *wai khru* among this particular community of healers.

Scholars consider notions of "tradition" and "lineage" to be socially constructed fictions, less transmissions from the past than products of the ways in which the past is remembered and recreated in the present.[31] The *wai khru* gives us a window into how Chiang Mai healers literally make the past come alive. It is conventional for TTM and *nuat boran* practitioners of all types to refer to Jīvaka and the rishis as the founders of Thai medical traditions, and to speak of themselves as the beneficiaries of a lineage of teachers who preserved and transmitted their knowledge across the millennia. The participants in the Old Medicine Hospital's celebration gathered on that Thursday morning to honor and give thanks to that entire line of past teachers. But this was not simply to be done in the abstract. One of the *achan*'s chief responsibilities in the ceremony was to ritually make the teachers manifest in the courtyard. By invoking their presence, his task is to collapse the temporal distance between the teachers and the guests and make it possible for each participant to directly connect with the lineage in person and in real-time. The *achan*'s ability to make this connection possible for his guests confirms his legitimacy as inheritor of his father's lineage and his own place in the intergenerational chain of teachers.

The performance of the *wai khru* was also about demonstrating the *achan's* ability to harness different sources of ritual power and to direct these toward the group. Scholars have for many decades debated how to understand the complex relationship between Buddhism and spirit practices in Thai religion. Though various highly sophisticated models have been proposed, in the simplest terms, the argument has centered on the question of whether we should consider the Thai religious world as a single holistic episteme, or as some kind of mosaic of interlocking Buddhist, Brahmanical, Chinese, and "animistic" components.[32] While I would not presume that a single ritual can speak to the nature of Thai religion writ large, the Old Medicine Hospital's ceremony was divided into two phases that took place within distinct areas of the courtyard. This points, I believe, to an understanding on the part of the participants that more orthodox Theravada devotions belong to a different spatial and temporal sphere than the invocation of spirits for assistance in healing practice.[33] In my reading, the spatial separation of the *wai khru* served to emphasize the *achan*'s unique role as master of distinct ritual spheres: in the first half of the ceremony, he played the role of lay paterfamilias hosting monks to earn merit and protection; in the second, he demonstrated his ability to control and gain blessings from the spirit world. At the same time, I would emphasize that the role of *sai sin* as a conduit for protection and blessings across both spaces suggests a unified notion of ritual power bridging these spheres. By using *sai sin* and other paraphernalia to channel the powers harnessed in both ritual spaces toward his guests, the *achan* demonstrated his competence and legitimacy in both arenas.

Finally, I also see the *achan*'s role as host of the celebration as a concrete performance of his ability to provide social cohesion for the lineage. It was because of his leadership that these representatives from across the fractious spectrum of Chiang Mai healers could come together in a common cause, volunteer an immense amount of labor in preparing the space and offerings, and share together in the merits of the morning. Through these communal activities, the guests had the opportunity to build karmic bonds both with one another and with the *achan*. While there would no longer be a physical length of string connecting the community of practitioners once they left, the participants would carry memorabilia from the *wai khru* back to their own homes and schools. Fanning out across Chiang Mai and beyond, these consecrated objects would provide tangible memories and meaningful connections back to the ceremony. Insofar as they integrated those objects into their own personal daily *wai khru* rituals, practitioners would continue to direct their respect, honor, and good feelings back towards the *achan*, the school, and the lineage, and receive blessings and protections in return.

These three aspects—making the ancient teachers present, harnessing multiple types of ritual power, and providing social cohesion—are, in my reading, the chief functions of the *wai khru* for this community of healers. If the ceremony was successful, it will have offered an important counterweight against the cognitive dissonance inherent in the practice of a "traditional" medicine that everyone in Chiang Mai knows is more a product of government regulation, global tourism, and market competition than the wisdom of the ancients.[34] But these functions hinge on the participants placing their faith in the *achan*'s legitimacy as head of the lineage and ability to function as representative of the group. His security in that role is far from guaranteed. In large part, the success of this year's ceremony will be determined by the level of prosperity experienced by the participants in the coming year. If faith in the *achan*'s ability to provide those core functions breaks down for any reason, it will lead to the fracturing of the lineage as subgroups splinter off to rally around new leaders and ritual methods.[35]

In fact, an example of precisely that phenomenon was taking place on the very same day as the Old Medicine Hospital's fiftieth anniversary *wai khru*, on the other side of town. Another *achan*, a family member who had previously been highly placed within the administration of the Old Medicine Hospital, had very recently broken off to start his own competing *nuat boran* school for tourists. It is significant that this new school did not differentiate itself on matters of pedagogical style or therapeutic methods, both of which seemed to me to remain quite similar to those of its predecessor. Rather, this *achan*'s radical break from the Old Medicine Hospital community was made clear by the fact that his rival *wai khru* represented a near complete repudiation of the hospital's. He did not lead the ceremony himself; rather, he brought in a tiger skin-clad medium who channeled the spirit of a rishi. Instead of invoking the spirits into statues and transferring their blessings into food offerings, this medium offered more direct communion with the spirits by inducing a state of possession in the participants. In addition to other empowered objects to take home, the medium also gave willing participants *yan* tattoos that marked them as disciples of his lineage. The details of this second *wai khru* will have to be a story for another time, but this episode clearly demonstrates the fluid and contestational nature of lineage, and points to the great relevance of rituals "honoring the teachers" in negotiating identity politics and social relationships among healers in Chiang Mai.

## Notes

1.  This paper is based on events observed on June 21, 2012, but is informed by over 30 months of training and field study conducted from 1997–2012 among practitioners of Buddhism and traditional medicine in Thailand. The school discussed in this paper was the site at which I first encountered TTM and *nuat boran* in 1997, and I consider its current director, who plays a major role in this paper, to be a mentor. I also wish to thank another of my principal informants on Thai medical and religious culture, Wit Sukhsamran, who although not present at the ritual described here has given invaluable assistance during other phases of my fieldwork.

2.    A review of the scholarly literature on the history of TTM and some com-
      ments about my experience with contemporary practice are available in
      C. Pierce Salguero, *Traditional Thai Medicine*, 2nd ed. (Bangkok: White
      Lotus Press, 2016). See also Komat Cheungsathiansap and Muksong
      Chatchai, eds, *Phromdaen khwamru prawattisat kanpaet lae satharanasuk
      thai* [The State of Knowledge of the Thai History of Medicine and the
      Health Care System] (Bangkok: Health Systems Research Institute, 2002);
      Viggo Brun, "Traditional Thai Medicine," in *Medicine Across Cultures:
      History and Practice of Medicine in Non-Western Cultures*, ed. Helaine
      Selin and Hugh Shapiro (Boston: Kluwer Academic Publishers, 2003),
      115–32; Vincent J. Del Casino, Jr., "(Re)placing Health and Health Care:
      Mapping the Competing Discourses and Practices of 'Traditional' and
      'Modern' Thai Medicine," *Health & Place* 10 (2004): 59–73, which focuses
      specifically on Chiang Mai; Junko Iida, "The Revival of Thai Traditional
      Medicine and the Promotion of Thai Massage: The Reaction of Villagers
      in Northern Thailand," *Southeast Asian Studies* 44, no. 1 (2006): 78–96;
      Junko Iida, "The Sensory Experience of Thai Massage: Commercialization,
      Globalization, and Tactility," in *Everyday Life in Asia: Social Perspectives
      on the Senses*, ed. Devorah Kalekin-Fishman and Kelvin E.Y. Low
      (Surrey: Ashgate, 2010); Junko Iida, "Holism as a Whole-body Treatment:
      The Transnational Production of Thai Massage," *European Journal of
      Transnational Studies* 5, no. 1 (2013): 81–111; Junko Iida, "The Efficacy
      of Thai Massage for Urban Middle Class in Contemporary Thailand:
      Discourse, Body Technique, and Ritualized Process," *Senri Ethnological
      Reports* 120 (2014): 121–39.
3.    See overview of fundamental TTM doctrines in Jean Mulholland, "Thai
      Traditional Medicine: Ancient Thought and Practice in a Thai Context,"
      *Journal of the Siam Society* 67, no. 2 (1979): 80–115; Somchintana
      Thongthew-Ratarasarn, *The Principles and Concepts of Thai Classical
      Medicine* (Bangkok: Thammasat University, 1996); Salguero, *Traditional
      Thai Medicine*, 41–52.
4.    Historical documents concerning medicine in Siam are unavailable prior to
      the Ayutthaya period (1351–1767), and the relevant manuscripts from the
      latter have yet to be catalogued, much less examined in critical detail. For
      a brief history of TTM, see Salguero, *Traditional Thai Medicine*, 1–32.
      For an outline of the compilation of the TTM corpus in the nineteenth
      and twentieth centuries, see Jean Mulholland, *Medicine, Magic, and Evil
      Spirits* (Canberra: Australian National University, 1987), 7–19.
5.    For a history of the tensions between Western and traditional models in
      the nineteenth and twentieth centuries, see Davisakd Puaksom, "Of Germs,
      Public Hygiene, and the Healthy Body: The Making of the Medicalizing
      State in Thailand," *Journal of Asian Studies* 66, no. 2 (2007): 311–44;
      Del Casino, "(Re)placing Health and Health Care."

6.   In the interests of full disclosure, I should note that I myself am implicated in the popularization of TTM and *nuat boran* in the US in the early 2000s through a series of popular guides to the Thai healing arts I wrote prior to becoming an academic.

7.   For discussion of the range of practitioners in the Thai health care landscape, see Ruth-Inge Heinze, "Nature and Function of Some Therapeutic Techniques in Thailand," *Asian Folklore Studies* 36, no. 2 (1977): 85–104; Louis Golomb, *An Anthropology of Curing in Multiethnic Thailand* (Urbana: University of Illinois Press, 1985); Louis Golomb, "The Interplay of Traditional Therapies in South Thailand," *Social Science & Medicine* 27, no. 8 (1988): 761–8; Heinze, "The Relationship Between Folk and Elite Religions: The Case of Thailand," in *The Realm of the Sacred: Verbal Symbolism and Ritual Structure*, ed. Sitakant Mahapatra (Calcutta: Oxford University Press, 1992), 13–30; Salguero, *Traditional Thai Medicine*. The current paper is part of a series that will explore the activities of various types of healers in the city based on my field study.

8.   GPS coordinates: 18.771826, 98.978437.

9.   www.thaimassageschool.ac.th, accessed Oct. 18, 2013.

10.   See discussion of rituals honoring teachers among practitioners of various traditional arts in Michael Smithies and Euayporn Kerdchouay, "The *Wai Kru* Ceremony of the *Nang Yai*," *Journal of the Siam Society* 62, no. 1 (1974): 143–7; Rosalind C. Morris, *In the Place of Origins: Modernity and Its Mediums in Northern Thailand* (Durham, NC: Duke University Press, 2000), 107ff; Bussakorn Binson, "The Role of Food in the Musical Rites of the *Lanna* People of Northern Thailand," *Rian Thai: International Journal of Thai Studies* 2 (2009): 45–69. Ceremonies honoring teachers from Thai elementary schools, muay thai matches, and many other settings are readily found by searching for the keyword "wai khru" on www.YouTube.com.

11.   See discussion and comparison of these versions in Kenneth G. Zysk, "Studies in Traditional Indian Medicine in the Pāli Canon: Jīvaka and Āyurveda," *Journal of the International Association of Buddhist Studies* 5, no. 1 (1982): 70–86; Zysk, *Asceticism and Healing in Ancient India: Medicine in the Buddhist Monastery* (Delhi: Motilal Banarsidass, 1998), 52–61, 120–7; more detailed discussion of the Chinese version of the text in C. Pierce Salguero, "The Buddhist Medicine King in Literary Context: Reconsidering an Early Example of Indian Influence on Chinese Medicine and Surgery," *History of Religions* 48, no. 3 (2009): 183–210. English translation of the Pāli source is available in I.B. Horner, *The Book of the Discipline (Vinaya-Piṭaka)*, vol. IV (Oxford: Pali Text Society, 2000), 379–97; of Tibetan in F. Anton von Schiefner, *Tibetan Tales Derived from Indian Sources: Translated from the Tibetan of the Kah-Gyur* (London: Kegan Paul, 1906), 75–109; of Sanskrit in Gregory Schopen, "The Training and Treatments of an Indian Doctor in a Buddhist Text: A Sanskrit

Biography of Jīvaka," in *Buddhism and Medicine: An Anthology of Premodern Sources*, ed. C. Pierce Salguero (New York: Columbia University Press, 2017), 184–204.

12.  For discussion of the *doṣa* in Pāli and other early Indian texts, see Hartmut Scharfe, "The Doctrine of the Three Humors in Traditional Indian Medicine and the Alleged Antiquity of Tamil Siddha Medicine," *Journal of the American Oriental Society* 119, no. 4 (1999): 609–29; for Chinese Buddhist texts, see C. Pierce Salguero, "Understanding the *Doṣa*: A Summary of the Art of Medicine from the *Sūtra of Golden Light*," in *Buddhism and Medicine: An Anthology of Premodern Sources*, ed. C. Pierce Salguero (New York: Columbia University Press, 2017), 30–40.

13.  These are *Phaetsat sangkhro* 2.5 and 2.7, cited in Mulholland, "Thai Traditional Medicine," 113.

14.  This pantheon has been discussed in Peter A. Jackson, "Royal Spirits, Chinese Gods, and Magic Monks: Thailand's Boom-time Religions of Prosperity," *South East Asia Research* 7, no. 3 (1999): 245–320; Pattana Kitiarsa, "Beyond Syncretism: Hybridization of Popular Religion in Contemporary Thailand," *Journal of Southeast Asian Studies* 36, no. 3 (2005): 461–87; Ara Wilson, "The Sacred Geography of Bangkok's Markets," *International Journal of Urban and Regional Research* 32, no. 3 (2008): 631–42.

15.  I have posted a video of the founder of the Old Medicine Hospital leading a 10-minute daily *wai khru* ceremony in its entirety at http://asianmedicine zone.com/southeast-asia/wai-khru/, filmed in 2004, posted May 3, 2009, last accessed Feb. 26, 2017.

16.  On *yan*, see François Bizot, "Notes sur les *yantra* bouddiques d'Indochine," in *Tantric and Taoist Studies in Honour of R.A. Stein*, ed. Michel Strickmann (Brussels: Institut Belge des Hautes études Chinoises, 1981), 155–91; Donald K. Swearer, *Becoming the Buddha: The Ritual of Image Consecration in Thailand* (Princeton: Princeton University Press, 2004), 63–73; Barend Jan Terwiel, *Monks and Magic: Revisiting a Classic Study of Religious Ceremonies in Thailand* (Copenhagen: Nordic Institute of Asian Studies, 2012), 77–90; Joanna Cook, "Tattoos, Corporeality and the Self: Dissolving Borders in a Thai Monastery," *Cambridge Anthropology* 27, no. 2 (2008): 20–35.

17.  These practices among spirit mediums in Chiang Mai are one of the main subjects of Morris, *In the Place of Origins*. On possession in the context of healing, see also Sangun Suwanlert, "Phii Pob: Spirit Possession in Rural Thailand," in *Culture-Bound Syndromes, Ethnopsychiatry, and Alternate Therapies: Volume IV of Mental Health Research in Asia and the Pacific*, ed. William P. Lebra (Honolulu: University of Hawai'i Press, 1976), 68–87; Heinze, "The Relationship Between Folk and Elite Religions"; Heinze, *Trance and Healing in Southeast Asia Today*, 2nd ed. (Bangkok: White Lotus Press, 1997).

18. The majority of the non-Thai participants in the ceremony were part of my nine-person party, which included my family members, friends, and colleagues from the US.

19. The symbolic significance in northern Thailand of some of these foods is briefly discussed in Binson, "The Role of Food."

20. On *bai si*, see Phya Anuman Rajadhon, "The Khwan and Its Ceremonies," *Journal of the Siam Society* 50 (1965): 119–64; Ruth-Inge Heinze, *Tham Khwan: How to Contain the Essence of Life, a Socio-Psychological Comparison of a Thai Custom* (Singapore: Singapore University Press, 1982), 69–75.

21. On spirit houses, see Phya Anuman Rajadhon, "Chao Thi and Some Traditions of Thai," *Thailand Culture Series* 6 (1956): 119–64; Peter A. Reichart, and Pathawee Khongkhunthian, *The Spirit Houses of Thailand* (Bangkok: White Lotus, 2007).

22. Compare with Swearer, *Becoming the Buddha*, 83–6; Morris, *In the Place of Origins*, 107 ff.

23. On the use of *sai sin* in other rites, see Heinze, *Tham Khwan*, 76–84; Swearer, *Becoming the Buddha*, 77–121.

24. See especially Stanley Jeyaraja Tambiah, *Buddhism and the Spirit Cults in North-East Thailand* (Cambridge: Cambridge University Press, 1970), 195–222; Swearer, *Becoming the Buddha*, 88–94, 115–18; Justin Thomas McDaniel, *The Lovelorn Ghost and the Magical Monk: Practicing Buddhism in Modern Thailand* (New York: Columbia University Press, 2011), 72–120; Terwiel, *Monks and Magic*, 209–13; Justin Thomas McDaniel, "The Verses on the Victor's Armor: A Pāli Text Used for Protection and Healing in Thailand," in *Buddhism and Medicine: An Anthology of Premodern Sources*, ed. C. Pierce Salguero (New York: Columbia University Press, 2017), 358–62.

25. See the discussion in Tambiah, *Buddhism and the Spirit Cults*, 53–7, 141–51.

26. The logic of the invocation of the spirits into the statues on the altar is similar to rituals involving Buddha statues described in Swearer, *Becoming the Buddha*, 108–15. On the potency of images in Buddhism, see also Koichi Shinohara, ed., *Images, Miracles, and Authority in Asian Religious Traditions* (Boulder: Westview Press, 1998), especially the chapters by Robert Brown.

27. Translation by Tevijjo Yogi, personal communication, used with permission. See Salguero, *Traditional Thai Medicine*, 36–40, 78–81.

28. Various practices involving the *khwan*, including the binding of the wrists, are discussed in Rajadhon, "The Khwan and its Ceremonies"; Heinze, *Tham Khwan*, 69–75; Tambiah, *Buddhism and the Spirit Cults*, 223–51; Barend Jan Terwiel, "The Tais and Their Belief in Khwans: Towards Establishing an Aspect of 'Proto-Tai' Culture," *South East Asian Review* 3, no. 1 (1978): 1–16.

29.   On Thai amulets, see Phya Anuman Rajadhon, "Thai Charms and Amulets," *Journal of the Siam Society* 52 (1964): 171–97; Stanley Jeyaraja Tambiah, *The Buddhist Saints of the Forest and the Cult of Amulets* (Cambridge: Cambridge University Press, 1984); M.L. Pattaratorn Chirapravati, *Votive Tablets in Thailand: Origin, Style, and Uses* (Kuala Lumpur: Oxford University Press, 1997); McDaniel, *The Lovelorn Ghost*, 189–212; Terwiel, *Monks and Magic*, 69–77. While most observers have discussed Thai amulets in association with forces of commercialization and commodification, McDaniel points to the role of amulets in creating memories and communities—"the cherishing (not just the collecting)" (p. 192)—which is more relevant in the present case.

30.   The empowerment of medicine via the invocation of deities has parallels in many other Buddhist societies (see, e.g., Frances Garrett, "The Alchemy of Accomplishing Medicine (*sman sgrub*): Situating the Yuthok Heart Essence (*G.yu thog snying thig*) in Literature and History," *Journal of Indian Philosophy* 37 (2009): 207–30 for a description of the Tibetan rite).

31.   See, e.g., John McRae, *Seeing through Zen: Encounter, Transformation, and Genealogy in Chinese Chan Buddhism* (Berkeley: University of California Press, 2004); Steven Engler and Gregory P. Grieve, eds, *Historicizing "Tradition" in the Study of Religion* (Berlin: Walter de Gruyter, 2005); Volker Scheid, "Chinese Medicine and the Problem of Tradition," *Asian Medicine: Tradition and Modernity* 2, no. 1 (2006): 59–71.

32.   Highlights in this debate include Barend Jan Terwiel, "A Model for the Study of Thai Buddhism," *Journal of Asian Studies* 35, no. 3 (1976): 391–403; A. Thomas Kirsch, "Complexity in the Thai Religious System: An Interpretation," *Journal of Asian Studies* 36, no. 2 (1977): 241–66; Kitiarsa, "Beyond Syncretism"; Terwiel, *Monks and Magic*, 1–20. Kitiarsa provides an extensive review of the preceding literature and articulates the argument for using the concept of hybridization. In my view, however, the most successful attempt to explain the range of Thai religious expressions is McDaniel's *The Lovelorn Ghost*, which succeeds precisely because it turns away from modeling epistemes in favor of thick description of repertoires of practice.

33.   Note, however, that this is not a critique of heterodoxy such as described in Donald K. Swearer, "Aniconism Versus Iconism in Thai Buddhism," in *Buddhism in the Modern World: Adaptations of an Ancient Tradition*, ed. Steven Heine and Charles S. Prebish (New York: Oxford University Press, 2003), 9–25.

34.   See works by Iida cited in note 2.

35.   Note that it is not uncommon for practitioners to identify as members of more than one lineage, particularly when having studied with more than one teacher. It is therefore entirely possible for them to attend more than one *wai khru* ceremony without any implication of competition.

# Bibliography

Abou Zahr, Carla Wardlaw, and Tessa Wardlaw. "Trends in Maternal Mortality in the 1990s." *Bulletin of the World Health Organization* 79 (2001): 561–8.

Aldrich, Robert. "Imperial *mise en valeur* and *mise en scène*: Recent Works on French Colonialism." *The Historical Journal* 15, no. 4 (2002): 917–36.

Amrith, Sunil. *Decolonising International Health: India and Southeast Asia, 1930–65*. Basingstoke: Palgrave Macmillan, 2006.

Andaya, Barbara, and Leonard Andaya. *A History of Malaysia*. Basingstoke: Palgrave, 2001.

Anderson, Warwick. *Colonial Pathologies: American Tropical Medicine, Race, and Hygiene in the Philippines*. Durham: Duke University Press, 2006.

––––––. "Science in the Philippines." *Philippine Studies* 55, no. 3 (2007): 285–316.

––––––. "Pacific Crossings: Imperial Logics in United States, Public Health Programs." In *Colonial Crucible: Empire in the Making of the Modern American State*, ed. Alfred W. McCoy and Francisco A. Scarano. Madison: University of Wisconsin Press, 2009, 227–87.

Anderson, Warwick, and Hans Pols. "Scientific Patriotism: Medical Science and National Self-Fashioning in Southeast Asia." *Comparative Studies in Society and History* 54, no. 1 (2012): 93–113.

Andrews, Bridie, and Andrew Cunningham. *Western Medicine as Contested Knowledge*. Manchester: Manchester University Press, 1997.

Apple, Michael W. *Ideology and Curriculum*. London: Routledge & Kegan Paul, 1979.

Apple, Michael W., and Kristen L. Buras, eds. *The Subaltern Speak: Curriculum, Power, and Educational Struggles*. New York: Routledge, 2006.

Apthorpe, Raymond. "Coda: With Alice in Aidland: A Seriously Satirical Allegory." In *Adventures in Aidland: The Anthropology of Professionals in International Development*, ed. David Mosse. New York/Oxford: Berghahn Books, 2011, 199–220.

Arnold, David, ed. *Imperial Medicine and Indigenous Societies*. Manchester: Manchester University Press, 1988.

––––––. *Colonizing the Body: State Medicine and Epidemic Disease in Nineteenth-Century India*. Berkeley: University of California Press, 1993.

————, ed. *Warm Climates and Western Medicine*. Amsterdam: Rodopi, 1996.

————. "Tropical Governance: Managing Health in Monsoon Asia, 1908–1938." *ARI Working Paper*, No. 116 (2009).

Asad, Talal. "The Concept of Cultural Translation in British Social Anthropology." In *Writing Culture: The Poetics and Politics of Ethnography*, ed. James D. Clifford and George E. Marcus. Berkeley: University of California Press, 1986, 141–64.

Aso, Michitake. "Patriotic Hygiene: Tracing New Places of Knowledge Production about Malaria in Vietnam, 1919–75." *Journal of Southeast Asian Studies* 44 (2013): 423–43.

Aso, Michitake, and Annick Guénel. "The Itinerary of a North Vietnamese Surgeon: Medical Science and Politics during the Cold War." *Science, Technology & Society* 18 (2013): 291–306.

Attewell, Guy. *Refiguring Unani Tibb: Plural Healing in Late Colonial India*. New Delhi: Orient Longman, 2007.

Au, Sokhieng. *Mixed Medicines: Health and Culture in French Colonial Cambodia*. Chicago: University of Chicago Press, 2011.

Balbuena, Nenita. "Assessment and Evaluation of the Pre-project Activities, WHO Mission Report to Maternal & Child Health including Birth Spacing Project." Manila: World Health Organization, 1991.

Bannerman, Robert H., John Burton, and Wen-Chieh Chen. *Traditional Medicine and Health Care Coverage: A Reader for Health Administrators and Practitioners*. Geneva: World Health Organization, 1983.

Banpasirichote, Chantana. "The Indigenization of Development Process in Thailand: A Case Study of the Traditional Medical Revivalist Movement (Thai Massage)." PhD diss., University of Waterloo, 1989.

Baradat, R. "Conditions d'élevage au Cambodge: A. – 5$^e$ secteur vétérinaire." *Bulletin Economique de l'Indochine* 4, no. 3 (1937): 547–56.

————. "La foire de Prek-Khpop." *Bulletin Economique de l'Indochine* 42 (1939): 230–59.

Basalla, George. "The Spread of Western Science." *Science* 156, no. 3775 (5 May 1967): 611–22.

Bashford, Alison. *Imperial Hygiene: A Critical History of Colonialism, Nationalism, and Public Health*. Basingstoke: Palgrave MacMillan, 2004.

Bastos, Cristiana. "Teaching European Medicine in 19th Century Goa: Local and Colonial Agendas." In *Contesting Colonial Authority: Medicine and Indigenous Responses in Nineteenth- and Twentieth-Century India*, ed. Poonam Bala. New York: Lexington Books, 2012, 13–28.

Bauche, J. "Rapport sur le service vétérinaire, zootechnique et des épizooties de l'Indo-chine." *Bulletin Economique de l'Indochine* 11 (1908): 600–77.

Bergeon, P. "Les maladies du bétail au Tonkin." *Revue de Médecine Vétérinaire Exotique* 5 (1932): 23–32.

Bergeon, P., and J. Cèbe. "Au sujet de la vaccination antipestique: Expériences faites au laboratoire de l'Ecole Vétérinaire de l'Indochine à Hanoi en 1929." *Bulletin Economique de l'Indochine* 33 (1930): 434B–445B.

Bernad, Miguel S.J. *Filipinos in Laos, with "Postscripts" by J. "Pete" Fuentecila.* New York: Mekong Circle International, 2004.

Beveridge, William. *Influenza: The Last Great Plague: An Unfinished Story of Discovery.* New York: Prodist, 1977.

Bijker, J. *Rapport der Commissie tot Voorbereiding eener Reorganisatie van den Burgerlijken Geneeskundigen Dienst.* Batavia: Landsdrukkerij, 1908.

Binson, Bussakorn. "The Role of Food in the Musical Rites of the *Lanna* People of Northern Thailand." *Rian Thai: International Journal of Thai Studies* 2 (2009): 45–69.

Birn, Anne-Emanuelle, Yogan Pillay, and Timothy H. Holtz. "The Historical Origins of Modern Public Health." In *Textbook of International Health: Global Health in a Dynamic World.* New York: Oxford University Press, 2009, 17–60.

Bizot, François. "Notes sur les *yantra* bouddiques d'Indochine." In *Tantric and Taoist Studies in Honour of R.A. Stein*, ed. Michel Strickmann. Brussels: Institut Belge des Hautes Études Chinoises, 1981.

Blin, J. "Note sur des vaccinations anticharbonneuses et sur le trypanosome des mammifères." *Bulletin Economique de l'Indochine* 5 (1902): 585–8.

Blin, J., and Carougeau. "La septicémie hémorragique aiguë des buffles." *Bulletin Economique de l'Indochine* 6 (1903): 60–74.

Bollet, Alfred Jay. *Plagues and Poxes: The Impact of Human History on Epidemic Disease.* New York: Demos, 2004.

Bonner, Thomas Neville. *Becoming a Physician: Medical Education in Britain, France, Germany, and the United States, 1750–1945.* Baltimore: Johns Hopkins Press, 2000.

Bonneuil, Christophe, and Patrick Petitjean. "Les chemins de la création de l'ORSTOM, du Front Populaire à la Libération en passant par Vichy." In *Les sciences colonials: Figures et institutions*, ed. P. Petitjean. Paris: ORSTOM Editions, 1996, 113–61.

Bradley, D.B. "Siamese Theory and Practice of Medicine." *Sangkhomsaat Parithat (Social Science Review)* 5 (1967): 103–19.

Brocheux, Pierre. *Une histoire économique du Viet Nam 1850–2007: La palanche et le camion.* Paris: Les Indes Savants, 2009.

Brocheux, Pierre, and Daniel Hémery. *Indochine, la colonisation ambigüe, 1858–1954.* Paris: La Découverte, 2001.

Brooks, Jane, and Anne Marie Rafferty. "Degrees of Ambivalence: Attitudes towards Pre-registration University Education for Nurses in Britain, 1930–1960." *Nurse Education Today* 30 (2010): 579–83.

Brown, Colin. "The Influenza Pandemic of 1918 in Indonesia." In *Death and Disease in Southeast Asia: Explorations in Social, Medical and Demographic*

*History*, ed. Norman Owen. Singapore: Oxford University Press, 1987, 235–56.

Brun, V., and T. Schumacher. *Traditional Herbal Medicine in Northern Thailand*. Bangkok: White Lotus, 1994.

Brush, Barbara L. "The Rockefeller Agenda for American/Philippines Nursing Relations." In *Nursing History and the Politics of Welfare*, ed. Anne Marie Rafferty, Jane Robinson, and Ruth Elkan. London: Routledge, 1997, 540–55.

Brush, Barbara L., and Julie Sochalski. "International Nurse Migration: Lessons from the Philippines." *Policy, Politics, & Nursing Practice* 8, no. 1 (2007): 37–46.

Budick, Sanford. "Crises of Alterity: Cultural Untranslatability and the Experience of Secondary Otherness." In *The Translatability of Cultures: Figurations of the Space Between*, ed. Sanford Budick and Wolfgang Iser. Stanford: Stanford University Press, 1996, 1–22.

Bui Van Y. "Public Health Support for Lao Friends During the Resistance Against the French." In *History of Vietnam-Laos Laos-Vietnam Special Relationship 1930–2007, Memoirs I*. Hanoi: National Political Publishing House, 2012, 243–8.

Burnet, F.M., and Ellen Clark. *Influenza*. Melbourne: Macmillan, 1942.

Burns, Adam D. "Winning 'Hearts and Minds': American Imperial Designs of the Early Twentieth and Twenty-First Centuries." *History and Policy*. http://www.historyandpolicy.org/policy-papers/papers/winning-hearts-and-minds-american-imperial-designs-of-the-early-twentieth-a.

Byerly, Carol. *Fever of War: The Influenza Epidemic and the US Army during World War I*. New York: New York University Press, 2005.

Chauveau, Sophie. *L'invention pharmaceutique: La pharmacie Française entre l'etat et la société au XXe siècle*. Paris: Sonéfi-Synthélabo, 1999.

Chen, Hsiu-Jane. *"Eine strenge Prüfung Deutscher Art": Der Alltag der Japanischen Medizinausbildung im Zeitalter der Reform von 1868 bis 1914*. Husum: Matthiesen Verlag, 2010.

Cheyfitz, Eric. *The Poetics of Imperialism: Translation and Colonization from The Tempest to Tarzan*. New York: Oxford University Press, 1991.

Cochran, Sherman G. *Chinese Medicine Men: Consumer Culture in China and Southeast Asia*. Cambridge: Harvard University Press, 2006.

Conklin, Alice. *A Mission to Civilize: The Republican Idea of Empire in France and West Africa, 1895–1930*. Stanford: Stanford University Press, 1997.

Chaninthon Rattanasakon, Raphiphan Janthanalat, Latda Naemjai, and Phailin Siarunothai. "Phatthanakan khong Kanbanthuek lae Kanthaithot Khwamru thang Kanphaet Phaen Thai." In *Kanbantuek lae Kanthaithot Khwamru thang Kanphaet Phaen Thai*, ed. Saowapha Phonsiriphong and Phonthip Usurat. Bangkok: Mahidol University, 1994, 5–73.

Cheungsathiansap Komat, and Muksong Chatchai. *Phromdaen khwamru prawattisat kanpaet lae satharanasuk thai.* Bangkok: Health Systems Research Institute, 2002.

Chirapravati, M., and L. Pattaratorn. *Votive Tablets in Thailand: Origin, Style, and Uses.* Kuala Lumpur: Oxford University Press, 1997.

Choquart, Lucien "Les marchés de bestiaux et le commerce du bétail au Tonkin." PhD diss., École Nationale Vétérinaire d'Alfort, 1928.

Choy, Catherine Ceniza. *Empire of Care: Nursing and Migration in Filipino American History.* Durham: Duke University Press, 2003.

Cohen, E. *Thai Tourism: Hill Tribes, Islands and Open-Ended Prostitution.* Bangkok: White Lotus, 1996.

Cohen, P.T. "Buddhism, Health and Development in Thailand from the Reformist Perspective of Dr. Prawase Wasi." In *Health and Development in Southeast Asia,* ed. P. Cohen and J. Purcal. Canberra: Australian Development Studies Network, 1995.

Collier, Richard. *The Plague of the Spanish Lady: The Influenza Pandemic of 1918–19.* New York: Atheneum, 1974.

Connerton, Winifred. "Have Cap, Will Travel: U.S. Nurses Abroad 1898–1917." PhD diss., University of Pennsylvania, 2010.

Conti, M.P. "Note sur les dix premières années de l'action vétérinaire au Laos." *Revue de Médecine Vétérinaire Exotique* 5 (1932): 80–3.

Coutant, Francis. "An Epidemic of Influenza at Manila, PI." *Journal of the American Medical Association* 71 (1918): 1566–7.

Craig, David. *Familiar Medicine: Everyday Health Knowledge and Practice in Today's Vietnam.* Honolulu: University of Hawaii Press, 2002.

Crosby, Alfred. *America's Forgotten Pandemic: The Influenza of 1918.* New York: Cambridge University Press, 1989.

Cueto, Marcos, and Steven Palmer. *Medicine and Public Health in Latin America: A History.* New York: Cambridge University Press, 2015.

Đàng, Thùy Trâm. *Last Night I Dreamed of Peace: The Diary of Dang Thuy Tram.* New York: Harmony Books, 2007.

Darwin, John. *The Empire Project: The Rise and Fall of the British World-System, 1830–1970.* Cambridge: Cambridge University Press, 2009.

Davis, Diana K. "Prescribing Progress: French Veterinary Medicine in the Service of Empire." *Veterinary Heritage* 29 (2006): 1–7.

———. "Brutes, Beasts and Empire: Veterinary Medicine and Environmental Policy in French North Africa and British India." *Journal of Historical Geography* 34 (2008): 242–67.

De Bevoise, Ken. *Agents of Apocalypse: Epidemic Disease in the Colonial Philippines.* Princeton: Princeton University Press, 1995.

De Jesus, Vicente. *Quarterly Report of the Philippine Health Service* (for the First, Second, Third and Fourth Quarters). Manila: Bureau of Printing, 1919.

_____. *Report of the Philippine Health Service, 1919*. Manila: Bureau of Printing, 1920.

_____. *Report of the Philippine Health Service, 1922*. Manila: Bureau of Printing, 1923.

Del Casino Jr., Vincent J. "(Re)placing Health and Health Care: Mapping the Competing Discourses and Practices of 'Traditional' and 'Modern' Thai Medicine." *Health & Place* 10 (2004): 59–73.

Dela Cruz, Arleigh Ross D. "Animal Contagions and Control Policies as Disasters: Filipino Vulnerability to Livestock Diseases and American Disease Control Policies, 1898–1934." Paper presented at the IAHA Conference, Solo, Indonesia, July 2–5, 2012.

Del Tufo, Vincent. *Malaya Comprising the Federation of Malaya and the Colony of Singapore: A Report on the 1947 Census of the Population*. London: Crown Agents for the Colonies, 1949.

Dervaux, Auguste. "L'élevage des animaux domestiques en Annam." PhD diss., Faculté de Médecine de Paris, 1929.

Dickson, H.P. *The Badge of Britannia: The History and Reminiscences of the Queen Elizabeth's Overseas Nursing Service, 1886–1966*. Edinburgh: Pentland Press, 1990.

Dinh-Chinh-Vu. "L'élevage bovin au Viêt Nam." PhD diss., Faculté de Médecine et de Pharmacie de Lyon, 1955.

Doel, H.W. van den. *Het Rijk van Insulinde: Opkomst en Ondergang van een Nederlandse Kolonie*. Amsterdam: Prometheus, 1996.

Dooley, Tom. *Dr. Tom Dooley's Three Great Books: Deliver Us from Evil, The Edge of Tomorrow [and] The Night They Burned the Mountain*. New York: Farrar, Straus & Cudahy, 1960.

Douarche, E. "Les bovins d'Indochine." *Bulletin Economique de l'Indochine* 5 (1902): 689–705.

Dreckmeier, G.J. "Zendingsarts op Java." In *'En Nog Steeds Hebben Wij Twee Vaderlanden': Op Avontuur in Nederlands-Indië*, ed. Carolijn Visser and Sasza Malko. Amsterdam: Meulenhoff, 2001.

Engler, Steven, and Gregory P. Grieve. *Historicizing "Tradition" in the Study of Religion*. Berlin: Walter de Gruyter, 2005.

Espinosa, Mariola. *Epidemic Invasions: Yellow Fever and the Limits of Cuban Independence, 1878–1930*. Chicago: University of Chicago Press, 2009.

Ettling, John. *The Germ of Laziness: Rockefeller Philanthropy and Public Health in the New South*. Cambridge: Harvard University Press, 1981.

Evanno, Charles. "Les entreprises d'élevage au Tonkin." *Bulletin Economique de l'Indochine* 41 (1938): 335–44.

Evans, Grant. *The Last Century of Lao Royalty. A Documentary History*. Chiang Mai: Silkworm Books, 2009.

Executive Committee of the Eighth Congress of the Far Eastern Association of Tropical Medicine. *Siam in 1930: General and Medical Features* (reprint). Bangkok: White Lotus, 2000.

Fabian, Johannes. *Language and Colonial Power: The Appropriation of Swahili in the Former Belgian Congo, 1880–1938*. Cambridge: Cambridge University Press, 1986.

Fajardo, Jacobo. *Report of the Philippine Health Service, for the Fiscal Year from January 1 to December 31, 1924*. Manila: Bureau of Printing, 1925.

———. *Report of the Philippine Health Service, for the Fiscal Year from January 1 to December 31, 1925*. Manila: Bureau of Printing, 1926.

———. *Report of the Philippine Health Service, for the Fiscal Year from January 1 to December 31, 1926*. Manila: Bureau of Printing, 1927.

Fakultas Kedokteran. *Report on the Development of Medical Education at the School of Medicine University of Indonesia Djakarta*. Djakarta: Fakultas Kedokteran, 1960.

Famin, P. *Au Tonkin et sur la frontière du Kwang-Si*. Paris: Challamel, 1895.

Fang, Xiaoping. *Barefoot Doctors and Western Medicine in China*. Rochester: University of Rochester Press, 2012.

Farley, John. *To Cast Out Disease: A History of the International Health Division of Rockefeller Foundation, 1913–51*. Oxford: Oxford University Press, 2003.

———. *Brock Chisholm, the World Health Organization, and the Cold War*. Vancouver: University of British Columbia Press, 2008.

Faure, Olivier. *Les Français et leur médecine au XIXe siècle*. Paris: Belin, 1993.

Fee, Elizabeth, and Roy M. Acheson. "Introduction." In *A History of Education in Public Health: Health that Mocks the Doctors' Rules*, ed. Elizabeth Fee and Roy M. Acheson. Oxford: Oxford University Press, 1991, 1–14.

Feunteun, L.M. "Concours interprovincial d'élevage de My-Tho (Cochinchine) 1937." *Bulletin Economique de l'Indochine* 41 (1938): 115–20.

Finer, David, Torston Thuren, and Goran Tomson. "TET Offensive: Winning Hearts and Minds for Prevention: Discourse and Ideology in Vietnam's 'Health' Newspaper." *Social Science and Medicine* 47 (1998): 133–45.

Fowler Wright, E.M. "The Singapore General Hospital." *Nursing Times* (1941): 765–6.

Fox, Renée C. *The Sociology of Medicine: A Participant Observer's View*. Englewood Cliffs: Prentice Hall, 1957.

———. *Experiment Perilous: Physicians and Patients Facing the Unknown*. Glencoe: Free Press, 1959.

———. *Essays in Medical Sociology: Journeys into the Field*. New York: Wiley, 1979.

Frieson, Kate. "Sentimental Education: *Les Sages-Femmes* and Colonial Cambodia." *Journal of Colonial History and Colonialism* 1 (2000): 18–33.

Gabe, J. and M. Calnan. "The Limits of Medicine: Women's Perception of Medical Technology." *Social Science and Medicine* 28 (1989): 223–31.

Garrett, Frances. "The Alchemy of Accomplishing Medicine (*sman sgrub*): Situating the Yuthok Heart Essence (*G.yu thog snying thig*) in Literature and History." *Journal of Indian Philosophy* 37 (2009): 207–30.

Gealogo, Francis. "The Philippines in the World of the Influenza Pandemic of 1918–19." *Philippine Studies* 57 (2009): 261–92.

Geest, Sjaak van der, and Susan Whyte. "The Charm of Medicines: Metaphors and Metonyms." *Medical Anthropology Quarterly* 3 (1989): 345–67.

Geest, Sjaak van der, Susan Whyte, and Anita Hardon. "The Anthropology of Pharmaceuticals: A Biographical Approach." *American Review of Anthropology* 25 (1996): 163–4.

German, R.L. *Handbook to British Malaya*. London: Malayan Civil Service, 1927.

Gilbert, L. "Annam, chapitre II: Animaux domestiques et sauvages." *Bulletin Economique de l'Indochine* 28 (1925): 126–32.

Golomb, Louis. *An Anthropology of Curing in Multiethnic Thailand*. Urbana: University of Illinois Press, 1985.

———. "The Interplay of Traditional Therapies in South Thailand." *Social Science & Medicine* 27 (1988): 761–8.

Good, Byron J., and Mary-Jo DelVecchio Good. "'Learning Medicine': The Constructing of Medical Knowledge at Harvard Medical School." In *Knowledge, Power and Practice: The Anthropology of Medicine and Everyday Life*, ed. Shirley Lindenbaum and Margaret Lock. Berkeley: University of California Press, 1993, 81–107.

Gordin, Michael D. *Scientific Babel: How Science Was Done Before and After Global English*. Chicago: University of Chicago Press, 2015.

Goscha, Christopher E. *Vietnam: Un etat né de la guerre, 1945–1954*. Trans. Agathe Larcher. Paris: Colin, 2011.

Gourou, Pierre. *L'utilisation du sol en Indochine française*. Paris: Hartmann, 1940.

Great Britain Ministry of Health. *Reports on Public Health and Medical Subjects no. 4: Report on the Pandemic Influenza 1918–19*. London: His Majesty's Stationery Office, 1920.

Greger, Michael. *Bird Flu: A Virus of Our Own Hatching*. New York: Lantern Books, 2006.

Guénel, Annick. "La lutte antivariolique en Extrême-Orient: Ruptures et continuité." In *L'Aventure de la Vaccination*, ed. Anne-Marie Moulin. Geneva: Fayard, 1996, 83–94.

———. "The Conference on Rural Hygiene in Bandung of 1937: Towards a New Vision of Health Care?" In *Global Movements, Local Concerns. Medicine and Health in Southeast Asia*, ed. Laurence Monnais and Harold J. Cook. Singapore: NUS Press, 2012, 62–80.

Halpern, Joel M. *Aspects of Village Life and Culture Change in Laos*. New York: Council on Economic and Cultural Affairs, 1958.

Hardy, G., and Ch. Richet. *L'alimentation indigène dans les colonies Françaises*. Paris: Vigot Frères, 1933.

Harianto, Mus. *Peringatan 90 Tahun Pendidikan Dokter di Surabaya*. Surabaya: Fakultas Kedokteran Universitas Airlangga, 2003.

Harrison, Mark. *Public Health in British India: Anglo-Indian Preventive Medicine 1859–1914*. Cambridge: Cambridge University Press, 1994.

————. *Diseases and the Modern World: 1500 to the Present*. Cambridge: Polity, 2004.

Havard-Duclos, B. "Possibilités d'amélioration et de développement de l'élevage en Indochine." *Bulletin Economique de l'Indochine* 42 (1939–40): 1125–70; 43 (1): 12–45; 43 (2): 213–58.

Havinden, Michael, and David Meredith. *Colonialism and Development: Britain and its Tropical Colonies, 1850–1960*. London: Routledge, 1996.

Heinze, Ruth-Inge. "Nature and Function of Some Therapeutic Techniques in Thailand." *Asian Folklore Studies* 36 (1977): 85–104.

————. *Tham Khwan: How to Contain the Essence of Life, a Socio-Psychological Comparison of a Thai Custom*. Singapore: Singapore University Press, 1982.

————. "The Relationship Between Folk and Elite Religions: The Case of Thailand." In *The Realm of the Sacred: Verbal Symbolism and Ritual Structure*, ed. Sitakant Mahapatra. Calcutta: Oxford University Press, 1992.

————. *Trance and Healing in Southeast Asia Today*. Bangkok: White Lotus Press, 1997.

Heiser, Victor. *An American Doctor's Odyssey: Adventures in Forty-five Countries*. New York: Norton and Co., 1936.

Hennessy, Deborah, Carolyn Hick, and Harni Koesno. "The Training and Development of Needs of Midwives in Indonesia." *Human Resources for Health* 4 (2006): 1–12.

Hernando, Eugenio. "Management of Communicable Diseases." In *Philippine Health Service Health Bulletin No. 21*. Manila: Bureau of Printing, 1919.

Hesselink, Liesbeth. *Healers on the Colonial Market: Native Doctors and Midwives in the Dutch East Indies*. Leiden: KITLV, 2011.

Hewa, Soma. *Colonialism, Tropical Disease and Imperial Medicine: Rockefeller Philanthropy in Sri Lanka*. Lanham: University Press of America, 1995.

Hien, Tan S. "Memoirs of Tan S. Hien." In *Memoirs of Indonesian Doctors and Professionals: More Stories that Shaped the Lives of Indonesian Doctors*, ed. Tjien Oei. Bloomington: Xlibris Corporation, 2010, 134–56.

Hoang, Bao Chau, ed. *Vietnamese Traditional Medicine*. Hanoi: The Gioi, 1999.

Hoang, Bao Chau. "The Revival and Development of Vietnamese Traditional Medicine: Towards Keeping the Nation in Good Health." In *Southern Medicine for Southern People: Vietnamese Medicine in the Making*, ed. Laurence Monnais-Rousselot, C. Michele Thompson, and Ayo Wahlberg. Newcastle upon Tyne: Cambridge Scholars, 2012, 113–52.

Hobsbawm, E. 1983, "Introduction." In *The Invention of Tradition*, ed. E. Hobshawm and T. Ranger. Cambridge: Cambridge University Press, 1–14.

Holland, Stephen, Chansy Phimphachanh, Catherine Conn, and Malcolm Segall. *Impact of Economic and Institutional Reforms on the Health Sector in*

*Laos: Implications for Health System Management.* Brighton, Sussex: Institute of Development Studies, 1995.

Hope-Simpson, R. Edgar. *The Transmission of Epidemic Influenza.* New York: Plenum Press, 1992.

Horner, I.B. *The Book of the Discipline (Vinaya-Piṭaka), vol. IV.* Oxford: Pali Text Society, 2000.

Hsu, E. *The Transmission of Chinese Medicine.* Cambridge: Cambridge University Press, 1999.

————. "The History of Chinese Medicine in the People's Republic of China and Its Globalization." *East Asia Science, Technology and Society: An International Journal* 2 (2009): 464–5.

Hubac, A. *Hygiène et maladies des animaux expliquées au paysan Annamite: Nói về vệ sinh và các bệnh loài vật nuôi.* Hanoi: Imprimerie Tonkinoise, 1925.

Hull, Terence H. "Conflict and Collaboration in Public Health: The Rockefeller Foundation and the Dutch Colonial Government in Indonesia." In *Public Health in Asia and the Pacific: Historical and Comparative Perspectives*, ed. Milton J. Lewis and Kerrie L. MacPherson. London: Routledge, 2008, 139–52.

Hydrick, J.L. *Intensive Rural Hygiene Work and Public Health Education of the Public Health Service of Netherlands India.* Batavia: Author, 1937.

Iida, Junko. *The "Revival" of Thai Traditional Medicine and Local Practice: Villagers' Reaction to the Promotion of Thai Massage in Northern Thailand.* 9th International Conference on Thai Studies, Northern Illinois University, DeKalb, Illinois, 2005.

————. *Tai Massaji no Minzokushi: "Tai-shiki Iryo" Seisei Katei ni okeru Shintai to Jissen* [Ethnography of Thai Massage: Body and Practice in the Process of the Creation of Thai Traditional Medicine]. Tokyo: Akashi Shoten, 2006.

————. "The Revival of Thai Traditional Medicine and the Promotion of Thai Massage: The Reaction of Villagers in Northern Thailand." *Southeast Asian Studies* 44 (2006): 78–96.

————. "The Sensory Experience of Thai Massage: Commercialization, Globalization, and Tactility." In *Everyday Life in Asia: Social Perspectives on the Senses*, ed. Devorah Kalekin-Fishman and Kelvin E.Y. Low. Surrey: Ashgate, 2010.

————. "Holism as a Whole-body Treatment: The Transnational Production of Thai Massage." *European Journal of Transnational Studies* 5 (2013): 81–111.

————. "The Efficacy of Thai Massage for Urban Middle Class in Contemporary Thailand: Discourse, Body Technique, and Ritualized Process." *Senri Ethnological Reports* 120 (2014): 121–39.

Irvine, W. "The Thai-Yuan 'Madman' and the 'Modernizing, Developing Thai Nation' as Bounded Entities under Threat: A Study in the Replication of a Single Image." PhD diss., University of London, 1982.

Jackson, Peter A. "Royal Spirits, Chinese Gods, and Magic Monks: Thailand's Boom-time Religions of Prosperity." *South East Asia Research* 7 (1999): 245–320.

Jacotot, Henri. *Instituts Pasteur d'Indochine. La peste bovine en Indochine.* Saigon: Imprimerie nouvelle Albert Portail, 1931.

———. "La situation de l'élevage indochinois au début du siècle et à la fin de la Deuxième Guerre Mondiale." *Revue d'Elevage et de Médecine Vétérinaire des Pays Tropicaux* 1 (1947): 287–94.

Janetta, Ann. *The Vaccinators: Smallpox, Medical Knowledge, and the Opening of Japan.* Stanford: Stanford University Press, 2007.

Jauffret, R. "L'école vétérinaire de l'Indochine: Son but, son organisation, ses résultats, son avenir." *Bulletin Economique de l'Indochine* 46 (1943): 351–62.

Johnson, Niall, and Juergen Mueller. "Updating the Accounts: Global Mortality of the 1918–1920 'Spanish' Influenza Pandemic." *Bulletin of the History of Medicine* 76 (2002): 105–15.

Jordan, Edwin. "The Present Status of the Influenza Problem." *American Journal of Public Health* 15 (1925): 943–7.

Jose, Ricardo. "The Philippine National Guard and World War I." *Philippine Studies* 36 (1988): 275–99.

Katz, Robert. "Influenza 1918–1919: A Study in Mortality." *Bulletin of the History of Medicine* 48 (1974): 416–22.

———. "Influenza 1918–1919: A Further Study in Mortality." *Bulletin of the History of Medicine* 51 (1977): 617–19.

Keyes, Charles F. *Thailand: Buddhist Kingdom as Modern Nation State.* Boulder: Westview, 1987.

Killingray, David. "The Influenza Pandemic of 1918–19 in the British Caribbean." *Social History of Medicine* 7 (1994): 59–87.

Kirsch, A. Thomas. "Complexity in the Thai Religious System: An Interpretation." *Journal of Asian Studies* 36 (1977): 241–66.

Kitiarsa, Pattana. "Beyond Syncretism: Hybridization of Popular Religion in Contemporary Thailand." *Journal of Southeast Asian Studies* 36 (2005): 461–87.

Komatra Chuengsatiansup. *Alternative Health, Alternative Sphere of Autonomy: Cheewajit and the Emergence of a Critical Public of Thailand.* 7th International Conference on Thai Studies, Amsterdam, 1999.

Kramer, Paul A. "Race, Empire and Transnational History." In *Colonial Crucible: Empire in the Making of the Modern American State*, ed. Alfred W. McCoy and Francisco A. Scarano. Madison: University of Wisconsin Press, 2009, 199–209.

La Loubère, S. *The Kingdom of Siam*. Oxford: Oxford University Press, 1969.

Lahille, Abel. "Le lait et les laiteries de Saigon." *Bulletin Economique de l'Indochine* 22 (1919): 199–213.

Landais, Etienne. "Sur les doctrines des vétérinaires coloniaux Français en Afrique noire." *Cahiers de Sciences Humaines* 26 (1990): 33–71.

Landon, K.P. *Siam in Transition: A Brief Survey of Cultural Trends in the Five Years since the Revolution of 1932*. Santa Barbara: Greenwood Press, 1968.

Langford, J.M. *Fluent Bodies: Ayurvedic Remedies for Postcolonial Imbalance*. Durham: Duke University Press, 2002.

Lao Family Welfare Association. *Family Planning (Vang phen khob khoua)*. Pamphlet, no publication details, undated.

*Laos: Mil neuf cent cinquante*. No publication details, undated.

Lapeyre, Jaime. "'The Idea of Better Nursing': The American Battle for Control over Standards of Nursing Education in Europe, 1918–1925." PhD diss., University of Toronto, 2013.

Latour, Bruno. *Science in Action: How to Follow Scientists and Engineers through Society*. Cambridge: Harvard University Press, 1987.

Lawrence, Mark Atwood. *Assuming the Burden of Europe and the American Commitment to the War in Vietnam*. Berkeley: University of California Press, 2005.

Leavitt, Judith Walzer, and Ronald L. Numbers, eds. *Sickness and Health in America: Readings in the History of Medicine and Public Health*. Madison: University of Wisconsin Press, 1978.

Le Louët, G. "L'élevage des bovidés en Cochinchine." *Bulletin Economique de l'Indochine* 31 (1928): 111–19.

———. "Consommation du bétail en Indochine." *Bulletin Economique de l'Indochine* 34 (1931): 1102B–13B.

———. "Essai sur les possibilités de l'élevage industriel du bétail en Indochine." *Bulletin Economique de l'Indochine* 34 (1931): 555B–72B.

———. "La production animale en Indochine." *Exposition coloniale internationale – Congrès de la production animale et des maladies du bétail* (1931): 107–25.

———. "La production animale en Indochine." *Revue de Médecine Vétérinaire Exotique* 5 (1932): 144–56.

Lebouc. "Rapports des chefs des services vétérinaires des divers pays de l'Union pour l'année 1933. II. Annam." *Bulletin Economique de l'Indochine* 37 (1934): 312–24.

Lee Yong Kiat. "The Origins of Nursing in Singapore." *Singapore Medical Journal* 26 (1985): 53–60.

———. "Nursing and the Beginnings of Specialised Nursing in Early Singapore." *Singapore Medical Journal* 46 (2005): 600–9.

Lees, Lynn Hollen. "Being British in Malaya." *Journal of British Studies* 48 (2009): 76–101.

Lentz, Christian Cunningham. "Mobilizing a Frontier: Dien Bien Phu and the Making of Vietnam, 1945–1955." PhD diss., Cornell University, 2011.

Lepinte, F. "Rapport sur le service vétérinaire, zootechnique et des épizooties de l'Indo-Chine." *Bulletin Economique de l'Indochine* 11 (1908): 462–85.

Lepinte, L., E. Douarche, and J. Bauche. "Rapport sur le charbon bactéridien au Tonkin." *Bulletin Economique de l'Indochine* 6 (1903): 628–37.

———. "Rapport sur le service vétérinaire, zootechnique et des épizooties." *Bulletin Economique de l'Indochine* 11 (1908): 600–93.

Lesch, John. *The First Miracle Drugs: How the Sulfa Drugs Transformed Medicine*. New York: Oxford University Press, 2007.

Lewis, David. "International Development and the 'Perpetual Present': Anthropological Approaches to the Re-historicization of Policy." *European Journal of Development Research* 21 (2009): 32–46.

Lewis, Milton, and Kerrie L. MacPherson, eds. *Public Health in Asia and the Pacific: Historical and Comparative Perspectives*. New York: Routledge, 2007.

Lichtenfelder, W. "Rapport sur les cultures et l'élevage dans la haute-région du Tonkin." *Bulletin Economique de l'Indochine* 5 (1902): 804–13.

Liew, Kai Khiun. "Terribly Severe Though Mercifully Short: The Episode of the 1918 Influenza in British Malaya." *Modern Asian Studies* 41 (2007): 221–52.

———. "Wats and Worms: The Activities of the Rockefeller Foundation's International Health Board in Southeast Asia (1913–1940)." In *Global Movements, Local Concerns: Medicine and Health in Southeast Asia*, ed. Laurence Monnais and Harold J. Cook. Singapore: NUS Press, 2012, 43–61.

Litsios, Socrates. "The Long and Difficult Road to Alma Ata: A Personal Reflection." *International Journal of Health Services* 32 (2002): 709–32.

Liu, Lydia H. *Translingual Practice: Literature, National Culture, and Translated Modernity—China, 1900–1937*. Stanford: Stanford University Press, 1995.

Lo, Ming-cheng M. *Doctors within Borders: Profession, Ethnicity, and Modernity in Colonial Taiwan*. Berkeley: University of California Press, 2002.

Locher-Scholten, Elsbeth. "Door een gekleurde Bril…Koloniale Bronnen over Vrouwenarbeid op Java in de Negentiende en Twintigste Eeuw." In *Vrouwen in de Nederlandse Koloniën: 7ᵉ Jaarboek voor Vrouwengeschiedenis*, ed. Jeske Reijs et al. Nijmegen: SUN, 1986, 34–51.

———. *Women and the Colonial State: Essays on Gender and Modernity in the Netherlands Indies 1900–1942*. Amsterdam: Amsterdam University Press, 2000.

Long, John D. *Annual Report of the Philippine Health Service, Fiscal Year 1915*. Manila: Bureau of Printing, 1916.

———. *Quarterly Report of the Philippine Health Service* (for the first, second, third, and fourth quarters 1918). Manila: Bureau of Printing, 1918.

Long, John D., and Vicente de Jesus. *Report of the Philippine Public Health Service Fiscal Year 1918*. Manila: Bureau of Printing, 1919.

Lubis, Firman. *Jakarta 1960-an: Kenangan Semasa Mahasiswa*. Jakarta: Masup, 2008.

Ludmerer, Kenneth. *Time to Heal: American Medical Education from the Turn of the Century to the Era of Managed Care*. New York: Oxford University Press, 1999.

MacDonald, Helen. *Human Remains: Episodes in Human Dissection*. Carlton, VIC: Melbourne University Press, 2005.

MacLeod, Roy, and Milton Lewis, eds. *Disease, Medicine, and Empire: Perspectives on Western Medicine and the Experience of European Expansion*. London: Routledge, 1988.

————. "Preface." In *Disease, Medicine, and Empire: Perspectives on Western Medicine and the Experience of European Expansion*, ed. Roy MacLeod and Milton Lewis. London: Routledge, 1988, x–xii.

Malarney, Shaun Kingsley. "Germ Theory, Hygiene, and the Transcendence of 'Backwardness' in Revolutionary Vietnam, 1954–60." In *Southern Medicine for Southern People: Vietnamese Medicine in the Making*, ed. Laurence Monnais-Rousselot, C. Michele Thompson, and Ayo Wahlberg. Newcastle upon Tyne: Cambridge Scholars Publishing, 2012.

Manderson, Lenore. "Race, Colonial Mentality and Public Health in Early Twentieth Century Malaya." In *The Underside of Malaysian History: Pullers, Prostitutes, Plantation Workers*, ed. P.J. Rimmer and L.M. Allen. Singapore: Singapore University Press, 1990, 193–4.

————. *Sickness and the State: Health and Illness in Colonial Malaya, 1870–1940*. Cambridge: Cambridge University Press, 1996.

Markel, Howard, Alexandra Stern, Alexander Navarro, and Joseph Michalsen. *A Historical Assessment of Nonpharmaceutical Disease Containment Strategies Employed by Selected US Communities during the Second Wave of the 1918–1920 Influenza Pandemic*. Ann Arbor: University of Michigan Center for the History of Medicine, 2006.

Marks, Shula. *Divided Sisterhood: Race, Class and Gender in the South African Nursing Profession*. Basingstoke: Macmillan, 1994.

Marr, David. "Vietnamese Attitudes Regarding Illness and Healing." In *Death and Disease in Southeast Asia: Explorations in Social, Medical and Demographic History*, ed. Norman G. Owen. Oxford: Oxford University Press, 1987.

McCormick, Thomas. "From Old Empire to New: The Changing Dynamics and Tactics of American Empire." In *Colonial Crucible: Empire in the Making of the Modern American State*, ed. Alfred W. McCoy and Francisco A. Scarano. Madison: University of Wisconsin Press, 2009.

McCoy, Alfred W. "Policing the Imperial Periphery: Philippine Pacification and the Rise of the US National Security State." In *Colonial Crucible: Empire in the Making of the Modern American State*, ed. Alfred W. McCoy and Francisco A. Scarano. Madison: University of Wisconsin Press, 2009, 106–15.

McCoy, Alfred W., Francisco A. Scarano, and Courtney Johnson. "On the Tropic of Cancer: Transitions and Transformations in the US Imperial State." In *Colonial Crucible: Empire in the Making of the Modern American State*, ed. Alfred W. McCoy and Francisco A. Scarano. Madison: University of Wisconsin Press, 2009, 3–33.

McDaniel, Justin Thomas. *The Lovelorn Ghost and the Magical Monk: Practicing Buddhism in Modern Thailand*. New York: Columbia University Press, 2011.

———."The Verses on the Victor's Armor: A Pāli Text Used for Protection and Healing in Thailand." In *Buddhism and Medicine: An Anthology*, ed. C. Pierce Salguero. New York: Columbia University Press, 2017, 358–62.

McGann, Susan. "Collaboration and Conflict in International Nursing, 1920–39." *Nursing History Review* 16 (2008): 29–57.

McGann, Susan, Anne Crowther, and Rona Dougall. *A History of the Royal College of Nursing, 1916–90: A Voice for Nurses*. Manchester: Manchester University Press, 2009.

McHale, Shawn. *Print and Power: Confucianism, Communism, and Buddhism in the Making of Modern Vietnam*. Honolulu: Hawaii University Press, 2004.

McRae, John. *Seeing through Zen: Encounter, Transformation, and Genealogy in Chinese Chan Buddhism*. Berkeley: University of California Press, 2004.

Meij-de Leur, A.P.M. van der. *Van Olie en Wijn: Geschiedenis van Verpleegkunde, Geneeskunde en Sociale Zorg*. Amsterdam/Brussels: Agon Elsevier, 1974.

Merton, Robert K., George G. Reader, and Patricia L. Kendall. *The Student-Physician: Introductory Studies in the Sociology of Medical Education*. Cambridge: Harvard University Press for the Commonwealth Fund, 1957.

Messer, Adam. "Effects of the Indonesian National Revolution and the Transfer of Power on the Scientific Establishment." *Indonesia* 58 (1994): 41–68.

Ministry of Health, Laos. *National Birth Spacing Policy*. Vientiane: Ministry of Health, 1995.

———. *Regulations on Maternal and Child Healthcare*. Vientiane: Ministry of Health, 2004.

———. *Reproductive Health Policy*. Vientiane: Ministry of Health, 2005.

———. *Strategy and Planning Framework for the Integrated Package of Maternal Neonatal and Child Health Services, 2009–2015*. Vientiane: Ministry of Health, 2009.

———. *Midwives in Lao PDR: Scaling up Skilled Birth Attendance: Putting Midwives at the Community Level towards Achieving MDGs for Mothers and Children: Report 2012*. Vientiane: Ministry of Health and UNFPA, 2012.

————. *Lao PDR Lao Social Indicator Survey (LSIS) 2011–12*. Vientiane: Ministry of Health, 2012.

Ministry of Health, Vietnam. *Draft Report on the Health Situation for the First Health Conference, 1–12 October 1979* (*Hang lay-ngane saphap viak-ngane sathalanasouk you kong-pasoum-nyai khang thi 1, tae 1-12 toula 1979*). Hanoi: Ministry of Health, 1979.

Monnais, Laurence. *Médecine et Colonisation: L'Aventure Indochinoise 1860–1939*. Paris: CNRS Editions, 1999.

————. "La médicalisation de la mère et de son enfant: L'exemple du Vietnam sous domination Française, 1860–1939." In *Children's Health Issues in Historical Perspective*, ed. Cheryl Krasnick Warsh and Veronica Strong-Boag. Waterloo: Wilfried Laurier University Press, 2005.

————. "De la reproduction d'une idéologie à la naturalisation d'un système: Essai sur la médecine 'moderne' au Viêt nam avant la Deuxième Guerre Mondiale." *Outre-mers: Cahiers d'Histoire* 352 (2006): 171–208.

————. "Traditional, Complementary and Perhaps Scientific? Professional Views of Vietnamese Medicine in the Age of French Colonialism." In *Southern Medicine for Southern People: Vietnamese Medicine in the Making*, ed. Laurence C. Monnais, C. Michele Thompson, and Ayo Wahlberg. New-castle upon Tyne: Cambridge Scholars Publishing, 2012, 61–84.

Monnais, Laurence, C. Michele Thompson, and Ayo Wahlberg, eds. *Southern Medicine for Southern People: Vietnamese Medicine in the Making*. Newcastle upon Tyne: Cambridge Scholars Publishing, 2012.

Monnais, Laurence, and Harold J. Cook, eds. *Global Movements, Local Concerns: Medicine and Health in Southeast Asia*. Singapore: NUS Press, 2012.

Monnais, Laurence, and Hans Pols. "Health and Disease in the Colonies: Medicine in the Age of Empire." In *The Routledge History of Western Empires*, ed. Robert Aldrich and Kirsten McKenzie. New York: Routledge, 2014, 270–84.

Monnais, Laurence, and David Wright, eds. *Doctors beyond Borders: The Transnational Migration of Physicians in the Twentieth Century*. Toronto: University of Toronto Press, 2016.

Moore, Alex. *Un Américain au Laos aux débuts de l'aide Américaine (1954–1957)*. Paris: L'Harmattan, 1995.

Morin, H.G., H. Jacotot, and J. Genevray. "Les Instituts Pasteur d'Indochine en 1934." *Archives des Instituts Pasteur d'Indochine* 20 (1934): 427–509.

Morris, Rosalind C. *In the Place of Origins: Modernity and Its Mediums in Northern Thailand*. Durham: Duke University Press, 2000.

Morton, Gladys. "The Pandemic Influenza of 1918." *Canadian Nurse* 69 (1973): 25–7.

Mulholland, Jean. "Thai Traditional Medicine: Ancient Thought and Practice in a Thai Context." *Journal of the Siam Society* 67 (1979): 80–115.

———. *Medicine, Magic, and Evil Spirits*. Canberra: Australian National University, 1987.

———. "Congenital Disease and Birthdays in Thai Traditional Medicine." In *Proceedings of the International Conference on Thai Studies*, 1987, 225–30.

Nathan, J.E. *The Census of British Malaya, 1921*. London: Waterlow and Sons, 1922.

National Statistics Centre. *Lao Reproductive Health Survey 2005*. Vientiane: National Statistics Centre and UNFPA, 2007.

National Statistics Centre/Lao Women's Training Centre/UNFPA. "Report on the Fertility and Birth Spacing Survey in Lao PDR (LFPSS)." Vientiane: UNFPA, 1995.

Neelakantan, Vivek. "The Campaign against the Big Four Endemic Diseases and Indonesia's Engagement with the WHO during the Cold War, 1950s." In *Public Health and National Reconstruction in Southeast Asia: International Influences, Local Transformations*, ed. Liping Bu and Ka-Che Yip. Abingdon: Routledge, 2014, 154–74.

———. "Health and Medicine in the Soekarno Era: Social Medicine, Public Health and Medical Education, 1949–1967." PhD diss., University of Sydney, 2014.

Neill, Deborah. *Networks in Tropical Medicine: Internationalism, Colonialism, and the Rise of a Medical Specialty, 1890–1930*. Stanford: Stanford University Press, 2012.

Ninh, Kim Ngoc Bao. *A World Transformed: The Politics of Culture in Revolutionary Vietnam, 1945–1965*. Ann Arbor: University of Michigan Press, 2002.

Nivat, Dhani. "The Inscriptions of Wat Phra Jetubon." In *Collected Articles by H.H. Prince Dhani Nivat*. Bangkok: The Siam Society, 1969, 5–28.

Nguyen, Vinh-Kim. "Antiretroviral Globalism, Biopolitics, and Therapeutic Citizenship." In *Global Assemblages: Technology, Politics, and Ethics as Anthropological Problems*, ed. Aihwa Ong and Stephen J. Collier. Oxford: Blackwell Publishing, 2005.

Oosterhuis, Harry, and Frank Huisman. "The Politics of Health and Citizenship: Historical and Contemporary Perspectives." In *Health and Citizenship: Political Cultures of Health in Modern Europe*, ed. Frank Huisman and Harry Oosterhuis. London: Pickering and Chatto, 2014, 1–40.

Osborn, June, ed. *History, Science and Politics: Influenza in America, 1918–1976*. New York: Prodist, 1977.

Osborne, Michael A. *The Emergence of Tropical Medicine in France*. Chicago: University of Chicago Press, 2014.

Ovesen, Jan, and Ing-Britt Trankell. *Cambodians and Their Doctors: A Medical Anthropology of Colonial and Post-Colonial Cambodia*. Copenhagen: NIAS Press, 2010.

Owen, Norman G., ed. *Death and Disease in Southeast Asia: Explorations in Social, Medical and Demographic History*. Singapore: Oxford University Press, 1987.

Padua, Regino. "Preliminary Analytic Study on the Measure of the Force of Mortality during the Last Decade in the Philippines." *Journal of the Philippine Islands Medical Association* 5 (1925): 4–16.

Paker, Sahila. *Translations: (Re)Shaping of Literature and Culture*. Istanbul: Boğaziçi University Press, 2002.

Palmer, Steven. *From Popular Medicine to Medical Populism: Doctors, Healers, and Public Power in Costa Rica, 1800–1940*. Durham: Duke University Press, 2003.

———. *Launching Global Health: The Caribbean Odyssey of the Rockefeller Foundation*. Ann Arbor: University of Michigan Press, 2010.

Pârlog, Hortensia, Pia Brînzeu, and Aba-Carina Pârlog. *Translating the Body*. Munich: Lincom Europa, 2007.

Pasuk Phongphaichit. *Massage garu: Thai no Keizai Kaihatsu to Shakai Henka* [From Peasant Girls to Bangkok Masseuses], translated into Japanese by N. Tanaka. Tokyo: Dobunkan, 1980.

Pati, Biswamoy, and Mark Harrison, eds. *Health, Medicine, and Empire: Perspectives on Colonial India*. Hyderabad: Orient Longman, 2001.

Patterson, K. David, and Gerald Pyle. "The Geography and Mortality of the 1918 Influenza Pandemic." *Bulletin of the History of Medicine* 65, no. 1 (1991): 4–21.

Patterson, R. "Dr. William Gorgas and His War with the Mosquito." *Canadian Medical Association Journal* 141, no. 6 (1989): 599.

Pennapa Subcharoen. *Sen Jut lae Rok nai Thritsadi Kannuat Thai* [Lines, Points and Diseases in the Theory of Thai Massage]. Bangkok: Rongphim Ongkan Songkhro Thahan Phan Suek, 1995.

———. *Prawat lae Wiwatthanakan Kanphaet Phaen Thai* [The History and Development of Thai Traditional Medicine]. Bangkok: Chi Hua Printing, 1995.

Pennapa Subcharoen, and Daroon Pechprai. "Present Status of Traditional Medicine in Thailand." In *The Proceedings of International Seminar on Traditional Medicine*. N.p., 1995, 3–9.

Philavong, Khamphienne, Somboune Phomtavong, and Saysavanh Ngonvorarath. "Issues and Challenges of Public Health of 21st Century of Lao People's Democratic Republic." In *Issues and Challenges of Public Health in the 21st Century*, ed. Khairuddin Yusof, Wah-Yun Low, Siti Norazah Zulkifli, and Yut-Lin Wong. Kuala Lumpur: University of Malaya Press, 1996.

Philippine Health Service. *Proposed Sanitary Code Prepared for General Use in the Philippine Islands*. Manila: Bureau of Printing, 1920.

Philippine Islands Census Office. *Census of the Philippine Islands*. Manila: Bureau of Printing, 1920–21.

Philips, Howard, and David Killingray, eds. *The Spanish Influenza Pandemic of 1918–1919: New Perspectives*. London: Routledge, 2003.

Phraxayavong, Viliam. *History of Aid to Laos: Motivations and Impacts*. Chiang Mai: Silkworm Books, 2009.

Phua Kai Hong. "The Development of Health Services in Malaya and Singapore, 1867–1960." PhD diss., London School of Economics, 1987.

Pierce, John R. *Yellow Jack: How Yellow Fever Ravaged America and Walter Reed Discovered Its Deadly Secrets*. Hoboken: Wiley, 2005.

Pisani, Elizabeth. "Medicine for a Sick System." *Inside Indonesia*. http://www.insideindonesia.org/medicine-for-a-sick-system-2.

Pols, Hans. "Nurturing Indonesia: Medicine, Nationalism, and Decolonisation in the Dutch East Indies 1900–1950." Forthcoming, 2018.

Pool, D.I. "The Effects of the 1918 Pandemic of Influenza on the Maori Population of New Zealand." *Bulletin of the History of Medicine* 47 (1973): 273–81.

Population Council. "Studies in Family Planning: Family Planning Programs." *World Review 1974* 6, no. 8 (August 1975): 229.

Prakash, Gyan. *Another Reason: Science and the Imagination of Modern India*. Princeton: Princeton University Press, 1999.

Prathip Chumphon. *Prawattisat Kanphaet Phaen Thai: Kansyksa jak Ekasan Tamra Ya* [A History of Thai Traditional Medicine: A Study from the Texts of Pharmacopoeia]. Bangkok: Aakhiithai, 1998.

Price-Smith, Andrew. *The Health of Nations: Infectious Disease, Environmental Change, and Their Effects on National Security and Development*. Cambridge: MIT Press, 2002.

Puaksom, Davisakd. "Of Germs, Public Hygiene, and the Healthy Body: The Making of the Medicalizing State in Thailand." *Journal of Asian Studies* 66 (2007): 311–44.

Pyle, Gerald. *The Diffusion of Influenza: Patterns and Paradigms*. New York: Rowman and Littlefield, 1986.

Pyenson, Lewis. *Civilizing Mission: Exact Sciences and French Overseas Expansion, 1830–1940*. Baltimore: Johns Hopkins University Press, 1993.

Rafael, Vicente L. "The War of Translation: Colonial Education, American English, and Tagalog Slang in the Philippines." *Journal of Asian Studies* 74, no. 2 (2015): 283–302.

———. "Betraying Empire: Translation and the Ideology of Conquest." *Translation Studies* 8, no. 1 (2015): 82–93.

———. *Motherless Tongues: The Insurgency of Language amid Wars of Translation*. Durham: Duke University Press, 2016.

Rafferty, Anne Marie. "Internationalising Nursing Education during the Interwar Period." In *International Health Organisations and Movements, 1918–1939*, ed. Paul Weindling. Cambridge: Cambridge University Press, 1995, 266–82.

————. *The Politics of Nursing Knowledge*. London: Routledge, 1996.

Rajadhon, Phya Anuman. "Chao Thi and Some Traditions of Thai." *Thailand Culture Series* 6 (1956).

————. "Thai Charms and Amulets." *Journal of the Siam Society* 52 (1964): 171–97.

————. "The Khwan and Its Ceremonies." *Journal of the Siam Society* 50 (1965): 119–64.

Reichart, Peter A., and Pathawee Khongkhunthian. *The Spirit Houses of Thailand*. Bangkok: White Lotus, 2007.

Richardson, Ruth. *Death, Dissection and the Destitute*. Chicago: University of Chicago Press, 2000 [1987].

Roche, G. "Prophylaxie de la peste bovine en Cochinchine: Campagnes antipestiques de 1930–1931 et 1932." *Bulletin Economique de l'Indochine* 35 (1932): 793B–808B.

————. "Rapports des chefs des services vétérinaires des divers pays de l'Union pour l'année 1933." *Bulletin Economique de l'Indochine* 37 (1934): 312–33.

Rogaski, Ruth. *Hygienic Modernity: Meanings of Health and Disease in Treaty-Port China*. Berkeley: University of California Press, 2004.

Rongrian Ayurawet Witthayalai. *Rabiap Kan Sop Khao pen Naksueksa Ayurawet Witthayalai (Chiwakakomaraphat)* [Regulations of Entrance Examination for Ayurawet College]. Bangkok: Rongrian Ayurawet Witthayalai, 1997.

Rongrian Phaet Phaen Boran. *Rongrian Phaet Phaen Boran, Tamra Ya Sila Jaruek nai Wat Phrachetuphonwimonmangkhlaram (Wat Pho) Phranakhon* [Pharmacopoeia on the Inscription at Wat Pho]. Reprint. Nonthaburi: Khrongkan Prasanngan Phatthana Khrueakhai Samunphrai (Herbal Network Development Coordination Project), 1994 [1962].

Rosenkrantz, Barbara. *Public Health and the State: Changing Views in Massachusetts, 1842–1936*. Cambridge: Harvard University Press, 1972.

Ryan, Jennifer, Lincoln C. Chen, and Anthony J. Saich, eds. *Philanthropy for Health in China*. Bloomington: Indiana University Press, 2014.

Salguero, C. Pierce. "The Buddhist Medicine King in Literary Context: Reconsidering an Early Example of Indian Influence on Chinese Medicine and Surgery." *History of Religions* 48 (2009): 183–210.

————. "Mixing Metaphors: Translating the Indian Medical Doctrine Tridoṣa in Chinese Buddhist Sources." *Asian Medicine: Tradition and Modernity* 6 (2010): 55–74.

————. *Translating Buddhist Medicine in Medieval China*. Philadelphia: University of Pennsylvania Press, 2014.

————. *Traditional Thai Medicine*. Second Edition. Bangkok: White Lotus Press, 2016.

————. *Buddhism and Medicine: An Anthology of Premodern Sources*. New York: Columbia University Press, 2017.

Sappol, Michael. *A Traffic in Death: Bodies, Anatomy and Embodied Social Identity in Nineteenth-Century America*. Princeton: Princeton University Press, 2002.

Sarazin, Ch. "Le bétail indochinois sur les marchés de France et d'Extrême-Orient." *Bulletin Economique de l'Indochine* 19 (1916): 563–608.

Sardjito. *The Development of the Universitas Gadjah Mada (UGM)*. Jogjakarta: Universitas Gadjah Mada, 1956.

Sathaban Kanphaet Phaen Thai. *Sathaban Kanphaet Phaen Thai* [National Institute of Thai Traditional Medicine]. Ministry of Public Health, 1994.

————. *Kanphaet Phaen Thai: Kanphaet Baep Ong Ruam* [Thai Traditional Medicine: Holistic Medicine]. Bangkok: Rongphim Ongkan Songkhro Thahan Phan Suek, 1996.

————. *Kannuat Thai phuea Sukkhaphap* [Thai Massage for Health]. Bangkok: Loef and Lip Press, 1997.

————. *Chut Nithatsakan Kanphaet Phaen Thai* [Program of the Exhibition of Thai Traditional Medicine]. Bangkok: Rongphim Ongkan Songkhro Thahan Phan Suek, 1999.

————. "Understanding the *Doṣa*: A Summary of the Art of Medicine from the *Sūtra of Golden Light*." In *Buddhism and Medicine: An Anthology*, ed. C. Pierce Salguero. New York: Columbia University Press, 2017, 30–40.

Satrio, and Mona Lohanda. *Perjuangan dan Pengabdian: Mosaik Kenangan Professor Dokter Satrio, 1916–86*. Jakarta: Arsip Nasional Republik Indonesia, 1986.

Savang Prom-Tep. "Facteurs sociaux et religieux dans l'élevage au Cambodge." PhD diss., Faculté Mixte de Médecine et de Pharmacie de Toulouse, 1954.

Schaffer, Simon, Lissa Roberts, Kapil Raj, and James Delbourgo, eds. *The Brokered World: Go-Betweens and Global Intelligence, 1770–1820*. Sagamore Beach: Science History Publications, 2010.

Scharfe, Hartmut. "The Doctrine of the Three Humors in Traditional Indian Medicine and the Alleged Antiquity of Tamil Siddha Medicine." *Journal of the American Oriental Society* 119 (1999): 609–29.

Scheid, Volker. "Chinese Medicine and the Problem of Tradition." *Asian Medicine: Tradition and Modernity* 2, no. 1 (2006): 59–71.

————. *Currents of Tradition in Chinese Medicine, 1626–2006*. Seattle: Eastland Press, 2007.

Schein, H. "Recrutement et formation du personnel vétérinaire indigène en Indochine." *Revue de Médecine Vétérinaire Exotique* 1 (1928): 177–81.

Schein, H., and H. Jacotot. "La séro-infection: Vaccination préventive contre la peste bovine." *Archives des Instituts Pasteur d'Indochine* (1925): 48–56.

Schiefner, F. Anton von. *Tibetan Tales Derived from Indian Sources: Translated from the Tibetan of the Kah-Gyur*. London: Kegan Paul, Trench, Trübner & Co, 1906.

Schneider, William H. *Rockefeller Philanthropy and Modern Biomedicine: International Initiatives from World War I to the Cold War.* Bloomington: Indiana University Press, 2002.

Schopen, Gregory. "The Training and Treatments of an Indian Doctor in a Buddhist Text: A Sanskrit Biography of Jīvaka." In *Buddhism and Medicine: An Anthology of Premodern Sources*, ed. C. Pierce Salguero. New York: Columbia University Press, 2017, 184–204.

Scopaz, Anna, Liz Eckermann, and Matthew Clarke. "Maternal Health in Lao PDR: Repositioning the Goal Posts." *Journal of the Asia Pacific Economy* 16 (2011): 597–611.

Setyonegoro, R. Kusumanto, and W.R. Roan. *Traditional Healing Practices: Proceedings, Asean Mental Health Teaching Seminar on Traditional Healing, Jakarta, Indonesia, Dec. 3–9, 1979.* Jakarta: Ministry of Health, 1983.

Sherman, Irwin. *The Power of Plagues.* Washington: ASM Press, 2006.

Shinohara, Koichi. *Images, Miracles, and Authority in Asian Religious Traditions.* Boulder: Westview Press, 1998.

Shope, Richard. "Influenza: History, Epidemiology and Speculation." *Public Health Reports* 73 (1958): 165–79.

Siddiqi, Javed. *World Health and World Politics: The World Health Organization and the UN System.* Columbia: University of South Carolina Press, 1995.

Silverstein, Arthur. *Pure Politics and Impure Science: The Swine Flu Affair.* Baltimore: Johns Hopkins University Press, 1981.

Singaravélou, Pierre. "'L'enseignement supérieur colonial': Un état des lieux." *Histoire de l'éducation* (2009): 71–92.

Smith, Bruce Lannes. *Indonesian-American Cooperation in Higher Education.* East Lanning: Institute of Research on Overseas Programs, Michigan State University, 1960.

Smithies, Michael, and Euayporn Kerdchouay. "The *Wai Kru* Ceremony of the *Nang Yai.*" *Journal of the Siam Society* 62 (1974): 143–7.

Somadikarta, S., Tri Wahyuning, M. Irsyam, and Boen Sri Oemarjati. *Tahun Emas Universitas Indonesia: Dari Balai ke Universitas.* Jakarta: Universitas Indonesia Press, 2000.

Somchintana Thongthew Ratarasarn. "The Principles and Concepts of Thai Classical Medicine." PhD diss., University of Wisconsin, 1986.

Souvannavong, Oudom. "Une étude du problème medico sociale au Laos." PhD diss., University of Paris, 1949.

Spring, Catherine. *Maternal Mortality in Lao PDR: Population Study, 1991.* Vientiane: World Health Organization, 1991.

State Planning Committee. *National Population and Development Policy of the Lao PDR.* Vientiane: State Planning Committee, 1999.

Stein, Eric Andrew. "Vital Times: Power, Public Health, and Memory in Rural Java." PhD diss., University of Michigan, 2005.

————. "Hygiene and Decolonization: The Rockefeller Foundation and Indonesian Nationalism, 1933–1958." In *Science, Public Health, and the State in Modern Asia*, ed. Liping Bu, Darwin H. Stapleton, and Ka-Che Yip. New York: Routledge, 2012, 51–70.

Steiner, George. *After Babel: Aspects of Language and Translation*. 3rd ed. Oxford: Oxford University Press, 1998.

Stokvis-Cohen Stuart, N. "Nota betreffende de Noodzakelijkheid van Verbetering van de Ziekenzorg voor Javaansche Vrouwen." *Bulletin van den Bond van Geneesheeren in Ned.-Indië* 97 (1914): 1–13.

————. "Over Inlandsche Ziekenverpleging in Nederlandsch-Indië." *Indische Gids* 37 (1915): 791–804.

————. "Plan tot Instelling eener Wijkverpleging." *Bulletin van den Bond van Geneesheeren in Ned.-Indië* 151 (1916): 1–22.

————. *Ilmoe Pembĕla Orang Sakit*. Groningen: Wolters, 1928.

————. "Vrouwelijke Artsen voor Indië." *Nederlands Tijdschrift voor Geneeskunde* 74 (1930): 1268–71.

————. "Medisch-sociaal Werk in Indië." *Leven en Werken* 16 (1931): 471–93.

————. "Leven en Werken in Indië." *Tijdschrift voor Ziekenverpleging* 41 (1931): 140–4, 179–84, 230–7, 264–70, 298–305.

————. "Tropenleergang voor Verplegenden." *Tijdschrift voor Ziekenverpleging* 41 (1931): 43–5, 388–90, 511–14, 651–2; 42 (1932): 20–1.

Stuart-Fox, Martin. *Buddhist Kingdom, Marxist State: The Making of Modern Laos*. Bangkok: White Lotus, 1996.

Suchai Trirat. "Itthiphon Munlanithi Rokkifenloe to Rongrian Phaet Thai [The Influences of Rockerfeller Foundation on Thai Medical School]." *Warasan Sangkhomsat Kanphaet* [Journal of Social Science of Medicine] 1 (1978): 40–55.

Summers, Anne. *Angels and Citizens: British Women as Military Nurses, 1854–1914*. London: Routledge and Kegan Paul, 1988.

Sutphen, Mary P., and Bridie Andrews. *Medicine and Colonial Identity*. New York: Routledge, 2003.

Sut Saengwichian. "Jut Jop khong Phaet Phaen Boran lae Kanroemton khong Kanphaet Phaen Patjuban khong Thai [The End of Traditional Medicine and the Beginning of Modern Medicine in Thailand]." *Warasan Sangkhomsat Kanphaet* [Journal of Social Science of Medicine] 1 (1978): 20–8.

Suwanlert, Sangun. "Phii Pob: Spirit Possession in Rural Thailand." In *Culture-Bound Syndromes, Ethnopsychiatry, and Alternate Therapies: Volume IV of Mental Health Research in Asia and the Pacific*, ed. William P. Lebra. Honolulu: University of Hawai'i Press, 1976, 68–87.

Swearer, Donald K. "Aniconism versus Iconism in Thai Buddhism." In *Buddhism in the Modern World: Adaptations of an Ancient Tradition*, ed. Steven Heine and Charles S. Prebish. New York: Oxford University Press, 2003, 9–26.

————. *Becoming the Buddha: The Ritual of Image Consecration in Thailand.* Princeton: Princeton University Press, 2004.

Sweet, Helen, and Rona Dougall. *Community Nursing and Primary Healthcare in Britain in the Twentieth Century.* New York: Routledge, 2008.

Tambiah, Stanley Jeyaraja. *Buddhism and the Spirit Cults in North-East Thailand.* Cambridge: Cambridge University Press, 1970.

————. *World Conqueror and World Renouncer: A Study of Buddhism and Polity in Thailand against a Historical Background.* Cambridge: Cambridge University Press, 1976.

————. *The Buddhist Saints of the Forest and the Cult of Amulets.* Cambridge: Cambridge University Press, 1984.

Tapaniyakon, Yuwadi. "Wiwatthanakan thang Kanphaet Thai tangtae Samai Roemton jon thueng Sinsut Ratchakan Phrabatsomdetphrajunlajomklao-jaoyuhua [Development of Thai Medicine from the Beginning until the End of the Era of King Chulalongkorn]." MA thesis, Chulalongkorn University, 1979.

Terwiel, Barend Jan. "A Model for the Study of Thai Buddhism." *Journal of Asian Studies* 35 (1976): 391–403.

————. "The Tais and Their Belief in Khwans: Towards Establishing an Aspect of 'Proto-Tai' Culture." *South East Asian Review* 3 (1978): 1–16.

————. *Monks and Magic: Revisiting a Classic Study of Religious Ceremonies in Thailand.* Copenhagen: Nordic Institute of Asian Studies, 2012.

The World Bank. "Lao PDR Overview." In *The World Bank: Working for a World Free of Poverty.* http://www.worldbank.org/en/country/lao/overview.

Thompson, C. Michele. "Medicine, Nationalism, and Revolution in Vietnam: The Roots of a Medical Collaboration to 1945." *East Asian Science, Technology, and Medicine* 21 (2003): 114–48.

————. *Vietnamese Traditional Medicine: A Social History.* Singapore: NUS Press, 2015.

Thongthew-Ratarasarn, Somchintana. *The Principles and Concepts of Thai Classical Medicine.* Bangkok: Thammasat University, 1996.

Tiangco, Mamerto. *Almanake at Kalendario ukol sa Kalusugan sa mga taong 1919, 1920 at 1921 ng Kagawaran ng Sanidad ng Pilipinas.* Manila: Bureau of Printing, 1921.

Tognotti, Eugenia. "Scientific Triumphalism and Learning from Facts: Bacteriology and the 'Spanish Flu' Challenge of 1918." *Social History of Medicine* 16 (2003): 97–110.

Tomes, Nancy. *The Gospel of Germs: Men, Women, and the Microbe in American Life.* Cambridge: Harvard University Press, 1998.

Tomkins, Sandra. "The Failure of Expertise: Public Health Policy in Britain during the 1918–19 Influenza Epidemic." *Social History of Medicine* 5 (1992): 435–54.

Tran-Trong-Hieu. "Considérations sur l'élevage et l'amélioration du gros bétail au sud-Vietnam." PhD diss., Paris, 1962.

Truong, Thanh-Dam. *Sex, Money and Morality: Prostitution and Tourism in Southeast Asia*. London: Zed Books, 1990. Translated into Japanese by N. Tanaka and A. Yamashita as *Baishun: Sei Rodo no Shakai Kozo to Kokusai Keizai*. Tokyo: Akashi Shoten, 1993.

Turner, Karen Gottschang, and Hao Thanh Phan. *Even the Women Must Fight: Memories of War from North Vietnam*. New York: Wiley, 1998.

UNFPA. *(Draft) Family Planning Situation Analysis*. Vientiane: UNFPA, 2015.

UNICEF. *Children and Women in the Lao People's Democratic Republic*. Vientiane: UNICEF, 1992.

———. *Children and their Families in the Lao PDR*. Vientiane: UNICEF, 1996.

USAID. *Audit Report MCH Project 1971*. Washington: USAID, 1971.

———. *Audit Report: Maternal and Child Health Project*. Washington: USAID, 1973.

———. *Termination Report for Laos*. Washington: USAID, 1976.

Vann, Michael G. "Hanoi in the Time of Cholera: Epidemic Disease and Racial Power in the Colonial City." In *Global Movements, Local Concerns: Medicine and Health in Southeast Asia*, ed. Laurence Monnais and Harold J. Cook. Singapore: National University of Singapore Press, 2012, 150–70.

Vaughan, Megan. *Curing Their Ills: Colonial Power and African Illness*. Stanford: Stanford University Press, 1991.

Vidy, G. "La communauté indienne en Indochine." *Sud-Est*, Paris 6 (1949): 1–8.

Vogel, W.T. de. "Memorie betreffende den Burgerlijken Geneeskundigen Dienst." *Bulletin van den Bond van Geneesheeren in Ned.-Indië* 14 (1906): 17–45.

Wahlberg, Ayo. "A Revolutionary Movement to Bring Traditional Medicine Back to the Grassroots Level: On the Biopoliticization of Herbal Medicine in Vietnam." In *Global Movements, Local Concerns: Medicine and Health in Southeast Asia*, ed. Laurence Monnais and Harold J. Cook. Singapore: NUS Press, 2012, 207–25.

Wall, Rosemary. *The International Health Division's Views on Nursing Practice, Policy and Education in British Malaya*. Sleepy Hollow: Rockefeller Archive Center, 2010. http://www.rockarch.org/publications/resrep/wall.pdf.

Wall, Rosemary, and Anne Marie Rafferty. "Nursing and the 'Hearts and Minds' Campaign, 1948–1958: The Malayan Emergency." In *Routledge Handbook on the Global History of Nursing*, ed. Patricia D'Antonio, Julie Fairman, and Jean Whelan. New York: Routledge, 2013, 218–36.

Wan Faizah binti Wan Yusoff. "Malay Responses to the Promotion of Western Medicine, with Particular Reference to Women and Child Healthcare in the Federated Malay States, 1920–1939." PhD diss., University of London, 2010.

Warner, John Harley. "The Selective Transport of Medical Knowledge: Antebellum American Physicians and Parisian Medical Therapeutics." *Bulletin of the History of Medicine* 59 (1985): 213–31.

———. *Against the Spirit of System: The French Impulse in Nineteenth Century American Medicine*. Princeton: Princeton University Press, 1998.

Warner, John Harley, and James E. Edmonson. *Dissection: Photographs of a Rite of Passage in American Medicine, 1880–1930*. New York: Blast Books, 2009.

Weindling, Paul, ed. *International Health Organizations and Movements, 1918–1939*. New York: Cambridge University Press, 1995.

Weinstein, Louis. "Influenza 1918: A Revisit?" *New England Journal of Medicine* 294 (1976): 1058–60.

Wellington, John S., and Ruth Boak. "Medical Science and Technology." In *Indonesia: Resources and Their Technological Development*, ed. Howard W. Beers. Lexington: University of Kentucky Press, 1970, 165–73.

Wendland, Claire L. *A Heart for the Work: Journeys through an African Medical School*. Chicago: University of Chicago Press, 2010.

Whitehurst, Robert D. "Đặng Thùy Trâm and Her Family, Lives in Medicine." In *Southern Medicine for Southern People: Vietnamese Medicine in the Making*, ed. Laurence Monnais, C. Michele Thompson, and Ayo Wahlberg. Newcastle upon Tyne: Cambridge Scholars Publishing, 2012, 85–106.

WHO. *Human Resources for Health*. Vientiane: World Health Organization, 2007.

Wiegman, Nanny. "'De Verpleegster Zij in de eerste Plaats Vrouw van Karakter': Ziekenverpleging als Vrouwenzaak (1898–1998)." In *Gezond en Wel: Vrouwen en de Zorg voor Gezondheid in de 20ᵉ Eeuw*, ed. Rineke van Daalen and Marijke Gijswijt-Hofstra. Amsterdam: Amsterdam University Press, 1998.

Wilson, Ara. "The Sacred Geography of Bangkok's Markets." *International Journal of Urban and Regional Research* 32 (2008): 631–42.

Wilton, Peter. "Spanish Flu Outdid WWI in Number of Lives Claimed." *Canada Medical Association Journal* 148 (1993): 2036–7.

Woolcock, Michael, Simon Szreter, and Vijayendra Rao. "How and Why Does History Matter for Development Policy?" *Journal of Development Studies* 47 (2011): 70–96.

World Bank. *Lao PDR: Social Assessment and Strategy*. Washington DC: World Bank Human Resources Operations Division, Country Department 1, East Asia and Pacific Region, 1995.

Yap, Felicia. "Eurasians in British Asia during the Second World War." *Journal of the Royal Asiatic Society* 21 (2011): 485–505.

Yersin, A. "Fonctionnement de l'Institut Pasteur de Nha-Trang (Annam)." *Annales d'Hygiène et de Médecine Coloniales* 3 (1900): 506–20.

Yoddumnern, Benja. *The Role of Thai Traditional Doctors*. Bangkok: Institute for Population and Social Research, Mahidol University, 1974.

Zysk, Kenneth G. *Asceticism and Healing in Ancient India: Medicine in the Buddhist Monastery*. Delhi: Motilal Banarsidass, 1998.

# Contributors

**Michitake Aso** is Assistant Professor of the Global Environment in the History Department at the University at Albany, SUNY. Before landing in Albany, he completed a postdoctoral fellowship at the Asia Research Institute at the National University of Singapore. In 2014–15, he was a Fellow at the Institute for Historical Studies, University of Texas at Austin. He is currently finishing a book manuscript called *Forest without Birds: Rubber Plantations and the Making of Vietnam, 1897–1975*, which explores the transformation of environments, human health, and knowledge through the places and people involved in rubber production in Vietnam. His dissertation on French colonial Vietnam won the 2013 Young Scholar Prize of the International Union of the History and Philosophy of Science. He has recently published articles in *Modern Asian Studies*, *Journal of Southeast Asian Studies*, and *Science, Technology, and Society*. He teaches courses on global environmental history and Asian history.

**Francis A. Gealogo** is Associate Professor and immediate past chair at the Ateneo de Manila University in the Philippines. He obtained his academic degrees from the University of the Philippines, Diliman, where he taught for 13 years before transferring to Ateneo in 2000. His research interests include social and demographic history, history of medicine and public health, history of freemasonry, history of prisons and penology, and the history of the Iglesia Filipina Independiente—all focusing on the Philippines.

**Jenna Grant** is Assistant Professor in the Department of Anthropology at the University of Washington. Her research concerns biomedicine, technologies, global health, and visuality in Cambodia. Specific projects focus on HIV prevention clinical trials, medical imaging, malaria drug resistance, and experimental forms of ethnography.

**Annick Guénel** is a researcher at the Centre d'Asie du Sud-Est (CNRS/ EHESS), Paris. She has conducted research on colonial human and veterinary medicine in French Indochina. She is currently working on the history of malaria control in Vietnam from the beginning of the twentieth century to the present time.

**Liesbeth Hesselink** received her degree in history from the University of Leiden in 1972. After graduation, she worked as a secondary school teacher and a civil servant for the Ministry of Education, after which she commenced working for the municipality of Leiden. She also represented the Dutch Labour Party as a member of the City Council of the municipality of Leiden for eight years. After her retirement in 2009, she attained her doctorate with a dissertation entitled *Genezers op de Koloniale Markt: Inheemse Dokters en Vroedvrouwen in Nederlands Oost-Indië 1850–1915*, which was published by Amsterdam University Press. An English translation appeared two years later: *Healers on the Colonial Market: Native Doctors and Midwives in the Dutch East Indies* (Leiden: KITLV Press, 2011). Liesbeth has published on medicine, physicians, midwives, and nurses in the Dutch East Indies.

**Junko Iida** is Professor of Anthropology at the Comprehensive Education Center (Department of Social Work, Faculty of Health and Welfare) of the Kawasaki University of Medical Welfare in Japan. She received her PhD from the School of Cultural and Social Studies (National Museum of Ethnology, Osaka), Graduate University for Advanced Studies in 2003. She was a Visiting Research Fellow at the Institute of Social and Cultural Anthropology, University of Oxford, in 2006–07. Her research interests are in Thai Traditional Medicine and local healing practices in northern Thailand, and currently also in palliative care in Japan. Her recent publications include: "The Sensory Experience of Thai Massage: Commercialization, Globalization, and Tactility," in *Everyday Life in Asia: Social Perspectives on the Senses*, ed. D. Kalekin-Fishman and Kevin E.Y. Low (Ashgate, 2010); and "Holism as a Whole-body Treatment: The Transnational Production of Thai Massage," *European Journal of Transnational Studies* 5, no. 1 (2013).

**Laurence Monnais** is Professor of History and Canada Research Chair in Health Care Pluralism at Université de Montréal (Canada). Trained in colonial studies, then in medical humanities, she is a specialist on the sociocultural history of medicine and health in Southeast Asia (French Indochina and Vietnam) and on alternative and traditional medicines in a transdisciplinary and global perspective. She is also vice-president of HOMSEA (History of Medicine in Southeast Asia). Laurence Monnais is the author and co-editor of 7 books and more than 40 peer-reviewed articles and chapters primarily on the history of medicalization in Southeast Asia, colonialism and medicine, colonial and colonized physicians and pharmacists, the invention of traditional medicines, and, more recently, vaccine hesitancy.

**Vivek Neelakantan** earned a doctorate from the University of Sydney in 2014. His thesis examined Indonesia's relations with the WHO during the Cold War in the 1950s and 1960s. He is the author of "The Campaign against the Big Four Endemic Diseases and Indonesia's Relations with the WHO during the Cold War," ed. Liping Bu and Ka-Che Yip (Routledge, 2014). He has published on disease eradication in Indonesia, postcolonial science, and the appropriation and transformation of social medicine in a non-Western context. Vivek is on the advisory board of *Paramita: Historical Studies Journal*, published by Semarang State University, Indonesia and has served as a peer reviewer for leading journals such as *Medical History*, *Women's History Review*, and *Development and Change*. He is one of the founding members of the International Indonesian Forum for Asian Studies (IIFAS), which seeks to promote dialogue between academia and policy-making. He is on the Organising Committee of the IIFAS Inaugural Conference, "Creating ASEAN Futures 2015: Towards Connected Cross-Border Communities," hosted by Andalas University, Padang (Indonesia) in September 2015. Vivek's current research interests center on the history of postcolonial science and medicine in Southeast and South Asia. He is currently a Postdoctoral Fellow at the Indian Institute of Technology Madras (IITM), Chennai.

**Hans Pols** is Associate Professor in the Unit for History and Philosophy of Science at the University of Sydney. He is interested in the history of psychiatry and the history of medicine in the Dutch East Indies and Indonesia. He has published on the history of the American mental hygiene movement, colonial psychiatry in the Dutch East Indies, and the history of medicine in Indonesia. He is currently involved in a project on the recent history of Indonesian psychiatry.

**Anne Marie Rafferty CBE** is Professor of Nursing Policy at the Florence Nightingale Faculty of Nursing and Midwifery, King's College London. She is a nurse (BSc Edinburgh University); policy expert (Harkness Fellowship University of Pennsylvania); clinical researcher (MPhil Surgery), and historian (DPhil Modern History). She was Co-Director of the Centre for the Humanities and Health funded by the Wellcome Trust and Principal Investigator of the nursing strand, a colla-borative venture with historian of medicine Dr. Rosemary Wall and literary scholars Dr. Jessica Howell and Prof. Anna Snaith. She was made Commander of the British Empire in 2008 for exceptional services to health care and is recipient of the Nursing Times Leadership Award in 2014 and Health Services Journal Clinical Leaders Top 100 award in 2015.

**C. Pierce Salguero** is an interdisciplinary humanities scholar interested in the role of Buddhism in the cross-cultural exchange of medical ideas. He has a PhD in History of Medicine from Johns Hopkins University, and teaches Asian history, religion, and culture at Penn State University's Abington College, located near Philadelphia. The major theme in his scholarship is the interplay between the global transmission and local reception of Buddhist knowledge about health, disease, and the body. His recent monograph, *Translating Buddhist Medicine in Medieval China* (University of Pennsylvania Press, 2014) integrates methodologies from history, religious studies, translation studies, and literary studies, and explores the reception of Buddhist healing in medieval China. Before entering graduate school, Pierce spent several years studying Buddhist meditation, Thai therapeutic massage, and other Buddhist-inspired healing practices in northern Thailand. Though he now publishes pri-marily academic works, he previously authored several textbooks for practitioners of Thai medicine, and continues to create opportunities for dialogue between scholarly and non-scholarly audiences.

**Kathryn Sweet** received her PhD from the Department of History at the National University of Singapore (NUS) in 2015. Her dissertation research focused on the development of the biomedical health system in Laos, from French annexation in 1893 until 2000, and its long-term reliance on external assistance. She is based in Vientiane, Lao PDR, where she also works as a development practitioner.

**C. Michele Thompson** holds an MA in East Asian History from the University of Alabama and a PhD in Southeast Asian History from the

University of Washington. She is Professor of Southeast Asian History at Southern Connecticut State University. Her most recent publications include *Vietnamese Traditional Medicine: A Social History*, National University of Singapore Press, 2015; "Would a Saola by Any Other Name Still be a Saola: Appropriating Rare Animals, Expropriating Minority Peoples," in *State, Society and the Market in Contemporary Vietnam: Property, Power and Values*, ed. Hue-Tam Ho Tai and Mark Sidel; and "Tuệ Tĩnh Vietnamese Monk-Physician at the Ming Court," in *The Illustrated History of Chinese Medicine and Healing*, ed. Linda L. Barnes and T.J. Hinrichs. She is currently working on two main projects—one on the fourteenth-century Vietnamese Buddhist monk physician Tuệ Tĩnh, who was sent as a living present to the court of the Minh Dynasty with the Vietnamese tribute mission of 1385; and the other on the continuing cultural, environmental, and political effects of the discovery, in 1992, in the mountains of Vietnam of a very rare animal called the saola.

**Rosemary Wall** is a Senior Lecturer in Global History at the University of Hull. She is a historian of medicine, studying Britain and areas of British overseas settlement between 1880 and 1960. Her current project is an interdisciplinary book on British colonial nursing, co-authored with colleagues at King's College London and Texas A&M University. Publications on this theme include "Nursing and the 'Hearts and Minds' Campaign, 1948–1958: The Malayan Emergency," in *Routledge Handbook on the Global History of Nursing*, ed. Patricia D'Antonio, Julie Fairman, and Jean Whelan (New York: Routledge, 2013). Rosemary's previous project investigated the use of bacteriology in hospitals, workplaces, and local communities, and her book, *Bacteria in Britain, 1880–1939* (London: Pickering and Chatto), was published in 2013. Rosemary enjoys engaging with the public through museum exhibitions and talks, television and radio appearances, as well as co-designing an iPod app, "Navigating Nightingale," which provides an interactive tour of the banks of the River Thames in London and explores the history of London through Florence Nightingale's interests. Rosemary was educated at the University of Liverpool (BA) and Imperial College London (MSc and PhD). She has previously held postdoctoral research positions at the University of Oxford and King's College London, and a temporary lectureship at Imperial College London.

**John Harley Warner** is Avalon Professor of the History of Medicine at Yale University. He is Chair of the History of Medicine department at the Yale School of Medicine, and is Professor of History, of American Studies, and of the History of Science and Medicine. He received his PhD in 1984 from Harvard University, and from 1984–86 was a Post-doctoral Fellow at the Wellcome Institute for the History of Medicine in London. In 1986 he joined the faculty at Yale, where he teaches undergraduate, graduate, and medical students. His books include *The Therapeutic Perspective: Medical Practice, Knowledge, and Identity in America* (Harvard, 1986), *Against the Spirit of System: The French Impulse in Nineteenth-Century American Medicine* (Princeton, 1998), and (with James Edmonson) *Dissection: Photographs of a Rite of Passage in American Medicine* (Blast Books, 2009). He is co-editor (with Janet Tighe) of *Major Problems in the History of American Medicine and Public Health* (Houghton Mifflin, 2001), and (with Frank Huisman) of *Locating Medical History: The Stories and Their Meanings* (Johns Hopkins, 2004). His research focuses on the history of medicine in nineteenth- and twentieth-century United States, including medical education, and the transnational history of medical cultures since the late eighteenth century. Ongoing projects include a book tentatively titled *The Quest for Authenticity in Modern Medicine*.

# Index

Abendanon, J.H., 60
Abhay, Maniso, 129
Act for the Control of the Practice of the Healing Art (1936), Thailand, 278, 287
    amendment of, 284
*Actualités*, 198–9
*adat* (indigenous customs and law), 56, 60, 184
advertisements, for patent medicines, 255
Alma-Ata Declaration (1978), 281
American County Health nurses, 76
American model, of medical education, 8–9, 11, 13, 16–17, 188
    American training of British nurses, 76
    British attitudes towards, 76
    *versus* British model of nursing, 67
    in Indonesia, 174, 175–86
    in Malaya, 67, 73–80
    in Philippines, 74
    public health policy, 74
    "public-private" nexus on, 74
Amrith, Sunil, 74
animal breeding, 96, 104
    animal anatomy and physiology, 100
    cattle selection program for, 105
    crossbreeding, 105
    development of, 105
    European breeding centers, 108

health policies related to, 102
in Indochina, *see* Indochina, veterinary science and animal breeding in
methods of, 105
for milk production, 105
Sind-bred animals, 105
water buffalo, 97
animal diseases, 98–9
    bovine
        contagious diseases, 103
        hemorrhagic septicemia, 99
        pasteurellosis, 99
    communicable, 102
    culling of infected animals, 102
    epidemic outbreak, 101
    immunization against, 102
    medicine for prevention of, 95
    prophylaxis of, 100
    rinderpest epizootic, 99, 102
    sero-infection (serum-simultaneous vaccine), 102
    spread of epizootics, 102
    vaccinations, benefits of, 103
animal husbandry, 104
    development of, 106
animal medicine, 95
anti-hookworm campaigns (Rockefeller Foundation), 19
*Assistance Médicale Indigène* (AMI), 20, 199, 251, 254, 255
    doctors affiliated with, 260
    establishment of, 263

legislative and institutional
framework of, 252
shortcomings of, 259
Assistant Nurses
Assistant Nurses scheme, 83
Huggins' report on, 83
utility of, 83
Australian Aid, 178
Ayurawet College, Thailand, 281
bureaucratic (traditional medicine
revivalist) movement, 282
massage adopted by, 281
royal style massage, 281–2
Thai Massage Revival Project,
282–4
Ayurawet doctor, 281
Ayurveda, 274, 289
Ayurveda-Unani Tibb movement,
India, 22

bacteriological revolution of 1870s
and 1880s, 12
Barnes, Milford, 76–7, 81
BCG (anti-tuberculosis) vaccine, 254
*bidan* (traditional midwives), 73
biomedical drugs, *see* biomedicine
biomedicine, 5, 17, 19, 84, 281, 283
in Cambodia, 196, 198–9, 208–11
education in, 156
and medical diplomacy, 217–18
professional values of, 148
teaching of, 27–8
techno-centric, 84
in Vietnam, *see* socialist
biomedicine, in Vietnam
bio-security, 196
"black market" medicine, 195, 255,
257, 269n33
bovine
contagious diseases, 103
hemorrhagic septicemia, 99
pasteurellosis, 99, 103

British Malaya, nursing services in,
*see* nursing services, in British
Malaya
British model, of medical services
American training of British
nurses, 76
apprenticeship-style training, 77
Assistant Nurses scheme, 83
in British Malaya, *see* nursing
sevices, in British Malaya
*versus* North American nursing,
67
quality of public health nurse
training, 77
State Enrolled Nurses, 83
British Rushcliffe Committee on
the Training of Nurses in the
Colonies (1943–45), 82
Buddhist socialism, ideology of,
197
*Bulletin of the Association of Health
Workers*, 201
bureaucratic (traditional medicine
revivalist) movement, 282
Burns, Adam D., 75, 90n58

*Cambodge d'Aujourd'hui*, 198, 203,
204, 225n35
Cambodia, medical education in, 17
Cambodian-Soviet collaboration
on, 195
decolonization of, 199
language of medical training and
administration, 199
Soviet model of, 195
Cambodian health and medical
services, 194
advertising biomedical
commodities, 207
attention to hygiene, 209
biomedicine and nation-building,
197

biomedicine during the Sangkum, 198–9
Cambodian Pathology, 208, 210
enacting Cambodian biomedicine, 208–11
global health initiatives, 221
health education, 210
health system, 196
Khmer-Soviet Friendship Hospital (KSFH), *see* Khmer-Soviet Friendship Hospital (KSFH), Phnom Penh
Medical Association, 200
medical diplomacy, 196
medical education, *see* Cambodia, medical education in
National Ethics Committee for Human Research, 221
pharmaceutical industry, development of, 196
postcolonial biomedicine and medical diplomacy, 217–18
Royal Society of Medicine of Cambodia, 200
Sangkum modernity, 197–8
*Sangkum Reastr Niyum* (People's Socialist Community), domains of biomedicine, 198–9
doctors, 200
medical publications, 200–1
modernity, 197–8
Superior Health Council, 200
cattle diseases, *see* animal diseases
Chaichakan, Sintorn, 297
Chaichakan, Wasan, 298
character, notion of, 67
Chee, Kong Tet, 82–3
childcare centers, 131
childhood illnesses and immunization program, 131

China Medical Board, 16, 34n34, 174, 178–80, 188
Chinese Buddhist bodhisattva Guanyin (Th. Kuan Im), 299
Chinese traditional medicine, 22, 289
Chiwakakomaraphat (personal physician of Buddha), 284, 293n48
cholera epidemics, 19, 241
anti-cholera vaccination campaigns, 254
Choy, Catherine, 72, 75, 81, 87n8
coccobacillus, 99
Colombo Aid Plan for Southeast Asia, 84, 178
colonial medicines, 250, 259
meaning of, 266n1
vaccines, 254
Colonial Nursing Association (CNA), 68, 86
colonized (patient) agency, importance of, 265
Crowell, Elizabeth, 77, 91n76
cultural
brokers, 14, 72, 88n32
colonialism, 76

*Dân Y* (civilian medicine), 147, 150, 164
Darville, Elizabeth, 67, 79
challenges faced in nursing career, 68
experiences of working with British, 81
Rockefeller Foundation, 68
integration into hierarchical colonial society, 80–1
lecture on maternity and child welfare, 79
training on "curative and preventive work," 80

Davis, Diana, 95
Debusmann, Robert, 271n59
*dépôts de médicaments*, *see* medicine
   stores
devas (*tewada*), 299
de Vogel, W.Th., 39, 41, 49–50, 58,
   60
district nursing, 38, 49–51, 58
*Doctors within Borders* (Ming-Cheng
   Lo), 150
doctor-to-patient ratio, in Indonesia,
   185
*dokter djawa* (Western-trained
   Indonesian physician), 24, 42,
   45, 175
*Đông Y* (Eastern medicine), 148, 161
Dooley, Tom, 124
*doṣa*, 299
Douarche, E., 96
Doumer, Paul, 99
*dukun bayi* (traditional birth
   attendant), 15, 51, 56–7, 61, 184
*dusa* (sorrow/suffering), 242
Dutch East Indies Department of
   Public Health, 18
   Division of Medical-Hygienic
      Propaganda, 18
Dutch model, of medical education,
   11, 15–16
   Ethical Policy, 25, 40
   in Indonesia, 173–4, 175–86

Eastern medicine, 161
   components of, 162
   development of, 162
   incorporation with Western
      medicine, 163
   involvement of the Viet Minh
      in, 162
   position in socialist biomedicine,
      162

   role in Y50 medical education,
      163
   *thuốc bắc* (Northern medicine),
      162
   *thuốc nam* (Southern medicine),
      162
   in Vietnam, 161–2
Ecole de Médecine de Hanoi, 99
economic well-being, index of, 26
empowerment
   of medicine, 318n30
   of nurses, 75
essential care, idea of, 252
"ethical" medicines, 266n1
exorcists (*mo phi*), 297, 300

Faculties of Medicine and Pharmacy
   (University of Santo Tomas), 11
family planning services, 117–19,
   123, 128–9, 132
   National Birth Spacing Policy,
      Laos, 134
Federated Malay States (FMS), 11,
   13, 69
feminization, of nursing, 13, 67, 72,
   83
Filipino hygienic belief and behavior,
   19
Fitzgerald, Alice, 81
folk healers, 275, 286
Ford Foundation, 178
Foucault, Michel, 6
Four Body Elements, principle of,
   274–5, 277, 286, 288
Franco-Lao Treaty (1949), 123
free health care, idea of, 251
free medicines, distribution of, 203,
   252
French international network of
   physicians, 8
French West Africa (AOF), 107

Gates, Frederick, 76
Geneeskundige Hoogeschool (GHS),
    Batavia, 175–6
General Nursing Council, UK, 83
German model, of medical education,
    16, 173, 175
Goscha, Christopher, 149–50, 164
Gourou, Pierre, 97–8

Halpern, Joel, 124
Hanoi Medical University (HMU),
    8, 146
    authority over linguistics, 159–61
    biomedical doctors at, 148
    curriculum of, 151
        French language, 160
    Đội Điều Trị 5 (DDT5), 153
    Eastern medicine, 163
    entrance exam, 160
    female medical students, 158
    founding of, 151
    and French-controlled medical
        system, 151
    Hồ Đắc Di, 151
    lessons of colonial medicine, 156
    medical education at, 156–7
    militarization of, 164
    military medicine, study of, 151
    need of medical doctors due to
        Indochinese War, 151
    politics over medicine, 153–6
    professional competence of
        training students, 149
    public health issues, 157
    traditional medicine at, 150
    training in maternal health, 159
    Y50, 151–3, 166
Harrison, Francis Burton, 232
Havard-Duclos, 107–8
health beliefs and practices, 3
health care professionals
    indigenization of, 14

local healers, 2
    medical doctors, *see* medical
        doctors
    Western-trained, 2
health citizenship, 3, 10, 28
    public health education and,
        17–21
health, dealing with, 260–2
health education
    in Cambodia, 210
    programs for, 10
    in Vietnam, 251–3
    Western ideas of, 72
"Health for All," 281
health information, communication
    of, 7, 20, 231
health policy, 11, 27, 29, 74, 102,
    116, 130–1, 196, 220, 246, 252,
    287
health practices
    bad habits in terms of, 253
    self-medication and therapeutic
        pluralism, 265
health practitioners, 3
Heiser, Victor, 74, 76, 80–2
herbalists (*mo ya*), 245–6, 297
herbal remedies, 280, 283, 285–8
Hien, Tan S., 185
Hoad, William, 71–2
Hoàng, Bảo Châu, 148, 162–3
Hobsbawm, Eric, 289
Ho Chi Minh, 146–7, 151, 153–4
hookworm eradication, program for,
    78
Hoops, A.L., 76, 82
hospital care, 251–2
*Hospital Edicts*, 201
hospital nursing, 78
hospitals, on Java, 38–40
    course in sick-nursing, 39
    employment of nurses, 39
    governmental hospitals, 39
    nursing workforce, 39

Huard, Pierre, 155
Huggins, Donald, 83
human plague bacillus, discovery of,
    98
hygiene
    hygienic modernity, 25, 27
    Western ideas of, 55


Indian Nursing Association, 68
Indigenous Medical Assistance, *see*
    *Assistance Médicale Indigène*
    (AMI)
indigenous medical teachers, 5
Indochina, veterinary science and
    animal breeding in
    animal anatomy and physiology,
        100
    animal health policy, 102
    beef and buffalo meat
        consumption, 97
    brochure produced by the
        veterinary service, 103
    cattle trade, 98
    culling of infected animals, 102
    development of, 96
    domestic animals, exploitation
        of, 95
    Ecole de Médecine de Hanoi, 99
    epidemic outbreak, 101
    free cattle movement, 101
    immunization method, 102
    livestock improvement program,
        104–8
    mapping of breeding areas, 96–8
    Pasteur Institute in Nha Trang,
        100
    rational farming systems, 104
    resource management policies,
        95
    scientific achievements in, 99
    sero-infection (serum-
        simultaneous vaccine), 102

training, for veterinary service,
        98–103
    veterinary schools, 95
    water buffalo breeding, 97
Indochinese Communist Party (ICP),
    151
Indonesia, medical education in
    American model of, 174
    attrition rates, 190
    cohort-based teaching, 175, 180,
        190
    Cold War politics and, 179
    as component of nation-building,
        173
    Curriculum Development
        Committee, 181–2
    Dokter Djawa School, 175
    Dutch military actions, impact
        of, 177
    Dutch model of, 173
    Geneeskundige Hoogeschool
        (GHS), 176
    Indonesian Decree (1946) on, 178
    Indonesian Faculty of Medicine,
        177
    *Inlandsch Arts* (Native Physician),
        175
    medical curricula, 174, 177,
        180–2
    medium of instruction, 174
    Ministry of Education and
        Culture, 179
    MOUs with University of
        California Medical School,
        180
    need for medical manpower and,
        185
    Netherlands-Indies Physicians
        School (NIAS), 175–6
    Nooduniversiteit (Emergency
        University), Jakarta, 176
    problem-based experiential
        learning, 180

School for the Education of
   Native Physicians (STOVIA),
   175–6, 186
Soviet aid and, 178
Surabaya, 186–8
transition from the Dutch to the
   American model, 175–86
Universitas Airlangga (UNAIR),
   Surabaya, 174, 177
Universitas Indonesia (UI),
   Jakarta, 174, 177
   affiliation of the medical
      school at, 179
US technical assistance and, 178
Indonesia, medical system in
   *adat* (indigenous customs and
      law), 56
   district nursing, 49–51
   doctor-to-patient ratio in, 185
   hospitals, on Java, *see* hospitals,
      on Java
   medical education, 16
   midwifery training, 47–9
   physician in Semarang, 40–2
   position of young women and,
      44
   *Puskesmas* (public health
      centers), 190
   quality of health services, 186
   students' relationship with
      patients, 44
   training for female nurses, 44–7
influenza pandemic, in Philippines,
   19, 230
   anti-influenza activities, 234, 240
   'commandments' of healthy
      living, 244, 245
   contesting discourses on, 240–5
   control of, 231
   disinfection of infected premises,
      235
   education drive against, 238–40
   feature of, 230

information and education
      campaigns during, 235–8
   knowledge production and
      transmission, 243
   mortality figures, 230–1
   newspaper reports on, 235–8
   official reports on, 238–40
   Philippine General Hospital, 238
   public health
      delivery system, 245
      education campaigns, 232–5
      social and cultural practices, 234
      and social behavior of
         communities, 234
   spread of, 232–3
*Inlandsch Arts* (Native Physician),
   175
Institute of Higher Technology,
   Phnom Penh, 217–18
*Instituts Pasteur*, 190, 254
International Cooperation
   Administration (ICA), 180
International Planned Parenthood
   Federation, 129
invented tradition, 289

Jacotot, Henri, 95, 108–9
Jenney, E. Ross, 179
Jīvaka, story of, 299, 309

*kahirapan* (poverty/suffering), 242
Kampo, Japan, 22
karmic bonds, 312
Kemper, Jeltje de Bosch, 52
Ketusing, Uai, 281
Khmer socialism, ideology of, 197
Khmer-Soviet Friendship Hospital
   (KSFH), Phnom Penh, 17, 27,
   194, 196, 198–9, 217, 218
   construction of, 202
   financing and support of, 202

idea for, 202
medical care at, 202
opening of, 204
"17 April Hospital," 207
units of, 202
Khmer-Soviet medical journal, *see*
    *Medical-Surgical Review of*
    *the Khmer-Soviet Friendship*
    *Hospital, The*
King's College for Women and
    Bedford College, London, 77

language of instruction, 7–8, 45, 175
Lao Family Welfare Association
    (LFWA), 129
Lao Patriotic Front, 128
Lao Social Indicator Survey (LSIS),
    135
*La Santé Publique au Cambodge*, 201
Latour, Bruno, 150, 195, 210
League of Red Cross Societies, 77
Lentz, Christian, 157–8
leprosy treatments, 255
Lewis, David, 118
licensing system, for traditional
    doctors
    training period, 278
    types of, 278
lineage, notion of, 311
livestock
    farming, 109
    and range management, 95
local healers, 2, 165, 245–7, 286,
    288–9
London School of Hygiene and
    Tropical Medicine (LSHTM),
    79, 81
Lubis, Firman, 183

McNeill, Annabella, 76, 78–81
magicians (*mo saiyasat*), 297

*maladies sociales* (social diseases),
    252
malaria
    malarial zones, classification of,
        267n9
    rejection of quinine in prevention
        of, 254
    transmission, 80, 157, 252
Malayan Medical Services, 69, 82, 85
Malayan medical services, *see*
    nursing services, in British
    Malaya
*Manila Times, The*, 235–8
*mantri* midwives, 52
*mantri* nurse, 44, 47, 48, 50
    training for, 57
Massachusetts Institute of Technology
    (MIT), 78
Maternal and Child Health (MCH)
    Services project, Laos, 124
medical anthropology, 11, 156, 266
medical curriculum, 26, 177–8
    in Indonesia, 182, 189
    remodeling of, 16
    reorganization of, 180
    in US, 181, 186, 189
medical diplomacy, 196, 202
    postcolonial biomedicine and,
        217–18
medical doctors
    Ayurawet doctor, 281
    colonial doctors, 254
    political education of, 156
    Sino-Vietnamese therapists, 259,
        264
    traditional doctors, 278, 296
medical education, in Southeast Asia, 1
    American model of, 8–9, 11, 13,
        16–17
    in Cambodia, *see* Cambodia,
        medical education in
    concept of, 3
    cross-cultural transmission of, 8

Dutch colonial model of, 15–16, 175–86
in Dutch East Indies, 16
educational alliances, 16
European model of, 11
German model of, 175
in Indonesia, *see* Indonesia, medical education in
language of instruction, 7–8
in Malaya, 73–4
of medical practitioners, 10
midwifery program, 13, 25, 47–9
modernization of, 26
multiple meanings of, 23–9
national sensibilities in, 24
nursing training, 13, 25, 44–7
organization of, 14
postcolonial programs for, 10
and public health education, 2
Soviet model of, 17
in Surabaya, 186–8
vernacularization and the ambitions of, 7–10
in Vietnam, 8, 21, 150
dominance of French, 159
Westernization of, 2, 21–2
medical ethics, 11
medical indigeneity, politics of, 22
medicalization, definition of, 289n1
medical pluralism, practices of, 21, 255–6, 265
medical practitioners
education of, 10
European, 25
physician, in Semarang, 40
professional identity of, 11
shaping of, 10–17
training, for female nurses, 44–7
women medical practitioner-teachers, 25
medical precept, selective transmission of, 4–6, 182
medical specialties, 252, 257, 266n1

*Medical-Surgical Review of the Khmer-Soviet Friendship Hospital, The*, 25, 194–6, 204–7
authorship, patterns of, 205
biomedicine of, 220
on Cambodian medicine, geopolitics, and International Medical Science, 216–17
enacting Cambodian biomedicine in, 208–11
picturing Cambodian medicine in, 211–5
practice of biomedical knowledge, 221
Soviet mentorship, 205
topics in, 206
medical translation
colonialism and power differences, effects of, 2
process of, 1–2
medicines
advertisements for, 255
animal, 95
anti-bacterial sulfonamides, 253
antiseptic tablets, 256
biomedicine, *see* biomedicine
"black market," 195
chaulmoogra oil injections, 255
Chinese traditional medicine, 22, 260
colonial, 250
consumption of, 253
*Dân Y*, 150, 164
demanding, 255–8
*Đông Y*, 148
Eastern, *see* Eastern medicine
"ethical" medicines, 266n1
historical studies of, 6
military, 151
Northern, *see* Northern medicine
opotherapeutic drugs, 270n49
*Quân Y*, 150, 161, 164
quinine, 252–3, 254

reasons behind choosing, 258–64
  for dealing with health,
    260–2
  for therapeutic care, 258–60
  therapeutic relationship as
    confrontation, 262–4
rejecting, 254–5
Salvarsan (anti-infectious drug),
  267n13
scientific, 251
side effects of, 255
Sino-Vietnamese, 253, 260
socialist, 148
Southern medicine, *see* Southern
  medicine
*Tây Y*, 161
as tool of empire, 251
traditional medicine, *see*
  traditional medicine
Traditional Vietnamese Medicine
  (TVM), 148, 161, 163
vaccines, 254
  BCG (anti-tuberculosis), 254
medicine stores, 253, 259
midwives
  hospital-based, 121
  in Lao PDR, 117
  licensing system for, 278
  maternal health and birthing, 158
  midwifery school, 121–2
  on-the-job training, 122
  professional classifications, 127
  Skilled Birth Attendance
    Development Plan, 117
  status of, 133
  training of, 13, 25, 47–9, 79,
    122, 126, 132
    curricula for, 127
    in Universitas Indonesia (UI),
      Jakarta, 184
  in Vietnam, 158
military humanitarianism, 196
military medicine, 165, 167

differences between civilian and,
  164
*Quân Y*, 164
study of, 151
Millennium Development Goals
  (MDGs), 116
Minto, Lady, 68
*mise en valeur*, 95, 108, 251
*mo boran* (traditional doctor), 296,
  298
monk doctors, 275
Monnais, Laurence, 6, 20–1
Moore, Alex, 124

National Birth Spacing Policy (1995),
  Laos, 134
National Institute of Thai Traditional
  Medicine (NITTM), 285–6
National Reproductive Health Policy
  (2005), Laos, 134
Netherlands Indies Civil
  Administration (NICA), 176
Netherlands-Indies Physicians School
  (NIAS), 175, 186
Nightingale, Florence, 52
non-government organization (NGO),
  119, 282–3
Nooduniversiteit (Emergency
  University), Jakarta, 176
Northern medicine, 260
  practitioners of, 162
  *thuốc bắc*, 162
  yin and yang, theory of, 162, 163
*nuat boran*
  clinics, 298
  practitioners of, 297, 300
  school for tourists, 313
  success of, 297
  training, 296
nursing education, in Southeast Asia,
  13
  American style of, 14

British *versus* American model
of, 67
ethnicity and religion, influence
of, 15
training course, 44–7
nursing services, in British Malaya
American model of, 67, 73–80
British attitudes towards, 76
*bidan* (traditional midwives), 73
British model of, 67
cessation of recruitment of
British nurses, 84
character, notion of, 67
colonial nursing policy, history
of, 68
critique and Americanization of,
73–80
difficulties faced by British
nurses, 82
District Health Centers, 78
domestic sanitation and hygienic
living, 79
early colonial nursing, 69–73
employment of nurses, 68
Federated Malay States (FMS),
69
female nurses, 71–2
Heiser's survey on, 82
during Malayan Emergency
(1948–60), 84
Malayanization of, 84
Malayan Medical Services, 69
male nurses, 71, 84–5
pattern of nursing care, 71
Perak report (1893), 70
process of feminization of, 72
*versus* public health system in
Philippines, 72–5
recruitment of local female Asian
nurses, 72
stimulus for developing, 80
Straits Settlements, 13, 69–71,
73, 76, 78, 80, 83

subordination of Asian nurses, 82
training and prospects for Asian
nurses, 74
Unfederated Malay States
(UFMS), 69
and Western ideas of health
education, 72
nursing workforce
Asian nurses
prospects for, 74
training of, 74, 83
capacity-building and training, 14
college-based education, 77
*dukun bayi* (traditional birth
attendant), 15, 51, 56
employment of, 39
empowerment of, 75
European nurses, 46–7
feminization of, 13, 67, 72, 83
health-visiting for, 77
hospital training schools, 75
locally-trained, 14
*mantri* nurse, 44, 47, 48
Overseas Nursing Association
(ONA), 67
recruitment of, 68, 72, 84
on role of health education, 77
training of, *see* training, of nurses

on-the-job training, for midwives, 122
Operation Brotherhood, 119, 127,
131, 134
hospital network, 131
opotherapeutic drugs, 270n49
Overseas Nursing Association (ONA),
67

Pāli Vinaya (monastic disciplinary
code), 299
Pasteur Institute, Nha Trang, 95,
100–2

patient-doctor relationship, 185,
271n58
*penghulu* (religious civil servant), 49
Perak report (1893), 70
pharmaceutical industry
development of, 196
pharmaceuticals, *see* medicines
Western, 252
Pharmacie Chassagne, 256
*Pharmacopoeia of King Narai, The*
(1661), 274–5
Philippines, public health system in
American model, of medical
education, 74
American-style public health
nursing, 76
comparison with Malaya, 72–5
empowerment of nurses, 75
Filipino nurses, 75
"hearts and minds" strategy for,
75
hospital training schools, 75
legacy of Spanish colonization
and, 74–5
Philippine Medical School, 11
policy of attraction, 75
"public-private" nexus on, 74
quality of training of nurses, 75
vaccination program, 75
Phouma, Souvanna, 128
physician-and-patient relationships,
167
physician, in Semarang, 40–2
*dokter djawa* (Western-trained
Indonesian physician), 42, 45
Ethical Policy, 40–1
moral mission towards the
population, 41
political citizenship, 10
Prakash, Gyan, 2
Prawirohardjo, Sarwono, 180
*priyayi* (Javanese nobilities), 51–2, 55

prostitution
regulations against, 279
in Thailand, 278–9
protective tattoos (*mo sak yan*), 297
public health care system
dealing with, 260–2
Inspection of Health Services,
260
legislative frameworks dealing
with, 252
limitations of, 260
medicine stores, 253, 259
state quinine service, 252–3
therapeutic relationship in, 262–4
public health education
after World War II, 21
campaigns, 2, 4, 18, 232–5
and health citizenship, 17–21
initiatives for, 18
medical education and, 2
methods of, 12
prominence of teaching, 18
promotional techniques for, 4
promotion of, 55
use of force for imposition of,
17–18
in Vietnam, 21
Western medical practices, 20
public health initiatives
during Cold War, 84
colonial, 12
funding for, 84
public health nursing
American-style, 76, 77
Anglo-American collaboration
in, 77
in Britain, 77
and hospital nursing, 78
international courses in, 77
at King's College for Women
and Bedford College,
London, 77

matron, 82
RF survey of, 77
WHO interventions in, 84
*Puskesmas* (public health centers),
    190

*Quân Y* (military medicine), 150,
    161, 164
quarantine regulations, 9, 12

Rafael, Vicente, 2
Rama VI (King of Thailand), 280
recruitment, of nurses, 68, 72
    during Malayan Emergency
        (1948–60), 84
Red Cross, 41–2, 55, 77, 84, 238
Reed, Walter, 6
Regents of the University of
    California, 179–80
reproductive health services, 116
Rest & Recuperation (R&R)
    global market for, 279
    during Vietnam War, 279
*Revue Médico-Chirurgicale de
    l'Hôpital de l'Amitié Khméro-
    Soviétique, see Medical-Surgical
    Review of the Khmer-Soviet
    Friendship Hospital, The*
rinderpest (cattle plague), 99, 101–3,
    113n41
Rockefeller Foundation (RF), 12–13,
    67, 80, 174, 178–9, 188, 278
    on American style of nursing
        education, 14
    anti-hookworm campaigns, 19
    criticism of British health care
        system, 73
    Darville's experience of working
        with, 68
    educational projects launched
        by, 19

funding for
    medical education, 18
    rural health, 76
Health Units in the USA, 76
International Health Commission
    (IHC), 13, 73
Straits Settlement Rural Sanitation
    Campaign (SSRSC), 68
survey of public health nursing
    in Britain, 77
on Westernization of medical
    education, 22
Roosevelt, Theodore, 75
Rowell, J. Irvine, 71–2
Royal College of Nursing, London,
    77, 83
Royal Lao Government (RLG), 119,
    123–30, 141n53
royal physicians, 274–5, 277, 284,
    286
Royal Society of Medicine of
    Cambodia, 200–1
*ruesi datton* (therapeutic exercises),
    275
rural birth attendants (*accoucheuses
    rurales*), 123, 125, 128, 135
Russell, Paul, 78, 81

*Sakdina* (social hierarchy system in
    pre-modern Thailand), 274
*sakit* (disease/illness/suffering), 242
Salvarsan (anti-infectious drug), 253,
    257, 267n13
sanitary protection, 252
*san phraphum*, 303
Santoso, Slamet Iman, 184
Schein, Henri, 97, 101
School for the Education of Native
    Physicians (STOVIA), 175–7, 186
Science, Technology, and Society
    (STS), 150
scientific medicine, 246, 251, 267n3

seers/diviners (*mo du*), 297
self-education, 10
sero-infection (serum-simultaneous
vaccine), 102
*Service de Quinine d'État* (SQ), *see*
state quinine service
sex industry, in Thailand, 273
development of, 278
expansion of, 279
massage parlors, 279
prostitution, 278–9
regulations against, 279
Thai traditional massage and,
278–9
Shivagakomarpaj Traditional Thai
Medicine School, Chiang Mai,
297
Old Medicine Hospital, 297–8,
301–2, 308, 310–11, 313
Sihanouk, Norodom (Prince of
Cambodia)
abdication of the throne, 197
foreign policy, 197
ideology of, 197
national development agenda, 198
Sino-Vietnamese medicine, 253, 260,
269n38
Siriraj Hospital, Thailand, 277–8, 281
Faculty of Medicine, 282
Sister Tutor's diploma, 83
slash-and-burn agriculture, 97
Slocomb, Margaret, 197
smallpox vaccination, 185, 251, 254
Smart, A.G.H., 82–3
Smyth, Francis Scott, 178–9, 182, 186
socialist biomedicine, in Vietnam
Chinese supplies and medical
advisors, 155
*Dân Y* (civilian medicine), 150,
164
*Đông Y* (Eastern medicine), 148,
161
position of, 162

"feudal imperialist" medicine,
147
Hanoi Medical University
(HMU), *see* Hanoi Medical
University (HMU)
and how to be close to the
patient, 156–9
and importance of politics over
medicine, 153–6
during Indochinese War, 150
legacy of French colonial
medical education, 155
maternal health and birthing,
158
medical doctors, 149
midwives, 158
politics and practice of, 147, 155
professional competence in, 149
professional values of, 148
*Quân Y* (military medicine), 150,
161, 164
reorientation of, 161–4
Southern medicine in giving
birth, role of, 158
*Tây Y* (Western medicine), 161
and Traditional Vietnamese
Medicine (TVM), 148, 150
Y50 medical students, 146–8
socialist medicine, 147
function of, 157
practitioners of, 148
Society for the Promotion of Native
Nursing Practices, 54–5, 59
soul-doctors (*mo sukhwan*), 297
Southern medicine
involving local plants and herbs,
162
practitioners of, 162
role in giving birth, 158
*thuốc nam*, 162, 260
Souvannavong, Oudom, 124
Soviet model, of medical education,
17

Soviet Union, 147
  collaboration with Cambodia on
    medical education, 195
  loan to Indonesia, 178
spirit healers (*mo song*), 297
spirit houses, 303–4, 310
state quinine service, 252–3
Stokvis-Cohen Stuart, Nel, 7, 12–13,
    15, 25, 38, 40
  on district nursing service, 49
  endeavors to train Javanese
    women, 42–3
  on indigenous patterns of
    birthing and mothering, 60
  memorandums to Governor-
    General, 59
  outpatient clinic, 42
  Society for the Promotion of
    Native Nursing Practices,
    54–5, 59
  training of Javanese nurses, 24
    *dukun bayi*, 56
    midwifery training, 47–9
    in practice, 55–8
    problems encountered in, 44
    strategy for, 51–5
Straits Settlements, 13, 69–71, 73,
    76, 78, 80, 83
Stuart-Fox, Martin, 130
Subardjo, Achmad, 178
Surabaya, medical education in,
    186–8
  Dutch model of, 186
  Faculteit der Geneeskunde
    (Faculty of Medicine), 186
  history of, 186
  medical curriculum, 186–7
  Netherlands-Indies Physicians
    School (NIAS), 175, 186
  Universitas Airlangga (UNAIR),
    174, 186–7
    Student Senate of, 187
  University of California, 187

Sustainable Development Goals
    (SDGs), United Nations, 137

Taft, William H., 75
*Tamra Phra Osot Phra Narai, see
    Pharmacopoeia of King Narai,
    The* (1661)
Tantipidoke, Yongsak, 283
Taxila, India, 299
*Tây Y* (Western medicine), 161
Technical Cooperation Administration
    (TCA), America, 178
Thailand, medical education in
  Buddhist temples, involvement
    of, 22
  network of TTM schools, 23
  Old Medical Hospital School, in
    Chiang Mai, 22
  School and Association of
    Traditional Medicine, 22
  Thai massage, *see* Thai massage
  Traditional Thai Medicine (TTM),
    *see* Traditional Thai Medicine
    (TTM)
  *wai khru* ritual, *see wai khru*
    (worship teachers) ritual,
    Thailand
  Wat Pho, in Bangkok, 22, 275–7,
    280, 284, 286
Thai massage, 22
  biomedical professionals, 283
  in Chiang Mai, 297
  as cover for prostitution, 278–9
  flourishing of, 279–80
  folk/general style massage, 282
  legal status of, 280
  legitimacy of, 273
  popularity of, 279
  royal style massage, 281–2
  standardization of skills for,
    283
  standards of, 273

Thai Massage Revival Project,
282–4
objectives of, 284
three-level training course, 284
as tourist-oriented service, 278
*wai khru* (worship teachers)
ritual, 284
whole-body style of, 279
Thai traditional medicine, *see*
Traditional Thai Medicine (TTM)
therapeutic citizenship, in colonial
Vietnam, 21, 250
colonial health system, 252
colonial medicines and, 250
history of, 251–3
colonization, impact of, 251–3
health education, 251–3
importance of medication, 252
during interwar period, 252
manifestations of, 254–8
vietnamization, process of, 252
therapeutic education, 265–6
Theravada Buddhists, 299, 307
tourist industry, in Thailand, 23, 279
toxic substances, 252, 259, 263
legislation on, 267n8
traditional birth attendant (TBA), 15,
51, 121, 184
traditional doctors
disorganization of, 278
licensing system for, 278
*mo boran*, 296, 298
traditional medicine, 2
applied traditional medicine, 281
Ayurveda-Unani Tibb, India, 22
Buddhist temples, 22
bureaucratic (traditional medicine
revivalist) movement, 282
Chinese, 22
construction of, 22
definition of, 278
invention of, 21–3
Kampo, Japan, 22

knowledge of, 278
marginalization of, 278–80
publications on, 28
revivalist movements, 278, 280–4
Southeast Asian, 22
Thai massage, 22
Traditional Thai Medicine, *see*
Traditional Thai Medicine
(TTM)
Traditional Vietnamese Medicine,
*see* Traditional Vietnamese
Medicine (TVM)
training programs in, 22
Traditional Thai Medicine (TTM),
22–3, 28
Act for the Control of the
Practice of the Healing Art
(1936), 278, 284, 287
administration of, 296
administrative center of, 285
and adoption of Western
medicine, 277, 278
as ancient therapeutic art, 274
based on community culture, 282
bureaucratic (traditional medicine
revivalist) movement, 282
commercialization of, 273, 287–8
Coordination Centers, 286
courses on, 280
Decade of Thai Traditional
Medicine, 285
encounter with the West, 274–7
Four Body Elements, principle
of, 274–5, 277, 286
herbal remedies, 280
history of, 273, 286
inscriptions on the walls at Wat
Pho, 276
institutionalization of, 285–7
*kanphaet phaen boran*
(traditional medicine), 277
*kanphaet phaen patjuban*
(modern medicine), 277

legitimacy of, 273
literature on, 274
marginalization of, 278–80
massage practitioners (*mo nuat*),
    274
medical texts, compilation of,
    274–7
National Institute of Thai
    Traditional Medicine
    (NITTM), 285–6
as natural therapy, 287
*Pharmacopoeia of King Narai,
    The* (1661), 274–5
practitioners of, 300
principle of, 274
production rights of, 287–8
revivalist movements, 278, 280–4
royal physicians (*mo luang*), 274
*ruesi datton* (therapeutic
    exercises), 275
School and Association of
    Traditional Medicine, 280
Seventh National Economic and
    Social Development Plan
    (1992–96), 285
Siriraj Hospital, 277, 278, 281–2
Siriraj Medical School, 278
sources of, 275
South Asian medicine, influence
    of, 274–5
standards of, 273, 289
statues of hermits at Wat Pho,
    276
Ten Primary *Sen*, 286
traditional doctors
    disorganization of, 278
    licensing system for, 278
variety of knowledge in, 288–9
Traditional Vietnamese Medicine
    (TVM), 148, 161, 163
relationship between biomedicine
    and, 150
value of, 161

tradition, notion of, 311
training, of nurses, 44–7
    Anglo-American collaboration in,
        77
    apprenticeship-style, 77
    Asian nurses, 74, 83
    Assistant Nurses scheme, 83
    award of diploma, 47
        Sister Tutor's diploma, 83
    boarding school, 45–6
    British model of State Enrolled
        Nurses, 83
    college-based education, 77
    examination requirements, 47
    facilities for, 77
    female nurses, 44–7
    language of instruction, 45
    nursing schools, 83
    quality of, 75, 77
    in Singapore, 83
    supervision of, 46
    under-provision of, 83
tropical diseases, 194, 253
tropical medicine, 209
Truman, Harry, 178
    Point Four Program, 178
Tuân, Nguyễn Duy, 152
Tùng, Nguyễn Thúc, 155


Unfederated Malay States (UFMS),
    69–70, 73
United Nations Children's Emergency
    Fund (UNICEF), 84, 119, 131–2,
    281
United States Agency for
    International Development
    (USAID), 119, 188
    Maternal and Child Health/
        Family Planning project,
        127
    Public Health Division program
        in Laos, 127

Universitas Airlangga (UNAIR),
    Surabaya, 174, 186–7
    Student Senate of, 187
Universitas Indonesia (UI), Jakarta,
    174
    affiliation of the medical school
        at, 179
    goal of, 181
    American curriculum at, 184
    clinical instruction at, 183–4
    Department of Obstetrics and
        Gynecology, 184
    Faculty of Medicine, 180, 183
    physicians graduating from, 185
    problem-based experiential
        learning, 184
    switch from the Dutch to the
        American curriculum at,
        182
    teaching at premedical level,
        182
    training in
        *dukun bayis*, 184
        midwifery, 184
    vaccination campaigns, 185
University of California Medical
    School, 174, 180


vaccination campaigns, 9, 12, 75,
    183, 251
    anti-cholera, 254
    in Indonesia, 185
    against smallpox outbreak, 185,
        251, 254
vaccines, 20, 99, 102–3, 252, 254
*Vêò Sinh Báo: Journal de
    vulgarisation d'hygiène* (VSB),
    256
veterinary science
    animal medicine, 95
    auxiliary veterinarians, 100
    cattle diseases, 98

colonial veterinarians, in British
    India, 95
domestic animals, exploitation
    of, 95
epizootics, prevention of, 98
in Indochina, *see* Indochina,
    veterinary science and
    animal breeding in
schools for study of, 95
serotherapy, 99
training, for veterinary service,
    98–103
Vietnam
    administrative territories of, 96
    August Revolution of 1945, 152
    beef and buffalo meat
        consumption, 97
    Chinese supplies and medical
        advisors, 155
    coalition of anti-colonial forces,
        151
    "communization" of the medical
        services, 153–6
    dominance of French in medical
        education in, 159
    First Indochinese War, 151, 154
    Indochinese Communist Party
        (ICP), 151
    medical doctors, need for, 151
    medical education in, 8, 150
        public health care, 21
    midwives in, 158
    national health care system of,
        161
    rice cultivation, 97
    rubber plantations, 97
    slash-and-burn agriculture, 97
    socialist biomedicine in, *see*
        socialist biomedicine, in
        Vietnam
    therapeutic citizenship in, *see*
        therapeutic citizenship, in
        colonial Vietnam

veterinary science and animal
breeding in, *see* Indochina,
veterinary science and
animal breeding in
Viet Minh, objectives of, 165
vietnamization, process of, 252,
256
War of Resistance against French,
151

*wai khru* (worship teachers) ritual,
Thailand, 23, 284
*achan*, 308–13
analysis of, 310–13
ceremony of, 305–10
Chinese Buddhist bodhisattva
Guanyin, 299
daily ceremonies, 298–301
devotional activities, 304
*Jayaparittam* (Victory Paritta),
chanting of, 307
Jīvaka, story of, 299
*liang khru*, 301
*mo boran* (traditional doctor),
296
*nuat boran*, 303
clinics, 298
practitioners of, 297, 300,
311
school for tourists, 313
success of, 296–7
training, 296
as obligation for Thai healers,
298
Old Medicine Hospital, 297–8,
301–2, 308, 310, 313
*paritta* ritual, 306
performance of, 311
preparing for, 301–5
principal purpose of, 300
quasi-divine rishis, 300
*sai sin*, 305, 307, 309–10, 312

in Thai culture, 298
three-step process of, 301
Wasi, Prawet, 282–3
Wendland, Claire, 156, 166
Western health care, intermediaries
of, 53
Westernization of medical education
medical care, 9, 18
in Thailand, 22
Western therapies, demand for,
21
Western medicine, 161
incorporation of Eastern medicine
with, 163
involvement of the Viet Minh
in, 162
women's health, in Laos
childhood illnesses and
immunization program, 131
clinical health services, 127
colonial education system and,
122
under colonial rule (1904–50),
119–23
contraceptive prevalence rate,
117
in early Lao PDR period (1976–
90), 130–3
family planning services, 117–19,
128–9
adoption of, 123
concept of, 132
fertility rate, 117
free delivery, prospect of, 117
French assistance to the medical
school, 131
health budgets to cover, 117
Lao Family Welfare Association
(LFWA), 129
Lao Health Service, 123–4
Lao Medical Service, 119–21
Lao Ministry of Health, 119,
127, 130

Lao Social Indicator Survey
(LSIS), 135
"Liberated Zone" health staff,
129
Maternal and Child Health
(MCH) Services project, 124
maternal mortality rates, 116–17,
124
Medical Sciences Technicians'
School, 132
midwives, 117, 120
French, 122
hospital-based, 121
midwifery school, 121–2
on-the-job training, 122
professional classifications,
127
status of, 133
training of, 117, 122, 126–7,
132
Millennium Development Goals
(MDGs), 116, 119
National Birth Spacing Policy
(1995), 134
National Reproductive Health
Policy (2005), 134
nurseries and childcare centers,
131
Operation Brotherhood, 119, 127,
130–1, 134
hospital network, 131
Patriotic Lao Front health
services, 131
and practice of giving birth, 121
Primary Health Care (PHC)
policy, 130
quality of healthcare service,
135

in recent Lao PDR period
(1991–2012), 133–6
reproductive health services, 116
responsibility for, 123
risks of childbirth, 117
in Royal Lao Government period
(1950–75), 123–30
rural birth attendants
(*accoucheuses rurales*), 123
Skilled Birth Attendance
Development Plan, 117
social medicine policy, 125
"Strategy and Planning
Framework for the Integrated
Package of Maternal, Neo-
natal and Child Health
Services," 117
unassisted delivery, 117
USAID-funded programs for, 131
World Health Organization (WHO),
12, 14, 68, 119, 178, 296
funding for public health
programs, 84
interventions in public health
nursing, 84

xerophthalmia, problem of, 209
Xiaoping, Fang, 147

yellow fever, transmission of, 6, 12,
73
Yersin, Alexandre, 95, 98–9
yin and yang, theory of, 162, 163

zootechny, 95, 100, 107